Rethinking 'Classical Yoga' and Buddhism

Bloomsbury Advances in Religious Studies

Series Editors: Bettina E. Schmidt, Steven Sutcliffe and Will Sweetman

Founding Editors: James Cox and Peggy Morgan

Bloomsbury Advances in Religious Studies publishes cutting-edge research in the Study of Religion/s. The series draws on anthropological, ethnographical, historical, sociological and textual methods amongst others. Topics are diverse, but each publication integrates theoretical analysis with empirical data. The series aims to refresh the interdisciplinary agenda in new evidence-based studies of 'religion'.

American Evangelicals, Ashlee Quosigk
Appropriation of Native American Spirituality, Suzanne Owen
Becoming Buddhist, Glenys Eddy
Community and Worldview among Paraiyars of South India, Anderson H. M. Jeremiah
Conceptions of the Afterlife in Early Civilizations, Gregory Shushan
Contemporary Western Ethnography and the Definition of Religion, Martin D. Stringer
Cultural Blending in Korean Death Rites, Chang-Won Park
Free Zone Scientology, Aled Thomas
Globalization of Hesychasm and the Jesus Prayer, Christopher D. L. Johnson
Individualized Religion, Claire Wanless
Innateness of Myth, Ritske Rensma
Levinas, Messianism and Parody, Terence Holden
New Paradigm of Spirituality and Religion, Mary Catherine Burgess
Orthodox Christianity, New Age Spirituality and Vernacular Religion, Eugenia Roussou
Post-Materialist Religion, Mika T. Lassander
Redefining Shamanisms, David Gordon Wilson
Reform, Identity and Narratives of Belonging, Arkotong Longkumer
Religion and the Discourse on Modernity, Paul-François Tremlett
Religion as a Conversation Starter, Ina Merdjanova and Patrice Brodeur
Religion, Material Culture and Archaeology, Julian Droogan
Secular Assemblages, Marek Sullivan
Spirits and Trance in Brazil, Bettina E. Schmidt
Spirit Possession and Trance, edited by Bettina E. Schmidt and Lucy Huskinson

Spiritual Tourism, Alex Norman
Theology and Religious Studies in Higher Education, edited by D. L. Bird and Simon G. Smith
The Critical Study of Non-Religion, Christopher R. Cotter
The Problem with Interreligious Dialogue, Muthuraj Swamy
Religion and the Inculturation of Human Rights in Ghana, Abamfo Ofori Atiemo
UFOs, Conspiracy Theories and the New Age, David G. Robertson

Rethinking 'Classical Yoga' and Buddhism

Meditation, Metaphors and Materiality

Karen O'Brien-Kop

BLOOMSBURY ACADEMIC
LONDON • NEW YORK • OXFORD • NEW DELHI • SYDNEY

BLOOMSBURY ACADEMIC
Bloomsbury Publishing Plc
50 Bedford Square, London, WC1B 3DP, UK
1385 Broadway, New York, NY 10018, USA
29 Earlsfort Terrace, Dublin 2, Ireland

First published in Great Britain 2022
This paperback edition published 2023

A catalogue record for this book is available from the British Library.

A catalog record for this book is available from the Library of Congress.

ISBN: HB: 978-1-3502-2999-0
PB: 978-1-3502-3003-3
ePDF: 978-1-3502-3000-2
eBook: 978-1-3502-3001-9

Series: Bloomsbury Advances in Religious Studies

Typeset by Newgen KnowledgeWorks Pvt. Ltd., Chennai, India

Contents

List of tables viii
Preface ix
Acknowledgements x
List of abbreviations xii
Note on translation and transliterations xiv

Introduction: 'Classical yoga' and Buddhism: Debates, dialogue and intertextuality 1
1 *Mokṣa*, metaphors and materiality: Concepts and contexts of 'liberation' 21
2 Seeds of bondage and freedom: Eliminating the afflictions (*kleśa*s) in the *Pātañjalayogaśāstra* and the *Abhidharmakośabhāṣya* 49
3 The 'other' yoga *śāstra*: The *Yogācārabhūmiśāstra* 75
4 Pātañjala yoga and yogācāra: The cultivation of the counterstate 95
5 Who put the classical in 'classical yoga'? The inadequacy of an analytical category 113
Conclusion: Rethinking 'classical yoga' – a categorical paradigm shift? 143

Appendix 1: A note on the title *Pātañjalayogaśāstra* 155
Appendix 2: Classical Indian metaphor theory 157
Appendix 3: Structure of the *Yogācārabhūmiśāstra* 159
Notes 161
Bibliography 225
Index 253

Tables

2.1 *Pātañjalayogaśāstra* 2.4 and *Abhidharmakośābhāṣya* 5.1 65
2.2 *Pātañjalayogaśāstra* 2.4 and *Abhidharmakośābhāṣya* 2.36 68
4.1 The *kleśa*s and their counterstates in *Bodhisattvabhūmi* 1.12 98
4.2 Patañjali's seven stages of wisdom paraphrased (*Pātañjalayogaśāstra* 2.27) 107
4.3 Asaṅga's seven stages of contemplation (*Śrāvakabhūmi* 3.28.2.1.1–8) 108

Preface

This book began work as a study focused on the *Pātañjalayogaśāstra*. However, the more I read, the more I became drawn into its intertextual web and the contemporaneous Buddhist literature. Hence, I see this book as representing a synchronic slice of the field of conceptual thought in South Asia from the second to early fifth centuries CE, a discursive milieu that was co-constructed by different religio-philosophical groups. This book hopes to model fruitful methodological interactions between close literary reading and broader historical, cultural and material analysis – together with specific theoretical and philosophical tools such as conceptual metaphor theory, hermeneutics and decolonial thought. It is also intended that this book will be particularly useful to scholars and students trained primarily in the study of Hinduism but who would like to deepen their contextual knowledge of less familiar Buddhist material and its intersection with Pātañjala yoga. The field of the academic study of yoga has been a fast-developing one in recent years, and even as I draw a line under this book, I observe further relevant scholarship emerging into publication. Therefore, I hope to continue some strands of my research and to further develop lines of thought and conversations in future endeavours.

Acknowledgements

I would like to thank my editor at Bloomsbury, Lalle Pursglove, for taking on this title and Lily McMahon for her patience and stellar editorial support at each stage.

I have presented draft sections from this book at conferences in the past years and had valuable feedback from the scholarly community. In particular, I would like to thank the organizers of the 'Yoga Darśana, Yoga Sādhana' conference – Modern Yoga Research and especially Elizabeth de Michelis – held in Krakow in 2016, where I was able to present a paper that was eventually published in *Religions of South Asia* and formed a basis for the more developed Chapter 2 in this book. That early paper received several close readings from Dr Philipp Maas, which greatly improved it. I also benefited from engaging comments from respondents at the Spalding Symposium on Indian Religions at Oxford University in 2017, where I had encouraging questions from Dr Naomi Appleton, Dr Michael Allen and Dr Simon Brodbeck. At the Sanskrit Tradition in the Modern World conference in 2018, my research paper benefited from a critical response from Dr Matthew Clark and generous support from Dr Jacqueline Suthren Hirst.

Research for this book began at SOAS University of London, and I must especially thank Dr Theodore Proferes, Professor Ulrich Pagel and Dr James Mallinson for their expert and complementary guidance on the various specialist areas that I was interested in – early Hinduism, Buddhism, yoga philosophy and Sanskrit. I am also grateful to Professor Rupert Gethin and Professor Richard King for further comments and feedback on my doctoral work. The writing of this book was in part funded by the Ouseley Memorial Language Fund and by the Phiroz Mehta Trust. At SOAS, I was fortunate to be part of the development of the SOAS Centre of Yoga Studies from 2018 to 2019 with James Mallinson as director and to benefit from immersion in the many talks and events. My time there was also enriched by the scholarship, collegiality and inspiration of Dr Avni Chag, Dr Lidia Wojtczak and Ruth Westoby, with whom I enjoyed the ventures of the Sanskrit Reading Room and the International Indology Graduate Research Symposium.

I would also like to thank Dr Suzanne Newcombe for being a key advisor and colleague in my research journey for this book. And over my years of teaching, my thinking has benefited from discussions with my students at SOAS and the University of Roehampton. My colleagues at Roehampton have supported the completion of this book, and I would like to extend particular thanks to Professor Laura Peters, Dr Simonetta Calderini, Dr Sean Ryan and Dr John Moxon. Lastly, I would like to thank the Oxford Centre of Hindu Studies for support and Seth Powell at Yogic Studies for conversations on Patañjali at the American Academy of Religion Meeting in 2019 as well as overall encouragement and engagement with my work.

Finally, my family: my deepest gratitude to my mother Margaret O'Brien, who did not live to see this book in print, but knew all about it, to Tom O'Brien and Trevor O'Brien and to my amazing son, Zohar.

Abbreviations

AKBh	*Abhidharmakośabhāṣya*
AKK	*Abhidharmakośakārikā*
AN	*Aṅguttara Nikāya*
BG	*Bhagavad Gītā*
BhāvBh	*Bhāvanāmayī Bhūmiḥ*
BoBh	*Bodhisattvabhūmi*
Bv	*Buddhavaṃsa*
Bybh	*Buddhasenayogācārabhūmi*
DBS	*Daśabhūmikasūtra*
DDS	*Damoduoluo chan jing / Dharmatrāta Dhyānasūtra*
DN	*Dīgha Nikāya*
It	*Itivuttaka*
Ja	*Jātaka* and *Jātak'-aṭṭhakathā*
MB	*Mahābhārata*
MDh	*Mānavadharmaśāstra*
Mil	*Milindapañha*
MN	*Majjhima Nikāya*
MuU	*Muṇḍaka Upaniṣad*
MVB	*Mahāvibhāṣaśāstra*
NAS	*Nyāyānusāra*
NySBh	*Nyāyasūtrabhāṣya*
Pd	*Paramatthadīpanī*
PP	*Prakaraṇapāda*
PrU	*Praśna Upaniṣad*
Pv	*Pettavathu*
PYŚ	*Pātañjalayogaśāstra*
ṚV	*Ṛg Veda*
Saddhsu	*Saddharmasmṛtyupasthānasūtra*
SamāBh	*Samāhitabhūmi*
Śbh	*Śrāvakabhūmi*
SDhPu	*Saddharmapuṇḍarīka Sūtra*

SKK	*Sāṃkhyakārikā*
Sn	*Sutta Nipāta*
SN	*Saṃyutta Nikāya*
SNS	*Saṃdhinirmocanasūtra*
SPS	*Saddharmapuṇḍarīkasūtra*
SvU	*Śvetāśvatara Upaniṣad*
SYCB	*Saṅgharakṣa's *Yogācārabhūmi*
TAS	*Tattvārthasūtra*
Vin	*Vināya Piṭaka*
Vism	*Visuddhimagga*
Viv	*Vivaraṇa*
Vv-a	*Vimānavatthu-aṭṭhakathā*
YĀBh	*Yogācārabhūmiśāstra*
YBh	*Yogasūtrabhāṣya*
YS	*Yogasūtra*
YVc	*Yogaviṁśikā* commentary by Yaśovijaya

Note on translation and transliteration

Most primary source quotations are in Sanskrit, with some instances in Pāli. Diacritics are employed throughout. *Sūtra*s from the *Yogasūtra* are marked in bold to differentiate them from the commentary. Any unattributed translations are the author's.

Introduction

'Classical yoga' and Buddhism: Debates, dialogue and intertextuality

Introduction

The category of 'classical yoga' is most often associated with, or sometimes conflated with the *Yogasūtra* of Patañjali,[1] a text referred to in this study as part of the *Pātañjalayogaśāstra* (PYŚ) and dated from the fourth to early fifth century CE.[2] This book argues that we should widen the discursive context of the category of 'classical yoga' beyond the *Pātañjalayogaśāstra* to incorporate elaborations of yogic liberation from other contemporaneous texts, such as the Buddhist *Abhidharmakośabhāṣya* (AKBh) and the *Yogācārabhumiśāstra* (YĀBh). Once we have accepted that the current category of 'classical yoga' is inadequate in several key respects and should include Buddhist texts that discuss yoga, we can then turn our attention to the broader fallibility of 'classical yoga' as a categorical descriptor in academia. Arguably, it is time to replace the Eurocentric 'classical' with other emic signifiers from South Asian culture, and this book suggests some starting possibilities. The trajectory of this volume is to argue that (a) any narrow definition of 'classical yoga' as Hindu-only has excluded relevant textual sources that describe Buddhist yoga, (b) 'classical yoga' was not a *sui generis* category but was informed by the European cultural colonialist project,[3] and (c) in rethinking the place of Buddhist yoga in 'classical yoga', the latter category becomes even more untenable and inadequate.

Entanglements: The story so far

A significant body of scholarly work exists on the relationship between the *Pātañjalayogaśāstra* and Buddhist salvific thought. However, in many cases similarities between the two traditions have been broadly sketched. In other cases, excellent fine-tuned textual analysis is nonetheless limited in scope (to a single passage or a few *sūtras*) and thus draws necessarily narrowly focused conclusions. Furthermore, the analysis of Patañjali's interaction with Buddhist thought has typically concentrated exclusively on either the *Yogasūtra* (e.g. de La Vallée Poussin 1936) or the *Yogasūtrabhāṣya* (e.g. Frauwallner 1973; Wezler 1987).

Senart was one of the first Western scholars to write about Buddhist elements in the *Yogasūtra*[4] (Senart 1900), asserting that Buddhism itself evolved out of a proto-yoga tradition (Senart 1900: 348). He identified structural correlates between the *Yogasūtra* and Buddhist thought – including *yamas/niyamas* (restraints/observances) with *śīla* (ethical conduct) of Buddhism and shared ideas of *vairāgya* (non-attachment), the doctrines of impermanence and suffering and the focus on the elimination of *saṃskāras* (mental impressions) – and classified these ideas as part of a common heritage in India (Senart 1900: 349). Oldenberg highlighted the gap between the terminology of Pātañjala yoga and Sāṃkhya. His *Lehre der Upanishaden und die Anfänge des Buddhismus* proposed new ideas about the role of the *dhyānas* as a transmission from proto-yoga to Buddhism and of Sāṃkhya as the vehicle that conveyed this transmission (Oldenberg 1923). According to Keith, we can only understand the quasi-theistic notion of *īśvara* (Lord) in the *Yogasūtra* in the light of Mahāyāna Buddhism (Keith 1932: 434). And Heiler posited that yoga and Buddhism evolved from the same root, with Buddhist meditation heavily indebted to yogic methods (Heiler 1922: 43–51). De La Vallée Poussin drew on Senart's work to argue further that Buddhism was influenced by a proto-yoga tradition, claiming that the relationship between yoga and Sāṃkhya, although ancient, was not exclusive (de La Vallée Poussin 1937: 224). He states that Buddhism drew on a 'pure' tradition of yoga that was free from metaphysics and called this 'Buddhist yoga' (de La Vallée Poussin 1937: 226). In many respects, he argued, early Buddhism is the only lens through which we can view the proto-yoga tradition, which, apart from the *dhyānas*, has otherwise been lost (de La Vallée Poussin 1937: 230). De La Vallée Poussin located the origin of these elements of meditation not within Buddhism but in a shadowy historical realm of archaic-magic practices. Complementing Oldenberg's work, he claimed that the first three *pādas* of the *Yogasūtra* contain more than one hundred 'Buddhist' terms, fifty of which can be directly traced to Vasubandhu's *Abhidharmakośabhāṣya*.[5]

Another scholarly approach to account for the Brahmin-Buddhist 'mix' of Patañjali's work has been to identify sections of the *Yogasūtra* as Buddhist interpolations. Deussen initiated this type of analysis (Deussen 1914: 509–43),[6] which subsequently remained focused on two particular sections of the *Yogasūtra*. Hauer (1958), Frauwallner (1973) and Oberhammer (1977) all classified the *aṣṭāṅga* section (YS 2.28–3.7) as closely related to Buddhist thought.[7] The other section of the *Yogasūtra* identified as having Buddhist 'origins', in part or total, is the fourth *pāda*. Dasgupta, Keith, Deussen, Hauer and Frauwallner discuss this *pāda* (particularly YS 4.16–21) as responding to the consciousness-only (*cittamātra*) positions of Yogācāra[8] thought. Although such structuralist 'hacking' of texts has now been abandoned, the point remains that the *Pātañjalayogaśāstra* is a composite text.

In the late twentieth century, the vexed relationship of the *Yogasūtra* and Buddhism was revisited anew. There was a shift from making broad and general comparisons across 'terminology' (such as de La Vallée Poussin) or structural analyses (such as Deussen) to specific contextual investigations of particular *sūtras*. Bronkhorst argued that *dhyāna* in the *Yogasūtra* is a Buddhist technique, as is the use of *smṛti* to denote mindfulness (as opposed to the Brahmanic context of indicating non-*śruti* texts) (Bronkhorst 1993: 95); Buddhist meditation is especially visible in the 'Samādhi Pāda' of the *Yogasūtra*, namely 1.17–20 and 1.46–51 (Bronkhorst 1993: 74).[9] Bronkhorst has also noted a striking parallelism between the *Yogasūtrabhāṣya* and the *Abhidharmakoṣabhāṣya* in describing the *tanmātra* (subtle element) as an atom (Bronkhorst 2006: 306 fn. 18). Klostermeier's 1986 essay 'Dharmamegha samādhi: Comments on *Yogasūtra* IV, 29' traced the primary context of Patañjali's term *dharmamegha* to Buddhist sources. Cousins's 1992 paper, '*Vitakka/vitarka* and *vicāra*: Stages of *samādhi* in Buddhism and Yoga', argued that the use of the terms *vitarka* and *vicāra* in both Buddhism and Brahmanism reflects an interconnection between the two traditions that has gone largely unacknowledged (Cousins 1992). Cousins surveyed the register and common usage of *vitarka* and *vicāra* in Buddhist canonical literature. He then compared this discursive and paradigmatic context with that in the *Yogasūtra*, noting the similarity between the yogic *saṃprajñāta samādhi* (cognitive concentration) and the Buddhist *rūpa-jhāna*s (the *dhyāna*s in a progressive formula) (Cousins 1992: 147). Wezler's 1987 study of the *Yogabhāṣya* (YBh) examined the commentary to YS 2.28, which includes a list of nine causes (*kāraṇāni*) elaborated in relation to 'the methods of yoga'. He infers that *śāstra* references in the *Yogasūtrabhāṣya* point to prior philosophical teaching systems. From the way in which the nine causes are contextualized by the editor of the *Yogasūtrabhāṣya*, Wezler deduces that they belong to a system that is not compatible with Sāṃkhya. He, then, suggests that the author of the *Yogasūtrabhāṣya* is drawing on Buddhist models of ten causes, as found in Vasubandhu's *Madhyhāntavibhāgabhāṣya*[10] and Asaṅga's *Abhidharmasamuccaya*. Such lists appear also, in modified form, in the *Sarvitarkādibhūmi* and the *Bodhisattvabhūmi*, two of the 'books' of the *Yogācārabhūmiśastra* (Wezler 1987: 356, 375). In making modifications to the Buddhist list of causes, Patañjali consciously chose to employ the term *viyoga* (disjunction), which appears in the *Abhidharmasamuccaya* but not in the *Madhyhāntavibhāgabhāṣya* (Wezler 1987: 374). Overall, Wezler agrees with Frauwallner (1973) that Sarvāstivāda Buddhism influenced the *Yogasūtrabhāṣya* but adds that Yogācāra also played a role.

In a full-length study, Yamashita surveyed a range of Buddhist terms, ideas and quotations contained in both the *Yogasūtra* and *Yogasūtrabhāṣya* (Yamashita 1994). Noting that the ontology of the *Yogasūtra* differs from that of Sāṃkhya (Yamashita 1994: 1), Yamashita observed fragments of Sarvāstivāda texts in the *Yogasūtrabhāṣya*. He traced the theory of the appearance and disappearance of *dharmas* (the theory of change, or *tirobhāvāvirbhāva-vāda*) in *Yogasūtrabhāṣya* 4.12 to the Buddhist *Mahāvibhāṣā*. Somewhat confusingly, however, the passage describing this doctrine also appears in the *Abhidharmakośabhāṣya*, where Vasubandhu cites it as a view of the Sāṃkhya teacher Vārṣagaṇya (Yamashita 1994: 46–55). According to Yamashita, Vasubandhu presents the *Yogasūtra*'s definition of *pariṇāma* (change/ transformation), and Patañjali had previously used the Buddhist Sarvāstivāda position to construct his own theory of change: *Abhidharmakośabhāṣya* 3.50 and *Yogasūtrabhāṣya* 3.13 are almost identical in wording. Less convincingly, Yamashita identifies several terms in the *Yogasūtra* as distinctly Buddhist, notably *citta* and *kliṣṭa* (Yamashita 1994: 65, 82), and he also proposes that the *samādhi* of the YS is similar to both *samādhi* in Sarvāstivāda and *manaskāra* in Yogācāra (Yamashita 1994: 126). Yamashita compares the term 'yoga' in the *Yogasūtra* to the *samādhi* of the Vijñānavāda (Yogācāra) and the *samāpatti* of the Sarvāstivāda. Although some of Yamashita's broad claims were not substantiated (and represented a return to the terminological generalizations of earlier scholarship), this study provided interesting clues and directions that called for further research.

In *The Numinous and the Cessative in Indo-Tibetan Yoga* (Sarbacker 2005), Sarbacker devoted a chapter to Buddhism and classical yoga. He concludes that there is an overlap between *samādhi* in Pātañjala yoga and *samādhi* in Buddhist conceptions of *śamatha*. Sarbacker also posits that the four *samāpatti*s of *samprajñāta samādhi* in the first *pāda* of the YS correspond to the four Buddhist *dhyāna*s (Sarbacker 2005: 77–8). Elsewhere, Wujastyk's analysis of the foundational āyurvedic treatise the *Carakasaṃhitā* (*c.* first to second century CE) identified an 'archaic' eightfold yogic path to liberation that 'owed its origins to Buddhist traditions of cultivating *smṛti*' (Wujastyk 2012: 36). Furthermore, Wujastyk's 'Some Problematic Yoga Sutras and Their Buddhist Background' examines three Pātañjala *sūtra*s that appear to have their origins in Buddhist texts or discourse (Wujastyk 2018). Wujastyk's analysis in this article provides a valuable template for close, comparative reading.

In 2020, Maas's article 'Sarvāstivāda Buddhist Theories of Temporality and the Pātañjala Yoga Theory of Transformation (*pariṇāma*)'[11] examined two passages (YS 3.13 and AKBh 5.25) that reflect interaction between proponents of Sāṃkhya-Yoga on the one hand and Sautrāntika and Sarvāstivāda schools of Śrāvakayāna Buddhism on the other. Maas concurs with the view that the *Yogasūtra* contains polemics against the Yogācāra school of Mahāyāna Buddhism (which are unpacked for us by Saṅkara's *Vivaraṇa* commentary) (Maas 2013: 73)[12] but disputes Frauwallner's claim that YS 3.13 presents an inferior imitation or weak copy of an original Buddhist verse (Maas 2020: 965). Rather, Maas argues, Patañjali combined the Sarvāstivāda theories in a novel way to transpose them from a Buddhist position (conditioned factors are subject to transitoriness) to a Sāṃkhya-yoga position (the transformation of substance has a permanent substratum even through time). Positing direct engagement with Buddhist philosophers, Maas shows that *Yogasūtra* 3.13 rewords Vasubandhu's passage, reworks Dharmatrāta's theory of the momentariness of conditioned factors in the *Vibhāṣā* and modifies the theories of Ghoṣaka, Vasumitra and Buddhamitra. In Maas's conclusion, Patañjali's reformulation was used as a polemic device in order to reorient a Sarvāstivāda ontology towards Sāṃkhya (Maas 2020: 989).

A counterargument to the thesis of Buddhist elements in the *Yogasūtra* comes from Burley, who refutes the notion that Patañjali's fourth chapter, 'Kaivalya Pāda', positions itself as realist in contrast to the idealist Yogācāra school. Burley proposes that the framing of Patañjali's fourth *pāda* as an anti-idealist polemic was due to a later commentarial interpretation. The first writers to identify polemics against Buddhism in the *Pātañjalayogaśāstra* were the commentators

Vācaspatimiśra (ninth to tenth century CE) and Vijñānabhikṣu (fifteenth to sixteenth century CE) (respectively *Tattvavaisāradī* 4.14 and *Yogavārttika* 4.14). It was they who argued that the idealists identified by Patañjali at YBh 4.14 are the Vijñānavādins (Yogācāra). Burley concludes that Vācaspatimiśra and Vijñānabhikṣu misinterpreted Patañjali's text and that the anti-Buddhist interventions of subsequent commentators resulted in a 'philosophical vendetta … at the expense of accurate exegesis' (2007: 90).

Recently, there have been some distinctive hypotheses on the relationship of the *Pātañjalayogaśāstra* to Buddhism. In the introduction to his 2012 French translation of the *Yogasūtra* and *Yogasūtrabhāṣya*, Angot argued that the *Yogasūtra* was mostly written by a Buddhist author and that the last *pāda* and the commentary was written by a Hindu named Vyāsa in the sixth–seventh century, as a Brahmanic appropriation of a Buddhist text (Angot 2012: 24–34). Elsewhere, Squarcini asserted that the *Yogasūtra* is a Buddhist work that has an 'interdiscursive' relationship with the Brahmanical tradition, albeit primarily polemical (Squarcini 2016: xlix). Squarcini's translation of the *Yogasūtra* includes an index, which links words and phrases from the *Yogasūtra* to Buddhist texts (Squarcini 2016: 179–89). Both of these scholarly accounts dwell at one end of the spectrum of views on Pātañjala yoga as either Buddhist or Brahmin. Although there are problems with such arguments for a clear-cut Buddhist identity for 'Patañjali', there is interesting detail in these approaches. In particular, a long-standing scholar on this subject, Gokhale has recently published *The Yogasūtra of Patañjali: A New Introduction to the Buddhist Roots of the Yoga System* (2020), which offers a comparative reading of the *Yogasūtras* in the Buddhist context, exemplifying fine-grained commentarial analysis.

To add to this body of scholarship is a daunting task, but what is different in this present book is an evaluation of the *Yogasūtra* and the *Yogasūtrabhāṣya* together as a unitary composition, the *Pātañjalayogaśāstra* – an approach that by itself offers unprecedented access to the integrated conceptuality of Patañjali's text. Furthermore, this study seeks to generate new perspectives on the entanglement between Patañjali's discourse and that of contemporaneous Buddhism by engaging in systematic analysis using fresh methodology – literary intertextual analysis[13] combined with conceptual metaphor theory. The meaning of the term 'yoga' in the fourth to fifth centuries was not confined to the Brahmanic-Hindu context; the practice of yoga most likely evolved from a common *śramaṇa* background of asceticism (Bronkhorst 2007; Samuel 2008), and the discourse of yoga was employed by various communities in a shared religio-cultural environment (Bronkhorst 2006: 302). My broad aim, then, is to situate the *Pātañjalayogaśāstra* in a dialogic context with Buddhist material and to illuminate the integral role of such dialogue in the conceptual formation of classical yoga soteriology through metaphors. The specific question at the heart of this research is one that Larson posed in his 1989 essay 'An Old Problem Revisited, the Relation Between Sāṃkhya, Yoga and Buddhism'. Given the self-identification of the *Pātañjalayogaśāstra* as a text of Sāṃkhya philosophy, why does it contain so few Sāṃkhya terms and so many that are apparently Buddhist? (Larson 1989). Larson addressed this problem convincingly by reconstructing a series of partially documented oral debates (discussed below) that occurred between Sāṃkhya and Buddhist teachers, which, he argued, produced the shared terminology of the texts. Within the texts themselves, we can find evidence of such debates not only in direct refutations of rival religious positions but also in subtle layers of interaction embedded in conceptual expression. In particular, conceptual metaphors played a key role in determining how the *Pātañjalayogaśāstra*, a text that is evidently doctrinally Sāṃkhya, could nonetheless share soteriological terminology and goals with another school of thought, in this case Buddhist.

To address one further relevant issue in contemporary scholarship on the *Pātañjalayogaśāstra*: the work is widely held to be the first systematized account of yoga.[14] Although this *sūtra* text is preceded by nascent descriptions of yoga in the Brahmanic texts, these accounts are by no means systematic. Burley argues that some form of textual systematization, now lost, must have existed before the *Yogasūtra*. The way in which the text declares itself an 'exposition' (*anuśāsana*) at its beginning points to 'a pre-existing body of teaching' (Burley 2007: 27). Larson, Bhattacharya and Maas, on the other hand, concur that yoga only came into existence as a systematic philosophy around the time of the composition of the *Yogasūtra* (Larson and Bhattacharya 2008: 27; Maas 2013). This book follows Maas's proposal that an author-editor, or group thereof, combined centuries-old textual material with new compositions to create the *Pātañjalayogaśāstra* (Maas 2013: 69).

Defining 'yoga'

Classical 'yoga' is perhaps better understood as a soteriological discourse rather than a specific term, text, practice or entity since 'yoga' has always been a polysemous word. 'Yoga' in the Vedic sources gradually migrated from archaic generic meanings (loosely clustered around ideas of application, purpose, effort, conjoining, activation) towards an emerging set of specific soteriological meanings focused on meditation. Circa the sixth to fourth centuries BCE, the Sanskrit grammarian Pāṇini's list of verbal forms contains two for the root '*yuj*': '*yuji*' denotes 'joining' or 'uniting' (cognate with the English 'yoking') and '*yuja*' denotes 'concentration' in the sense of *samādhi*.[15] By the early Common Era, 'yoga' had a wide semantic field and could simultaneously signal a range of meanings, including apparently antonymic ones, such as 'bondage'[16] and 'liberation from bondage'.[17]

In the fourth to fifth centuries CE, proto-systems of 'yoga' had already been established in the Brahmanic and Sāṃkhya traditions. During the second half of the first millennium BCE, nascent systems of yogic meditation emerged in both the *Upaniṣads* and in the two sections of the *Mahābhārata* that deal with yoga, the *Bhagavad Gītā* and the 'Śānti Parvan' – these accounts all describe yoga in relation to Sāṃkhya.[18] We do not find consistent definitions of yoga in Brahmanism prior to the late Principal *Upaniṣads*. The word 'yoga' in Vedic culture was both generic and polyvalent. Even if there were strands of Vedic culture that reflected ascetic identities (such as the *muni*, the *vrātya*, the *yati*),[19] it is likely, as Bronkhorst has pointed out, that the most intense development of yoga as an ascetic practice geared towards spiritual liberation occurred in the renouncer (*śramaṇa*) communities of the north eastern subcontinent (Bronkhorst 2007). These *śramaṇa* communities evolved around the mid-first millennium BCE, possibly as a reaction towards increased urbanization, and from them emerged the religions of Buddhism and Jainism. By the start of the Common Era, then, there were several formative and coexisting strands of yoga discourse that were entangled. In addition to the Brahmanic forms of yoga described in the *Upaniṣads* and the *Mahābhārata*, there was a concurrent Buddhist discourse of yoga[20] called yogācāra.[21] This developed in early Mahāyāna meditation *sūtras* and was comprehensively described in Asaṅga's fourth-century treatise, the *Yogācārabhūmisāstra*.

The titular labels that a text grants itself are not always a guarantee of a text's thematic focus. For example, the *Yogasūtra* mentions yoga only three times and the *Yogabhāṣya* eight,[22] in contrast to the contemporaneous Buddhist *Laṅkāvatārasūtra* which mentions yoga more than fifty times (many of which references are to 'yoga discipline' – yogācāra – specifically). Likewise, while the importance of the Sāṃkhya frame of the *Pātañjalayogaśāstra* should not be underemphasized, neither should it be overplayed. The *Sāṃkhyakārikā* (SKK), the text with which the *Yogasūtra* is conventionally aligned, mentions yoga only once. The *Pātañjalayogaśāstra* refers to Sāṃkhya in its chapter colophons (in the title *Sāṃkhyapravacana*, 'The Sayings of Sāṃkhya', as a name for the *Yogasūtra*) and only twice more in the commentary text[23] – and not at all in the *sūtra*s themselves. In focusing more broadly on the soteriology of yoga, this book also addresses a text such as Vasubandhu's *Abhidharmakośabhāṣya*, which (unlike the *Pātañjalayogaśāstra* and the *Yogācārabhūmiśāstra*) does not purport to deal with the topic of yoga. However, even if the focus of the *Abhidharmakośabhāṣya* is not designated as 'yoga', a close reading of certain passages reflects a shared conceptual basis between the *Pātañjalayogaśāstra* and the *Abhidharmakośabhāṣya* in describing meditation practices that lead to spiritual liberation. More specifically, a complex of botanical and agricultural metaphors recurs across the *Abhidharmakośabhāṣya*, the *Pātañjalayogaśāstra* and the *Yogācārabhūmiśāstra*, respectively representing Sautrāntika, yoga and yogācāra ideas. This scheme of metaphors forms part of the broader soteriological paradigm of cultivation (*bhāvanā*), as a primary means to spiritual liberation. In particular, there is a conceptual resonance between the *Pātañjalayogaśāstra* and some key Sautrāntika and Sarvāstivāda ideas in the *Abhidharmakośabhāṣya*. Potentially, this stems from an entwinement of these two bodies of thought (Sautrāntika and Sarvāstivāda) in early yogācāra, as reflected in the first layers of the *Yogācārabhūmiśāstra*.

The resulting picture is of a yogic soteriology that is dialogically constructed across sectarian lines and compels us to review the issue of why, in scholarship, 'classical yoga' is still predominantly categorized as Brahmanic soteriology.[24] Going forward, it also prompts us to reassess what we include in the category of 'classical yoga' within the study of South Asian religions. Furthermore, the period during which the *Pātañjalayogaśāstra* was composed (*c.*325–425 CE – with some sections almost certainly being older) was against the general backdrop of the ascendant age of Buddhism in South Asia, providing a context for the hypothesis of conceptual influence from Buddhist soteriology in Patañjali's text.

Debate, doctrine and dialogue

In order to better understand how conceptual sharing might have occurred, it is necessary to paint a picture of the context of debate in the early Common Era. At the time of production of our texts (second to fifth centuries CE), the shared culture of debate ensured an intellectual milieu in which interaction between different schools of thought took place explicitly through refutation.

We cannot underestimate the significance of the role of debate in the transmission of ideas between schools of thought and communities in this period. As Gombrich reminds us, the Buddha's teachings began in an atmosphere of debate in which the Buddha was necessarily winning over converts from Brahmanism using the 'skilful means' of argument (Gombrich 1996: 1–26). In this respect, debate is built in to Buddhism. In the early centuries of the first millennium CE, there was also the broader formal context of philosophical debates at the royal courts (Bronkhorst 2006: 303). Biographical sources[25] claim that Vasubandhu partook in such debates. From these accounts, Anacker draws a picture of the intellectuals with whom Vasubandhu may have interacted, citing as possible contemporaries the poet Kālidāsa, the lexicographer Amarasiṃha and the Mīmāṃsā philosopher Śabara (Anacker 1984: 11). The stakes of philosophical debates were sometimes high, with material consequences such as punishments, beatings, and even death (Anacker 1984: 20). Although such debates were initially organized at court where participants from different schools were obliged by the king to engage with each other institutionally, these encounters became embedded in the scholarly culture, so that it became commonplace to critically refine one's own position by engaging with those of opponents (Bronkhorst 2006: 303).[26]

If oral debate was an inherent part of intellectual life in the first centuries of the Common Era, it also filtered into the literary apparatus of the written tradition, albeit less dynamically. The voluminous Sarvāstivāda *Mahāvibhāṣā*, which forms one basis for Vasubandhu's *Abhidharmakośabhāṣya*, is itself a systematic record of the debates that occurred in a conference called by the Emperor Kaniṣka *c.* the first to second century CE (Anacker 1984: 12). Those whose views are quoted include Dharmatrāta, Ghoṣaka, Vasumitra and Buddhadeva. Anacker notes, 'This tremendous work often reads like a committee report, with widely varying opinions being offered' (Anacker 1984: 12). The *Mahāvibhāṣā* shows acquaintance with Vaiśeṣika and Sāṃkhya (Bronkhorst 2006: 290),[27] and Vasubandhu refutes both the Sāṃkhyas and the Nyāya-Vaiśeṣikas in the *Abhidharmakośabhāṣya*[28] and the Sāṃkhyas in his *Paramārthasaptati*.[29] The *Sāṃkhyakārikā* closes by claiming that it is a distillation of the key points of the *Ṣaṣṭitantra* (a lost work) without the consideration of opponents' views (SKK 72), indicating that such views were originally laid out in the *Ṣaṣṭitantra*. Indeed, the Brahmanical *sūtra* format, as Tubb and Boose remind us, is essentially a remnant from oral presentation structured via logical argumentation, a 'series of signposts in an oral argument' (Tubb and Boose 2007: 1). In short, argumentative pluralism was built in to the philosophical texts of the early first millennium CE in India and as Pollock states: 'The classicity of Indian philosophy lies precisely in the development of reasoned argument in the face of wholesale conceptual assaults' (Pollock

2015). The three texts that I examine – the *Pātañjalayogaśāstra*, the *Yogācārabhūmiśāstra* and the *Abhidharmakośabhāṣya* – were produced within and against this backdrop of formal debate.

The degree to which intellectual identities, such as philosophical standpoints, were strictly tied to religious identities is not clear. Nicholson has argued that the traditional divisions between *āstika* and *nāstika* schools is better framed doctrinally as 'affirmer' and 'denier' rather than 'orthodox' and 'heterodox' (Nicholson 2010: 176–9). In his view, such school divisions showcase a medieval doxographic perspective that did not necessarily reflect complex and self-perceived doctrinal identities in the earlier periods. Although scholars retrospectively label the classical logicians as 'Buddhist logicians' or 'Nyāya logicians', for example, those figures may have understood themselves to be simply 'logicians'. Similarly, if we regard yoga as a philosophical training, as well as a soteriological one, then perhaps a yoga philosopher was first a foremost a philosopher and not an essentially 'Brahmin' or 'Buddhist' philosopher.[30] On the other hand, the following passages from the *Yogācārabhūmiśāstra* suggest clear sectarian identities for yoga in a soteriological context. In the commentarial section of the *Yogācārabhūmiśāstra*, the eighth chapter of the *Saṃdhinirmocanasūtra*[31] contains detail on yoga practice,[32] as well as a polemic against other ascetics who practice yoga. In the dialogue between the Buddha and the bodhisattva Maitreya, we are told,

> Then, on this occasion, the Lord made these statements: 'This exposition on Dharma and on Yoga, which is without fault, is for the higher good. Those who lean on the Dharma and who practice Yoga vigorously obtain enlightenment.
>
> Those who, in their own interest, reject Yoga and who, for the sake of liberation, scrutinize the Dharma, are as far from Yoga as the sky is from the earth. …
>
> For this reason, abandon refutation and idle debate, and increase your energy. In order to liberate gods and humans, devote yourself to Yoga'. (SNS 8: 40)[33]

This passage demonstrates that yoga was claimed by individual religions such as Buddhism, was doctrinally affiliated and was understood as a branch of the Buddha's *dharma*, or teaching. To underline this point, the same chapter closes:

> Then the bodhisattva Maitreya said to the Lord: 'Lord in this sermon of the *Saṃdhinirmocana*, what does one call this teaching? How is it apprehended?'
>
> The Lord responded: 'Maitreya: this is "The teaching of the explicit meaning of Yoga"'. (SNS 8.41)[34]

Such statements highlight how parts of the *Yogācārabhūmiśāstra* were as concerned with transmitting knowledge and systems of yoga as the *Pātañjalayogaśāstra*. These passages also highlight how the *Yogācārabhūmiśāstra* sets itself up as *the* authoritative exposition on yoga discipline.

In similar measure, the *Pātañjalayogaśāstra* contains a polemic against a Mahāyāna doctrine referred to as *cittamātra*, or mind-only.[35] The *sūtras* and commentary from PYŚ 4.14–23[36] address the relationship between mind (*citta*) and the external object, entailing a refutation of the Buddhist position[37] and concluding that those who believe that this world is mind-only are pitiable in their delusion.[38] The commentary to YS 4.23 leaves little doubt that it is a specific critique of the yogācāra doctrine – and most likely refers to the works of Vasubandhu or Asaṅga. Eventually, the Yogācāra epistemology was known by different names: not only *cittamātratā* ((the doctrine that) there is nothing but mind) but also *vijñānavāda* (consciousness doctrine) and *vijñaptimatratā* ((the doctrine that) there is nothing but representation). The first exposition of the doctrine of mind-only or representation-only[39] is commonly traced to Vasubandhu's works: *Vimśatikāvijñaptimatratāsiddhi*, *Triṃśikāvijnaptimatratā[siddhi]kārikā* and *Trisvabhāvanirdeśa*. However, Asaṅga also uses the term *cittamātra* in association with the theory of eight consciousnesses set forth in the *Viniścayasaṃgrahaṇī* portion of the *Yogācārabhūmiśāstra*, as well as in his other works, the *Mahāyānasaṃgraha* and *Mahāyānasūtrālaṅkāra*.[40] Indeed, the earliest use of the stock phrase associated with this doctrine – 'these three realms are nothing but mind' (*cittamātram idaṃ yad idaṃ traidhātukam*) – occurs in a Buddhist Sanskrit text no longer extant but which was translated into Chinese in 179 CE, the **Bhadrapālasūtra* (Schmithausen 1973: 246–7).[41] The same phrase subsequently appeared in both the *Daśabhūmikasūtra* (Rahder 1926: 49, 74)[42] and the *Saṃdhinirmocanasūtra* (Lamotte 1935: 90–1), works that are both important to understanding the *Yogācārabhūmiśāstra* (as we will see in Chapters 3 and 4).[43] Given the specificity of *cittamātra* as a label associated with early yogācāra, it is clear that Patañjali's polemic is directed at this stream of Buddhism specifically.

Larson's 'problem': Sāṃkhya, yoga and Buddhism

Of course, when examining the debates between Pātañjala yoga and the contemporaneous schools of Buddhism, any investigation must include the philosophy of Sāṃkhya[44] to which the *Pātañjalayogaśāstra* purports to adhere. Although many scholars have discussed the possible relationships between

Sāṃkhya and Buddhism, such studies can be supplemented and extended by further specific textual analysis. The arguments vary. Warder asks whether Sāṃkhya evolved not from the Vedic and Brahmanic traditions as largely supposed but rather from within the non-Vedic *śramaṇa* tradition (Warder 2000: 32–4). This view is echoed by Bronkhorst, who adds Vaiśeṣika to the mix; since systematic thinking began in Sarvāstivāda Buddhism (Bronkhorst 2006: 290), philosophical systems such as Sāṃkhya and Vaiśeṣika were closer to Buddhism than Vedic religion (Bronkhorst 2006: 287–8). In particular, Bronkhorst views Vaiśeṣika as influenced by Sarvāstivāda ontology, and Sāṃkhya as influenced by the culture of Greater Magadha.[45] Other scholars argue for an opposite direction of influence, that Buddhism may have evolved from Sāṃkhya (Garbe 1897: 12; Keith 1918: 20–8; Jacobsen 2008: 10). Chakravarti, too, proposes that the Vaibhāṣikas (the orthodox Sarvāstivādins) 'were more or less influenced by Sāṃkhya' in their ontology and speculates that 'the influence of Sāṃkhya upon the Abhidharma literature was brought about by scholars who had been previously adherents of Sāṃkhya' (Chakravarti 1975: 99 fn. 2). Chakravarti, then, posits an influx of Sāṃkhya scholars into Abhidharma at some point in time. Whatever the truth of these claims, we can certainly agree that ontological taxonomy is central to both Sāṃkhya, with its scheme of the constituents (*tattvas*), and Abhidharma Buddhism, with its complex classifications of the factors (*dharmas*).[46] Yet, as Bronkhorst emphasizes, something does not quite add up about the *Sāṃkhyakārikā* in relation to the textual impressions left by its predecessors in Sāṃkhya thought.

> Various early authors – most notable among them Bhartṛhari, Dharmapāla, and Mallavādin – attribute to Sāṃkhya a position which differs from the one which finds expression in the surviving Sāṃkhya works. According to them, Sāṃkhya looked upon substances as being collections of qualities. (Bronkhorst 2006: 288)[47]

It is clear that Sāṃkhya itself was in transition during, or just before, the period of the composition of the *Pātañjalayogaśāstra*, undergoing 'important changes' during the second to fourth centuries CE (Bronkhorst 2006: 288). Given that this transition overlaps with the window of time during which the *Pātañjalayogaśāstra* was compiled, it makes it increasingly problematic to state that it is a straightforward Sāṃkhya text, when we cannot be sure where Sāṃkhya itself stood at this point in time.

Larson's 1989 essay 'An Old Problem Revisited: The Relation Between Sāṃkhya, Yoga and Buddhism' still provides a rigorous investigation of the intellectual identity of the author of the *Yogasūtra* and its *bhāṣya*. And in assessing the relationship between Sāṃkhya and Buddhist philosophy in the fourth–fifth centuries, this present book must also revisit Larson's 'problem'.[48] Although the first surviving work of Sāṃkhya is the *Sāṃkhyakārikā*, produced in the fourth century CE, Larson believes that the lost *Ṣaṣṭitantra*[49] was the first systematic presentation of Sāṃkhya philosophy.[50] In speculating about the authorship of this lost treatise, he alights on Vārṣagaṇya as the most probable agent (Larson 1989: 133).[51] Thus the Sāṃkhya work of Vārṣagaṇya around the second century CE would have roughly coincided with the commentarial output of Sarvāstivāda Abhidharma (Larson 1989: 133). The parallel that Larson draws between Sāṃkhya and Abhidharma is not in terms of doctrine but rather the structural tendency towards systematic enumeration.[52] Since the terms of *ṣaṣṭitantra* are largely absent from the *Yogaśūtra*, while many more terms from Abhidharma Buddhism appear, 'there were two streams of early systematic philosophizing in India, namely Ṣaṣṭitantra of Sāṃkhya and the Abhidharma of Sarvāstivāda and Sautrāntika' (Larson 1989: 134): these two streams of soteriological thought were known as the *vijñāna* (knowledge-based) philosophy of Sāṃkhya and the *nirodha-samādhi* (cessative concentration) philosophy of Abhidharma (Larson 1989: 136).[53] In sum, the foundational work of Sāṃkhya (the lost *Ṣaṣṭitantra*) was produced in the heyday of Abhidharma commentarial output in the second century and appears to share some key philosophical features.

By looking into the historical record of debates, Larson proposed that Vindhyavāsin was the real 'author' of the *Sāṃkhyapravacanabhāṣya*, which somehow became mistakenly attributed to the grammarian Patañjali and renamed as the *Yogasūtrabhāṣya* (Larson 1989: 135). Larson thus identified three different interpreters of the Sāṃkhya *ṣaṣṭitantra* tradition: Vārṣagaṇya as the author of the lost *Ṣaṣṭitantra*, Īśvarakṛṣṇa as author of the later *Sāṃkhykārikā* and Vindhyavāsin (of whom no proven works are extant), who innovated around Sāṃkhya philosophy in dialogue with the Buddhists and possibly wrote the *Yogasūtrabhāṣya* (Larson 1989: 134).[54] Regarding the debates that occurred, this is how Larson sets up the order of events (Larson and Bhattacharya 2008: 41–2):

1. In the first to second century CE, Vārṣagaṇya creates the *Ṣaṣṭitantra*, based on an older version of this text.[55]
2. Sometime in the fourth century CE (300–350), Īśvarakṛṣna creates the *Sāṃkhyakārikā*, which purports to be a summary of the views of Vārṣagaṇya.

3. Vindhyavāsin, a Sāṃkhya teacher and follower of Vārṣagaṇya, becomes involved in a debate with the Buddhist Buddhamitra, one of the teachers of Vasubandhu. Vindhyavāsin wins and receives a prize from the king.[56]
4. In defence of his teacher, Vasubandhu launches a successful attack on Sāṃkhya in the form of an oral debate and a subsequent treatise, the *Paramārthasaptati*.[57]
5. Vindhyavāsin then revises Sāṃkhya to address Buddhist ideas and to defend it against new attacks. He not only influences the redactor of the *Yogasūtra* but also creates the *Yogasūtrabhāṣya* (the *Sāṃkhyapravacanabhāṣya*) to systematize and update yoga philosophy while also incorporating popular Buddhist language and ideas.

In short, Larson postulates that the *Yogasūtra* and its *bhāṣya* emerged from a dialogue between the Sāṃkhya thinker Vindhyavāsin and the Buddhist Vasubandhu. It was Vindhyavāsin who was responsible for the radical philosophical hybridity of the *Pātañjalayogaśāstra* and not Patañjali, who was merely a textual compiler in the shadows.[58] At the end of his article, Larson points towards the need for further understanding of the triadic relationship between yoga, Sāṃkhya and Abhidharma, and this is still a valid entreaty.

I concur that while Larson's broad assessment of the interaction between Sāṃkhya and Sarvāstivāda Abhidharma is highly plausible, there are several aspects that must be probed further, namely the ways in which this interaction occurred and the reasons why it occurred. Larson does not appear to distinguish between Sarvāstivāda and Sautrāntika thought, even though Sautrāntika positions are distinct soteriogically. Additionally, I would like to extend Larson's polyphonic 'mix' by including the vital influence of early yogācāra, which itself contained strands of Sarvāstivāda and Sautrāntika. Larson's identification of the Buddhist component of the *Pātañjalayogaśāstra* as 'Buddhist psychology and/or meditation theory' also merits rethinking. Such an analysis is somewhat limited because the *Pātañjalayogaśāstra* also includes Abhidharma and Sautrāntika ontology and epistemology. Overall, when assessing the intellectual, and particularly the soteriological, components of the *Pātañjalayogaśāstra*, we are looking at a dense myriad web of confluences and interactions that probably took many configurations, with ideas constantly moving back and forth across religious and philosophical demarcations.

The ontological debates

To date, analyses of the philosophical interaction between Pātañjala yoga and Buddhist traditions have focused primarily on epistemology.[59] For example, Sparham argued that yogācāra drew on proto-Sāṃkhya models of mind regarding a permanent mental substratum, which was then refashioned by yogācāra as the notion of storehouse-consciousness (*ālayavijñāna*) (Sparham 1993: 9–10). However, this present book highlights polemical interactions that have been less well examined, those in the domain of ontology. As I discuss in Chapter 1, ontological positions form a necessary basis for soteriology, theories of existential liberation. In our texts, this is clearly expressed using metaphors such as the seed, which proved particularly effective for constructing theories of being, becoming and transformation.

We have discussed Vārṣagaṇya as an important Sāṃkhya thinker from *c.* second century CE who may, or may not, have been the author of the lost *Ṣaṣṭitantra*. Vārṣagaṇya was also known to the Buddhists, as is evident from both the *Yogācārabhūmiśāstra* and the *Abhidharmakośabhāṣya*. In the *Savitarkādibhūmi* – one of the books of the *Yogācārabhūmiśāstra* – Vārṣagaṇya is named as an adherent of the doctrine that the effect pre-exists in the cause (*satkāryavāda*). This doctrine, central to Sāṃkhya ontology and casuality, holds that the effect pre-exists in the cause in a potential state and that change is then merely a transformation (*pariṇāma*) of what was already there.[60] Here, the doctrine of *satkāryavāda* is called the *hetuphalasadvāda* (the doctrine of the existence of the effect in the cause).[61]

> What is the doctrine of the existence of the effect in the cause? It is just as when some *śramaṇa* or *brāhmaṇa* holds this view or says this: the result exists (*vidyata*) in the cause solely as the eternal in eternal time or the perpetual in perpetual time. Such a one is a Vārṣagaṇya follower. (*Savitarkādibhūmi* 6.38) [62]

Indeed, Mikogami points out that the way in which Asaṅga systematically refutes the Sāṃkhya theory of *satkāryavāda* closely mirrors the structure of an argument in the *Sāṃkhyakārikā*, which defends this very position (Mikogami: 1969: 445). Mikogami concludes that the *Yogācārabhūmiśāstra* is therefore referring to the earlier work of Vārṣagaṇya (the *Ṣaṣṭitantra*), which predates the *Sāṃkhyakārikā*. The author of the *Sāṃkhyakārikā* (Īśvarakṛṣṇa) subsequently used Asaṅga's critique (in the YĀBh) to strengthen his own position (Mikogami 1969: 447). We also find reference to the followers of Vārṣagaṇya in the *Abhidharmakośabhāṣya*. Here, the dissident Sautrāntikas accuse the orthodox Vaibhāṣikas of running dangerously close to the Vārṣagaṇyas (i.e. the Sāṃkhyas) with their theory of dharma and temporality.[63] The Sautrāntikas also criticize the Vaibhāṣika notion of 'the three times'[64] as sounding like 'pre-existence' and bearing a resemblance to the Sāṃkhya doctrine of *satkāryavāda*.[65] In both Buddhist passages above, the name Vārṣagaṇya stands in for the Sāṃkhyas, and in both cases the particular doctrine of *satkāryavāda* is singled out for polemical comment. This reflects the interaction of the Abhidharma and Yogācāra schools with the ontology of Sāṃkhya, a conceptual web from which the *Pātañjalayogaśāstra* constructs its soteriology.

In fact, Vārṣagaṇya is only mentioned once in the *Pātañjalayogaśāstra* and then in relation to ontological matters (PYŚ 3.53). However, the doctrine of *satkāryavāda* is referenced indirectly in PYŚ 2.15 commentary in relation to *upādāna* (grasping/cause) and self.[66]

> Of these, *saṃsāra*, because it contains great suffering, is to be escaped. The cause of that which is to be escaped (i.e. suffering) is the conjunction of *pradhāna* (unmanifest Prakṛti) with Puruṣa. Escape (*hānam*) is when there is absolute cessation of the conjunction. The means of escaping is correct seeing. In correct seeing, the intrinsic nature of the one who escapes is not something that should be accepted or rejected: if it is rejected the consequence is the doctrine of its[67] annihilation, and if accepted (*upādāne*) the doctrine that it has a cause. When both [doctrines] are denied, the doctrine that it is eternal [follows]; this is correct seeing. (PYŚ 2.15)[68]

This passage argues that self is an eternal given and is not something that is 'caused' – which is in line with Sāṃkhya. The passage also functions as a refutation – two other doctrines are referred to and rejected – that the self can be annihilated or caused. The broader context of the passage appears to be a response to Buddhist doctrine in two ways. The first way is to refashion the four noble truths of Buddhism (suffering, the cause of suffering, cessation, the path) so that the Buddhist frame is, rather, filled with Sāṃkhya doctrinal content. Patañjali's second dialogic response appears to be a reference to the Buddha's rejection of two 'extreme' views: the doctrine of annihilation (*ucchedavāda*) and the doctrine of an eternal self (*śaśvatavāda*).[69] Thus Patañjali appropriates the Buddha's critique of the two extremes and makes it a critique of Buddhism itself. Often, schools did not have to be explicitly named in textual refutation; it was enough to refer to their doctrines alone.

The nature of philosophical debate in the early period means that we cannot regard our three texts as anything less than intertextual. If philosophical authors were not referring to each others' work via processes of refutation and co-option, they would have been going against the intellectual grain. Such sparring dialogues only partially reflect the need to distinguish one's position on the basis of difference. Rather, debates were used to explore the weaknesses in one's own argument in order to strengthen it for the next round. In the centuries preceding the final redactions of our three texts (PYŚ, YĀBh, AKBh), that is, in the second to third century CE, Sarvāstivāda Abhidharma was flourishing, and the first systematization of Sāṃkhya was taking place in Vārṣagaṇya's work. It seems likely that Sāṃkhya and Sarvāstivāda Abhidharma co-evolved in a milieu of debate, and this is certainly reflected in both schools' emphases on ontological categorization. Debate, then, was an environment in which difference cloaked similarity; on the surface these schools refuted each other, but in the detail of the debate they co-constructed their own concepts in partnership with their opponents.

The discursive correspondences between the *Pātañjalayogaśāstra* and the *Abhidharmakośabhāṣya* discussed in this book and in other studies (e.g. Maas 2020) suggest one of two things: either that both texts are crystallizations of the same milieu of live debate or that one author is consciously making intertextual revisions to the other's text as a form of refutation. A text that expresses refutation is an interesting case in literature. In live debate, there are always two sides and hence at least two audiences (in favour and against), but in textual accounts of such debates the audience is necessarily reduced to a single presence, the reader. In the case of the *Pātañjalayogaśāstra*, the intended audience of the text were Brahmin yogins (PYŚ 2.30–3).[70] However, if the refutational strategies of the *Pātañjalayogaśāstra* were to be truly effective, a point-by-point critique of the stock arguments of Abhidharma could have only been 'victorious' if the audience were already familiar with that doctrinal context. It leads to the question as to whether Patañjali's *sūtra* text was aimed at Brahmins who also knew the Abhidharma texts or whether there was a wider scholastic audience of Buddhists who were able to read, consult or listen to the *Pātañjalayogaśāstra*. Given the detailed correspondences of the *Pātañjalayogaśāstra* to instances of Sarvāstivāda and yogācāra discourse in the fourth to fifth centuries (discussed in Chapters 2, 3 and 4), one can suggest that the text's function was partly to serve as a record of structured refutations of Buddhist karma theory and path (*mārga*) systems to liberation. Patañjali also appears to co-opt certain argument forms, conceptual metaphors and rhetorical structures from the Buddhists and then to replace the metaphysics with those of Sāṃkhya. Whatever the direction of the intertextual borrowings, Patañjali was certainly familiar with the concepts of the Buddhist Sarvāstivāda and yogācāra milieux – and we must assume that his audience was too.

Joining the dots: 'Classical yoga' and 'Buddhist yoga'

There is somewhat of a scholarly divide between those who study 'classical yoga' and those who study 'Buddhist yoga'. To date, much of the scholarship on classical yoga has focused on the place of yoga within Brahmanical and early Hindu traditions. In this book, I demonstrate that integrating the findings of contemporary scholars in Buddhist studies within current research in 'classical yoga' scholarship generates a richer understanding of the discourse of historical yoga and of the character and evolution of yoga soteriology in the early Common Era. There is much analysis in recent scholarship on yogācāra and Sautrāntika that, when used to contextualize the *Pātañjalayogaśāstra*, can yield fresh and interesting insights about Pātañjala yoga.

In Buddhist studies, the label 'Buddhist yoga' is not widely used.[71] Rather the significance of the term 'yoga' in Buddhist texts is often absorbed into the general lexicon of spiritual practice. Tzohar, for example, translates the title *Yogācārabhūmi* as 'Levels of Spiritual Training' (Tzohar 2018: 9). A recent examination of yogācāra in Buddhism is Kragh's formidable edited volume, *The Foundation for Yoga Practitioners: The Buddhist Yogācārabhūmi Treatise and Its Adaptation in India, East India, and Tibet*. This impressive study runs to almost 1,500 pages and provides an in-depth account of the *Yogācārabhūmiśāstra* and its reception history. Yet of the thirty-five essays that analyse the subject matter of the text as 'yoga discipline' (yogācāra),[72] none explores yogācāra in relation to the contemporaneous Pātañjala yoga. Kragh – understandably given the breadth of his volume – restricts his analysis of yoga to 'the Buddhist parlance of the time' (Kragh 2013b: 30).

However, it is problematic to suggest that the meaning of the term 'yoga' in the *Yogācārabhūmiśāstra* pertains only to Buddhist contexts[73] – as it is reductive to restrict the semantic field of 'yoga' to Brahmanic *or* Buddhist discourse. Indeed, it is difficult to isolate any term as precisely or definitively 'Buddhist' and not also 'Jain' or 'Brahmanic' (e.g. the shared term for meditative absorption *jhāna*, *jhana*, *dhyāna*)[74] – such was the degree of interaction, conversion and confluence between these communities. Moreover, Sanskrit was a shared language for scholastic writing between Buddhists (Śrāvakayāna and Mahāyāna) and

Brahmins – and, from the time of Umāsvāti, for Jains too.[75] However, restricting a study of yoga to the 'classical' form of Patañjali or to a discrete Buddhist context is not unusual within the study of religions. This is, of course, reflective of how field-specialists within the study of religions have worked historically; religions and texts have been viewed as clearly delimited entities.[76] However, if we upscale our object of study from the religious text to religious discourse, we will see that discourse (being intertextual) cannot be so easily fenced off.

An effective methodology to address the limitations of disciplinary streamlining in the study of religious texts is intertextuality. This approach impacts upon the categorization of religious practice. In 'Nets of Intertextuality: Embedded Scriptural Citations in the *Yogācārabhūmi*', Skilling highlights the difficulties of categorizing schools of thought and proposes the importance of 'polylogue' (2013: 783). He debunks the categorical separation of Buddhist 'streams' such as 'Mainstream versus Mahāyāna' and declares, 'There was no Mainstream, there were only many streams' (Skilling 2013: 783). In accordance with his argument that there was not a monolithic Buddhism nor discrete Buddhist schools, I argue that there was not a singular tradition of classical yoga. Texts are not enclosed units of language and meaning but are rather entwined discussions within a wider field of discourse – and the discourse of yoga in fourth- to fifth-century South Asia was an entangled one. Thus, when we look back on distant history from such a removed vantage point how can we even be sure which living communities were the dominant proponents of the discourse of yoga? Perhaps, at certain points in the early Common Era, it was the Buddhists.

To sum up: when analysing yoga discourse in the early first millennium, we are compelled to consider not only the term 'yoga' itself but also standard synonyms such as *samādhi*, *dhyāna*, *bhāvanā* – and, of course, yogācāra. Therefore, a text does not have to refer explicitly to 'yoga' for it to share the same discourse or episteme as the *Pātañjalayogaśāstra*. The religio-philosophical milieu was one of vibrant dialogic interaction, and rival schools often critiqued each others' positions vigorously. When we consider the dialogic nature of lived philosophy together with the way in which *śāstra*s partly functioned as syntheses of prior textual knowledge, our reading approach cannot be other than 'intertextual'. Simply put, intertextual analysis helps us to access and understand the polyphonic cultural forum in which the discourse of yoga was co-constructed in the so-called classical period.

1

Mokṣa, metaphors and materiality: Concepts and contexts of 'liberation'

Introduction

Contrary to the perennial view on religion and philosophy,[1] yoga and meditation are not 'timeless, essential, universal' practices that have always existed unchanged across history. Rather, these practices were created and developed by humans in specific material contexts. It is those contexts that this chapter investigates by laying out some key material settings[2] for the early development of yoga and meditation schemes – contexts that affirm the interconnectedness of Buddhism and Brahmanism in this respect. Not only is it necessary to disrupt the 'timeless origins' narrative of yoga to gain a better understanding of its early beginnings, but we must also probe our very understanding of the embodied and mental reality of these practices and beliefs. What is one 'doing' when one follows a system of meditation to attain 'liberation' (*mokṣa* or *nirvāṇa*)? Models or paths of yoga and meditation are, in fact, complex systems of conceptual metaphors that are derived from bodily experiences of the material world. This chapter identifies some primary metaphors of mind and meditation in 'classical' Indic soteriology and then critically examines them to show how such metaphors were constructed within real-world agrarian and urban economies in the early first millennium CE. In brief, early meditation was materially determined, and textual metaphors tell us something about the material world in which they were produced. Since meditation schemes did not arise in a cultural vacuum, we can argue against the easy cultural transferability of such schemes across material contexts, time and space – for example, from the South Asian Gupta regime to contemporary global contexts. However, within the early Common Era itself – across religious communities – soteriologies were interlinked and metaphors were a basis of conceptual transference. Lastly, by establishing a framework of systematic connections between conceptual metaphors that were shared in

Sanskrit texts on yogic meditation, we can advance our understanding of possible shared material and geographical contexts for Brahmanical and Buddhist yoga.

In the following sections, I consider the role of metaphors within soteriology, specifically with regard to meditation, in order to argue that soteriology is necessarily constituted by conceptual metaphors. Then, I sketch a broad picture of the soteriological thinking around meditative cultivation (*bhāvanā*) in the early Common Era. *Bhāvanā*, I argue, can be understood as a complex 'orientational' metaphor that was mapped from the domain of botanical cultivation. This metaphorical complex was predominantly found within Buddhist discourse, and Patañjali enfolded aspects of Buddhist *bhāvanā* into his śāstric system of yoga.

What are conceptual metaphors?

The classical Indian theory of metaphor is often framed as one of ornament rather than function and will not be discussed here (but see Appendix 2 for a summary of the issues). Rather, this study employs a contemporary theory of metaphor as an analytical basis for approaching Indic thought. So why might metaphor be useful or relevant in understanding 'classical yoga' or the way in which Buddhism and Hinduism interacted? Until recent decades, the Western notion of metaphor has been framed primarily through the classical rhetorical theory of Aristotle, and defined as an aspect of figurative speech, conventionally contrasted with literal speech.[3] However, contemporary theories of metaphor have been wrought in many disciplines (such as linguistics, literature and philosophy), and this book draws on an understanding of metaphor that is derived more from cognitive linguistics than from classical rhetoric. Conceptual metaphor theory (part of a broader approach of cognitive metaphor theory)[4] was initiated by Lakoff and Johnson (Lakoff and Johnson 1980),[5] who proposed two fresh ideas: firstly that metaphors are an inherent cognitive reflex and not a linguistic one and secondly that metaphors are not only analogous but also contingent. According to this approach, figures of speech – such as metaphor and metonymy[6] – are not just about conveying ideas and nor are they ornamental literary devices. Rather, metaphors are unconscious and reflect how thinking and thought are fundamentally structured. Metaphors, then, are not a property of language or words but are a property of concepts – that is to say, we cannot form concepts without metaphors. As Lakoff and Johnson put it, 'our ordinary conceptual system, in terms of which we both think and act, is fundamentally metaphorical in nature' (Lakoff and Johnson 1980: 3).[7] Let us now survey some core principles of conceptual metaphor theory.

Domain-mapping

Lakoff and Johnson introduced the idea that metaphor is produced by 'domain-mapping'. This is the cognitive process by which one area of life (a domain)[8] is conceptualized in the terms of another, with the properties transferred from one domain to the other (Lakoff and Johnson 1980). People construct concepts, particularly abstract ones, by mapping their knowledge of more concrete domains to more abstract domains. Thus, two unconnected spheres of life are drawn together in a metaphor – qualities from a source domain are mapped to a target domain.[9] This process of connecting two domains in metaphor can be partially accounted for by similarity. Kövecses offers the example of a human life cycle (target) conceived of as a plant cycle (source).

> In both domains, there is an entity that comes into existence; it begins to grow and reaches a point in its development when it is strongest; then it begins to decline; and finally it goes out of existence. (Kövecses 2017: 18)

However, in conceptual theory, metaphor is understood to operate primarily not on the basis of analogy (as in the Aristotelian understanding), but often because the target and source domains are *not* alike. Domains are frequently connected by convention rather than inherent likeness.

In this study of domain-mapping in soteriological metaphors, I focus on the mapping of attributes from the domain of agricultural cultivation to the domain of spiritual cultivation. In this process, religious striving, particularly meditation, is conceptualized in the terms of crop cultivation. Such domain-mapping produces a conceptual pattern, and many conceptual patterns are shared between Brahmanism and Buddhism.

Selective editing

As Lakoff and Johnson point out, there are limits to the efficacy of a metaphor, and these are inherent in the nature of metaphor itself. The structuring of one concept using the qualities (semantic features) of another concept can only ever be a partial and not a complete process; otherwise, there would be a total identification between two 'objects' (Lakoff and Johnson 1980: 13). This means that the features of one domain are selectively edited in order to map them most effectively to the other domain. Such editing entails highlighting some qualities of the source domain and hiding others.[10]

Structural metaphor

Lakoff and Johnson identified types of metaphor that function differently. The simplest form is that of the structural metaphor, which is the basic association of two domains via a mapping of qualities. For example, in the metaphor LIFE IS A JOURNEY,[11] the abstract domain of life (target) is understood by mapping qualities from a more concrete domain (source), a journey. This basic structural metaphor can be seen in common expressions such as 'children need a good *start* in life' or 'death is the *end*'.

Complex metaphor

Structural metaphors can be combined to create compound or complex metaphors. An example of a compound metaphor is PURPOSEFUL LIFE IS A JOURNEY, which contains more than one metaphor. This compound is created by combining several related structural metaphors: LIFE IS A JOURNEY (see above), PURPOSE IS DESTINATION (e.g. 'getting one's career *on track*'; 'finding one's *direction* in life') and DIFFICULTIES ARE IMPEDIMENTS ('life is full of *obstacles*'; 'life has *bumps* in the road').

Primary metaphor

Primary metaphors are those that are generated by sensorimotor experience. An example of a primary metaphor is INTENSITY IS HEAT. This primary association is initially created by the sensorimotor experience of an increase of temperature in the body during intense emotional experiences. This primary association is then extended to apply to specific emotional experiences, such as ANGER IS HEAT or DESIRE IS FIRE. Examples of everyday sayings that express the underlying conceptual metaphor ANGER IS HEAT are 'you make my blood boil', 'letting off steam', 'he blew up at me', 'she lost her cool', 'hothead' and so on. Examples relating to DESIRE IS FIRE include 'burning up with desire', 'the fires of passion', 'love fizzled out', 'the spark of attraction' and so on.[12]

Orientational metaphors and image-schemas

Another type of metaphor is an orientational metaphor. An orientational metaphor expresses a whole system of concepts with regard to another system. Furthermore, orientational metaphors have a spatial dimension (Lakoff and

Johnson 1980: 14). This spatial aspect is expressed by developing metaphoric 'directions' for concepts. The classic example is that happy is conceived as 'up' and sad as 'down'. Thus, the linguistic expressions 'I am feeling upbeat' or 'I am feeling downcast' are part of a larger orientational metaphor that expresses a whole system of feelings. These orientational metaphors create large-scale interlocking systems such as ethics, emotions and values.[13]

An image-schema is the practical knowledge drawn from the physical domain (the body or the environment) and is based on 'recurring patterns of embodied experience' (Gibbs 2017: 23). An image-schema, then, is a preconceptual structure governed by bodily logic. Two common image-schemas are 'verticality' (which produces the metaphors HAPPY IS UP and SAD IS DOWN) or 'source-path-goal' (which produces LIFE IS A JOURNEY). As Gibbs states, 'image schemas can generally be defined as dynamic analog representations of spatial relations and movements in space' (Gibbs 2017: 23). The orientational metaphors HAPPY IS UP and SAD IS DOWN are initially produced by sensorimotor experience[14] but are then extended to produce abstract statements: 'good is up' and 'bad is down', 'more is up'[15] and 'less is down'; 'unknown is up' and 'known is down'; or 'virtue is up' and 'sin is down' (Lakoff and Johnson 1980: 19–20). Although the scope of these conceptual schemes is complex, there is an overall external systematicity[16] and coherence (Lakoff and Johnson 1980: 18).[17]

Metaphoric entailment

Cognitive metaphor theory maintains that a conceptual metaphor can influence or affect reality because of the way that we extend metaphors. For example, let us consider the common cross-cultural metaphor ANGER IS HEAT[18] or ANGER IS A FIRE, derived from the experiential sensation of raised temperature in the body during the mood of anger. The real-world knowledge that a fire can be extinguished produces the expectation that anger, like a fire, can be extinguished or quenched (i.e. it is not an eternal or incessant phenomenon and can be countered by a 'cooling' or 'cessative' agent). The conceptuality of ANGER IS HEAT can be logically extended to produce ANGER CAN BE QUENCHED. Thus, conceptual metaphors have real-world impacts:

> A major consequence of the idea that metaphors are conceptual in nature, i.e. that we conceive of certain things in metaphorical ways, is that, since our conceptual system governs how we act in the world, we often act metaphorically. (Kövecses 2017: 17)

In a conceptual metaphor, the possibilities of logical extension in the target domain are determined or shaped by the parameters of the source domain (and often informed by sensorimotor experience). Domain-mapping, then, is inferentially determined, is underpinned by an unconsciously reasoned process and is logically entailed.

To connect this example to the context of South Asian religion and philosophy, we can identify the central 'problem' of Buddhism as the 'fire' of suffering. The solution to this suffering is *nirvāṇa*, which literally denotes the quenching of a flame. Thus, this soteriological strand of Buddhism is underpinned by the primary (sensorimotor) metaphor INTENSITY IS HEAT, which is extended to SUFFERING IS FIRE, while the solution to this problem is logically entailed as NON-SUFFERING (LIBERATION) IS THE QUENCHING OF FIRE. The elements of Buddhist practice designed to facilitate liberation are, then, constructed in relation to these metaphorical concepts. Conceptual metaphor is informed by processes of reasoning: not only can conceptual metaphors be driven by analogical reasoning (in the mapping from the source to the target domain), but they are often underpinned by syllogistic structures of deductive reasoning and are therefore subject to logical entailment, as in the above example:

> Fire can be quenched
> Suffering is fire
> Therefore suffering can be quenched

Lakoff and Turner also note that in metaphor image-schemas 'the spatial logic of the image-schema is preserved by metaphorical mappings and becomes abstract logic in the nonspatial target domains' (Lakoff and Turner 1989: 100). This constraint produces logical consistency and is called the 'invariance principle' (Lakoff and Turner 1989).

'Live' and 'dead' metaphor

A standard distinction in the analysis of metaphors is that between creative metaphors and commonplace metaphors (or 'live' and 'dead' metaphors). Creative metaphors are those that are generated in a 'live' context, while commonplace metaphors are those that have become 'lexicalized' or 'conventionalized' through repeated use over time and so no longer have a conceptual link to the original metaphoric referent. These commonplace metaphors become so engrained in our thinking that we no longer notice them. The linguistic expressions 'a local *branch* of this organisation' and '*cultivating* business relationships' draw on tree and agriculture metaphors, while 'the *workings* of the mind' draws on the metaphor of the mind as a machine. These dead metaphors are so far removed in time from the historical contexts in which they were created that they are no longer perceived as metaphors but as literally descriptive language. Metaphors, then, play a role in the diachronic development of language, and the transition from a creative metaphor to a commonplace metaphor is one that can be traced (Allott 2010: 122). Therefore, analysing literary metaphors can support speculations about chronologies of texts, as a kind of supplement to the more explicit evidence of doctrinal developments or manuscript dating. The change from live to dead metaphors is also a process that we see in the transition from oral to written texts. The process is 'fossilization' of discourse; what began as oral teachings, mnemonic scriptures, epic recitation and live debates is frozen in time when committed to the written form. We would, then, expect to see many dead metaphors in written texts derived from oral culture.

Metaphors and soteriology

Soteriology is the theory or study of religious doctrines of 'salvation'. Although 'salvation' itself is an inherently Christian concept,[19] soteriology is an attempt to encapsulate the theories by which different religions define goals or 'success'. The end goals of different religions can be entirely at odds with each other; for example, the aspiration in Christianity towards 'a world without end' is in fact the very problem that Indic soteriology seeks to solve – escape from prolonged living in the form of reincarnation (Collins 2010: 31). Doctrinal statements such as the Buddhist 'All life is suffering' or the Brahmanic 'The self is misperceived' or the Jain 'The soul is in bondage' are formulations of an existential problem to which the various soteriologies are applied. Thus meditation, yoga[20] and other practices are abstracted from the concrete context of a human or social problem (in this time, in this place, for this person or society) and are offered as independent units of knowledge that represent universal solutions (true for all people, in all places, in all time). In his study of Theravada Buddhism, Gombrich defines soteriological religion as a matter of individual beliefs which are only secondarily connected to systems of ethics and right practices (Gombrich 1988: 26, 41). However, if we acknowledge the centrality of metaphor in soteriology, this undermines the notion that soteriology is a matter of individual belief; a metaphorical system can only operate in language on the basis of shared conceptuality. Viefhues-Bailey describes the role of metaphors in religion:

> Far from describing different types of religious entities, they are heuristic devices helping us organize the various functions that religious symbols and practices can and do play in the lives of practitioners. (Viefhues-Bailey 2017: 252)

Thus, belief in the efficacy of a particular soteriology is not simply a matter of private belief but one of shared conceptuality, as reflected in interwoven discourses of liberation within and between religious societies.

Since soteriology is particularly replete with abstract concepts such as self, soul, god, heaven, reincarnation, afterlife and so on, it follows that it should be a realm that is dense with conceptual metaphor. As Kövecses states, the typical direction of domain-mapping is from concrete to abstract, that is, from that which we know about to that which we do not know about (Kövecses 2017: 13). In other words, in dealing with the hidden (the self), the unknown (post-death states; god), the invisible (the soul) and the utopian (heaven), soteriology is always directed towards the temporally and spatially absent, the not-here and the not-now. Soteriological thinking is an aspiration towards immateriality and immortality and, as such, is a domain that is entirely abstract – there is no way to conceive of it other than through the concrete.

Metaphor in soteriology is not optional or ornamental, and we would be mistaken to think that a metaphor such as Patañjali's cloud of dharma, *dharmamegha*, used to describe a meditative state, is merely aesthetic embellishment. Of course, in a literary sense such elaborate description – in the Buddhist Mahāyāna *sūtra*s, for example – does add aesthetic value to a text. However, metaphor is also a structural expression of the deep semantic field of Indic soteriology in the early Common Era. To put it another way, soteriology in this period is structured by the domain-mapping of metaphor and is given meaning through metaphors.

In early South Asian religion and philosophy, soteriology was conceptualized primarily as attainment of 'liberation'. The metaphor SUCCESS IS LIBERATION was then used as a basis on which to construct other more complex metaphors. Jainism, Hinduism and Buddhism share a theory of emancipation from a wheel of earthly existence (*saṃsāra*) that is characterized by suffering and rebirth. Although these religions present diverse technical understandings of *mokṣa*,[21] nonetheless 'liberation' in some variant form is the prevalent conceptual goal.[22] Moreover, any doctrine of liberation is, by definition, metaphorical. In speaking of 'liberation of the soul' or 'escape from *saṃsāra*' or 'transcendental freedom', one is necessarily evoking metaphorical concepts such as the self/soul is 'caged', or the self/soul is 'bound' to a 'wheel' that rotates, or that the self/soul can somehow fly 'up' once 'unfettered'.[23] Key paradigms in Buddhism include enlightenment as 'awakening' (*bodhi*), the attainment of 'fruition' (*phalasamāpatti*), completing the 'path' (*mārga*) and, most famously, *nirvāṇa* as the quenching of a flame due to lack of fuel.[24] In all of the soteriological systems in this period, bodily practice is merely preparatory, while some form of meditation holds the key to liberation. Once we accept that soteriology itself is intrinsically metaphorical, then meditation, as the salvific method par excellence, is also by definition a metaphorical act.

Metaphor and meditation

In the Principal *Upaniṣads*, there is an evolution in the terminology used to denote the act of contemplation, a shift in usage from *upāsana* (veneration) in the early *Upaniṣads* to *dhyāna* (absorption) in the later *Upaniṣads*.[25] The root √*ās* in *upāsana* denotes both 'to venerate' and 'to take as' which can mean to 'take one thing to be the same as another. The term thus establishes equivalences between components of different spheres' (Olivelle 1998: 314). It seems, then, that the early act of contemplation or *upāsana*, rooted as it is in Upaniṣadic correspondences between self and cosmos, is a metonymic act, in the sense of substituting one thing for another. Roebuck highlights the associative dimension of *upāsana*, which renders it structurally similar to the texts' key principles of establishing conceptual relationship (*bandhu*) and connection (*upaniṣad*):

> Often the seeker is advised to contemplate something as a symbol or embodiment of something else, as in the first words of the *Chāndogya Upaniṣad*: 'One should contemplate the syllable OṂ as the Udgītha.' (Roebuck 2000: xxi)

However, *upāsana* and *dhyāna* are not identical actions. If *upāsana* is metonymic (and, as we can see in the above example of *oṃ*, at times synecdochical), then *dhyāna* is metaphoric, in that it deals with conceptual metaphors such as 'levels' of attainment, 'stages' of progress, the 'path' of practice, 'awakening' from spiritual sleep and so forth. Indeed, if we accept that 'mind' itself is a concept (Lakoff and Johnson 1980: 61), then meditation, which uses the mind to investigate the mind, is a reflexively conceptual act or process.

Stuart's analysis of the path of meditation in the Buddhist meditation text *Saddharmasmṛtyupasthānasūtra* (*Saddhsu*) (second to fourth century CE) concludes that there is a 'central importance of simile and metaphor in the meditative process' (Stuart 2015, 1: 197). He notes 'the fundamental role of simile and metaphor in the *Saddhsu*'s contemplative program' to allow the practitioner to maintain 'the traditional distinctions between material and immaterial categories' (Stuart 2015, 1: 162). This analysis hints at the binary structure of domain-mapping in conceptual metaphors: only two domains can be related at once, although later domains can of course be added by accretion (as in the case of orientational metaphors). The fundamental mapping of metaphor, however, remains binary. If we accept that acts of meditation are structured by metaphor, it follows that the structure of meditation is, in some sense, also binary.

Many forms of meditation that we encounter in early Brahmanic and Buddhist texts can be described as 'binary' in structure because meditation is often performed 'upon' something else, thus linking two domains (the source and the target), often that of the mental subjective sphere and that of the objective sphere. Objective or cognitive forms of concentration require an object of focus – be it a mantra, a *maṇḍala*, an image, an icon or a bodily function such as breathing. Paired techniques like scrutiny (of an object) (*vitarka*) and comprehension (of an object) (*vicāra*)[26] rely on mapping the qualities of an object to the domain of the mind in order that the object be fully known. This is sometimes described as the mind taking the form of the object; in this case the mind is understood to have an impressionable plasticity (e.g. PYŚ 1.1; PYŚ 1.4).[27] Other meditative methods, such as idealist forms of Buddhist Yogācāra, theorize that the direction of domain-mapping is the other way round: idealism understands the object as a mapping of the qualities that already exist in the mind to 'create' the domain of external reality. However, Saṅgharakṣa's **Yogācārabhūmi* (which I discuss in Chapter 3) includes metaphorical mapping of the qualities of the body to the domain of the mind: in the practice of yoga, the mind becomes supple and loses its hardness and becomes adaptable (SYCB 23, 215; Demiéville 1951: 413) – that is, the mind assumes the material qualities of the body. Equally, in meditation practice we are told that the body sits straight and the mind is 'not slack' (SYCB 8, 195–6; Demiéville 1951: 404). Another binary mapping occurs in the process of deity visualization, which is present in both early Mahāyāna meditation and in the devotion (*bhakti*) of the *Bhagavad Gītā*. By mapping qualities from the deity to oneself, one instantiates the presence of the divine (McMahan 2002: 152–8). But this is also a bidirectional process in that human attributes were first mapped to the bodhisattva or deity in order to create these anthropomorphic images.[28]

Meditation, then, is an act but also a process. The act of meditation rests on reified conceptual metaphors – after all, the mind does not actually contain seeds, nor does the mind ascend ladders or steps or become released from a confined space. But once the mind cognizes and visualizes its own meditative experience in terms of these qualities, it then processes the results of meditation in similar terms. Thus following an act of meditation, one might conceptualize that the 'weeds in the mind have been uprooted', or that one's 'mind is lighter in weight', or that the 'mind has been cleared of cloudy material'. Yet none of these changes have taken place materially. Nonetheless, the perception that they have is consequently translated back into real-world action: speaking more coherently, making sound decisions, displaying a calm attitude and so on. The point here is that domain-mapping is not just a one-way process – from mind to world or world to mind – but is a constantly accruing process of bidirectional reification of experience in relation to concepts.

To step away from meditation for a moment, let us return to a generic conceptual metaphor such as LIFE IS A JOURNEY, which is frequently used to structure theories of 'spiritual progress'. If one understands life in the terms of a journey (i.e. maps the qualities of a journey to a life), one might think of life as having a start and end point, having a destination, being consequential and linear, being subject to diversion and delay, containing the possibility of getting lost, requiring a map, being full of adventure or danger and whatever else is understood by the visceral experiences of 'going on a journey'. Understanding life in these terms then affects how one lives one life (i.e. the metaphorical understanding of one's own life shapes our choices and actions in the world).[29] Similarly, understanding meditation in conceptual terms (which is unavoidable) in turn affects how one lives one's life. Meditation then is an act (a process) of translating a conceptual metaphor into experience that effects real-world change. At the very least, such change takes place at the sensorimotor level of the individual body, and at a wider level such change takes place in individual actions, social conventions and cultural agreements.

'Yoga' as a metaphor

The central metaphor under discussion here is, of course, yoga itself. In its early Vedic context, the concept of yoga was structured by a range of metaphors generated by the pastoralist lifestyle of *yogakṣema*, a cyclical lifestyle of 'application' and 'rest' (or 'activation' and 'cessation').[30] In particular, 'yoga' was conceptualized in relation to the domain of the horse, which Witzel refers to as a 'prestige animal'.[31] Many of the early metaphors used to construct practices of yoga reflect this key material pastoralist context of animal husbandry: the chariot, the charioteer, holding the reins, reining in, yoking to the plough, tying the horse to the post and so on. Even the common understanding of yoga as 'joining' or 'union' is a metaphor: it most likely derives from the Vedic and epic image of *yogayukta*, 'joined to application' (of the animal to the plough) but which in soteriological terms comes to refer to the martial image of being 'hitched to a chariot' in White's interpretation (White 2009: 38–121), or 'yoga-harnessing' in Fitzgerald's translation (Fitzgerald 2012). This hitching is what the dying warrior is said to accomplish in the Vedas as he travels to the gateway of the sun to ascend to heaven and thereby seeks liberation from redeath (White 2009: 38–121). In early contexts, yoga is also understood as meditative 'concentration' (*samādhi*).[32] What was understood by *sam+ā√dhā* ('to put together') cannot, of course, be fully known.[33] However, we can speculate that there may be a connection to the common English translation of *samādhi* as 'concentration', which carries the sense of squeezing matter together or distilling a material essence in high strength.[34] Concentration is accompanied by purity (both in the sense of material density and high strength) in that concentration is the opposite of dilution and dispersion; and this notion of material purity complements concomitant notions of ritual purity (clean and unclean).[35]

These two simple understandings of the word yoga (as 'union' or 'concentration') reveal two underlying 'root' metaphors.[36] The metaphor of YOGA IS UNION maps the qualities of control (tight reins prevent the escape of the animal and ensure compliance) and harnessing power (yoking the animal to the plough is an effective agricultural strategy that yields high gains). The metaphor of YOGA IS CONCENTRATION maps the quality of compressing material in space (pulling together against the forces of dispersion) and the quality of purifying materiality (strengthening the material essence of a substance). These basic metaphors then become the ground for building more elaborate conceptual schemes, such as soteriology and philosophy. For example, Sāṃkhya philosophy (in the *Sāṃkhyakārikā* or *Pātañjalayogaśāstra*) draws on the metaphor of YOGA IS CONCENTRATION to elaborate the idea that the mind is material and is part of material reality (*prakṛti*); therefore, practice should concentrate the dispersed constituents (*tattva*s) back into one compressed reality, primordial matter (*mūlaprakṛti*). Another example is the Upaniṣadic description of yoga as control of unruly sense faculties that must be reined in or tied.[37] By the fourth to fifth century CE, the term yoga itself had layers of accretion of metaphorical meaning that had built up from the ancient period and in which simple structural metaphors had been combined to create a complex conceptual system.

Since domain-mapping in metaphor is a fundamentally binary way of thinking, these conceptual structures can also be seen to shape the emergence of dualist metaphysics such as the Upaniṣadic *ātman-brahman* (self-Self) or the Sāṃkhya *prakṛti-puruṣa* (materiality-consciousness). These core binary pairings in the conception of 'self' in relation to reality are metaphors. Mapping the self to the cosmos (as in *ātman-brahman*) is a fundamentally metaphorical act of understanding the abstract (cosmic *brahman*) through the concrete (personal self, *ātman*). And even though the dualist relationship of *prakṛti* and *puruṣa* purports to be categorical separation (i.e. ontological isolation, *kaivalya*), analysing this binary in terms of conceptual metaphor helps us to see the associative as well as the differential aspects of the relationship.

Bhāvanā: The metaphor of cultivation in early Indic soteriology

The process of domain-mapping can also be seen at work in the Indic connection of two spheres or practice: the domain of religious practice geared towards liberation and the domain of agriculture. In this metaphorical linking, the domain of liberation (success in religious practice) is conceptualized in the terms of agricultural methods and outcomes: preparing the soil, sowing seeds, nurturing the seed with water and light, tending the crop, harvesting the crop, enjoying the fruits of the harvest, experiencing abundance and so forth. This domain-mapping produces the conceptual scheme of spiritual cultivation (*bhāvanā*). *Bhāvanā* is a complex orientational metaphor that describes the practices that lead to liberation and it is in ample evidence in all three of the texts that I discuss in this book: the *Pātañjalayogaśāstra*, the *Abhidharmakośabhāṣya* and the *Yogācārabhūmiśāstra*. In this section, I establish a context for the development of religious praxis termed '*bhāvanā*' in the first half of the first millennium CE by showing that the image-schema of *bhāvanā* is derived from the practical knowledge of botanical cultivation. In particular I focus on rice cultivation practices and argue that these are central to the soteriological metaphors of *bhāvanā*.

Bhāvanā is the nominative form of a causative stem from the verbal root √*bhū*, meaning 'to be' or 'to become'. The causative form of √*bhū* is *bhāvayati*, 'to cause to come into being' or 'to bring into being'.[38] Given the causative sense of *bhāvanā*, 'cultivation' is an apt translation because it reflects the agency entailed in acts of cultivation. There are two main strands in the semantic development of *bhāvanā* during the early period, both of which represent 'production': immaterial production and material production. In the immaterial sense, *bhāvanā* refers to production in the mind – of ideas, visions, notions, views and so on – what

Collins refers to as 'mental culture' (Collins 1982: 111).[39] Important though this first sense of *bhāvanā* is, it is a second strand of meaning, that of material production, on which I will focus more closely. *Bhāvanā* also has in its ancient Vedic use a nuance of 'to grow, to thrive, to prosper', and this meaning is largely derived from the context of botanical cultivation.[40] According to Monier-Williams's analysis, *bhāvanā* stems from both √*bhā* 'to see' and √*bhū* 'to be' – and this accounts for the bifurcation in meanings of *bhāvanā*. I therefore suggest that we distinguish between the two semantic fields by referring to (a) *bhāvanā* as the production of 'seeing', that is, conjuring up visually, imagining, 'producing from thin air', and (b) *bhāvanā* as the production of 'growth' from a soil with the right conditions.[41]

Bhāvanā also relates to other derived forms of √*bhū*, such as *bhūmi* (ground, foundation),[42] *bhūti* (well-being, thriving, prosperity) and *bhāva* (state, condition). The most important of these three terms for our discussion is *bhūmi*, which denotes the material 'ground, soil, earth' but also the abstract 'foundation, stage'. In Buddhist soteriology, the *bhūmi*s, as stages on the path (*mārga*), form a key component of the broader image schema of *bhāvanā*. Cultivation in our sources often means 'mental cultivation' in particular, in which case *bhāvanā* can be a synonym for meditation or, indeed, yoga.[43] However, I will translate *bhāvanā* more generally as 'cultivation', partly to reflect that it can designate a wider set of practices beyond meditation and partly to keep its metaphoric function in the foreground.

Although the *Veda*s and *Upaniṣad*s used ecological cycles as a structuring principle for notions of redeath and rebirth, the most specific systematic development of *bhāvanā* is to be found in Buddhist texts. According to Frauwallner, the formal distinction between the path of vision (*darśanamārga*) and the path of cultivation (*bhāvanāmārga*) was innovated in Dharmaśrī's *Abhidharmasāra* (Frauwallner 1995: 192), which 'represents the earliest dogmatics of the Sarvāstivāda' (Frauwallner 1995: 151) and predates the canonical Sarvāstivāda *Jñānaprasthāna* (Frauwallner 1995: 152).[44] The distinction between *darśanamārga* and *bhāvanāmārga* is also central in the *Abhidharmakośabhāṣya* (AKBh 6.25–29) – and this is not surprising given that, in Frauwallner's estimation, the *Abhidharmakośabhāṣya* 'is ultimately nothing but an extended reworking of the Abhidharmasāra' (Frauwallner 1995: 152). In Sarvāstivāda thought, the two paths lead to abandonment (*heya*): *darśana* is abandonment that can be achieved by cognizing the four noble truths, and *bhāvanā* is mental cultivation, or repeated contemplation, thereupon to actualize.[45] The primary component of cultivation was meditation, and it enfolded both tranquility (*śamatha*) and insight (*vipaśyana*). This path was focused on concentration (*samādhi*) – thus the wisdom of cultivation (*bhāvanāmayī prajñā*) was also known as the wisdom born of concentation (*samādhija-prajñā*) (Dhammajoti 2009: 338). The complete eradication of the afflictions (*kleśa*s) and their traces (*vāsanā*s) occurs only at the diamond concentration (*vajropasamādhi*) stage of the path of cultivation. The afflictions abandoned at this stage are more persistent and tenacious than the ones abandoned in the path of sight (Dhammajoti 2009: 338).

In the Mahāyāna schemes of the ten stages (*daśabhūmi*s) (see Chapter 3), the first *bhūmi* corresponds to *darśanamārga* and the next nine to *bhāvanāmārga* – indicating that the *bhūmi*s themselves are closely related conceptually with cultivation. In Saṅgharakṣa's **Yogācārabhūmi*, there is a telling simile that explains the distinction between tranquility (*śamatha*) and insight (*vipaśyana*):

> Or, again tranquility is just like the act of a harvester who grabs the ears [of wheat] with his left hand, while insight is like the act of cutting [them] with a sickle in his right hand.[46]

Here, the agricultural simile is that of harvesting the crop, by cutting – *śamatha* gives access to the harvest, but only by *vispaśyana*, or cutting, can one obtain it. In metaphors, too, the qualities of labour and hard work are mapped from agriculture (source) to spirituality (target). Thus cultivation (*bhāvanā*) is understood as mental 'work' and spiritual 'labour', and certainly reflects adherence to a gradualist path rather than subitist. Cultivation of plants can never be a sudden or immediate process, but is rather a long-term investment, a waiting process that relies on consistent provision of the right conditions for growth.[47] Indeed, the outcome of cultivation (i.e. plant maturity or fruit) is never guaranteed and often requires skill and knowledge, accrued over successive cycles, to get right. In contrast, subitist soteriology is anything but 'hard work'. The early yogācāra alignment to gradualism continues prior understandings of yoga, which expound cumulative and labour-intensive approaches such as asceticism and austerity (*tapas*). Even the sixth to eighth century CE Jain *Yogabindu*, by Haribhadra, which lists five stages of yoga, counts the second stage as cultivation (*bhāvanā*) (Chapple 2003: 1–14). In contrast, the subitist approaches of tantra, Advaita Vedānta or rāja yoga propose divine grace, initiation, visions, *śaktipat*, the guru and so forth as functions that partly replace the idea of 'hard work' and one's own agency in the attainment of liberation.

We have established that basic conceptual metaphors arise from sensory experience in physical environments and from preconceptual structures (e.g. up/down) derived from visceral human practices and embodiment. We have also established that *bhāvanā* is a gradualist soteriology steeped in ideas of 'hard work'. In our texts, *bhāvanā* is not simply a structural metaphor but rather a complex scheme of metaphors. This scheme is composed of two complementary soteriological and hence ontological claims: CAPTIVITY IS [BEING] GROUNDED (as reflected in images of the seed) and LIBERATION IS [BEING] SKYWARD (as reflected in the cloud of dharma). These inferences are made not only on the basis of sensorimotor experience but also by mapping the system of botanical cultivation to create a new conceptual scheme of spiritual cultivation. *Bhāvanā* as a system of cultivation and liberation is designed to facilitate 'fantastical' escape from the ground, such as modes of ascension, merging in the sun or becoming a cloud.[48] Thus the realm of hard labour and toil on the ground is left behind. These soteriological metaphors of cultivation emerged against a backdrop of material agricultural practice and change. In order to understand this concept of 'work' and other technical concepts that are deeply embedded in *bhāvanā*, let us now turn to some historical context for agricultural cultivation around the turn of the Common Era.

In assessing the possible connections between the metaphorical complex of *bhāvanā* and historical agrarian societies in which such metaphors may have been generated, two regions are of particular interest: the Gangetic Plain (the Eastern part of which includes Magadha) and the north-western frontier region, which includes Kashmir and Gandhara. These two regions are relevant since they were particularly important in the development of the religio-philosophical strands that we are following: Sarvāstivāda Abhidharma, yogācāra, Sautrāntika, Pātañjala yoga and Sāṃkhya.[49]

Regions and rice-farming

Rice grain is the primary example of a crop seed cited in the *Pātañjalayogaśāstra* and the *Abhidharmakośabhāṣya* (see below). Therefore, the regions in which rice cultivation occurred are of interest to this study. In narrowing my focus on *bhāvanā* to rice-farming in particular, I am indebted to Potter,[50] who noted an elegant coordination of the image of the seed with the image of irrigation in the *Pātañjalayogaśāstra*:

> We have, then, in the Yoga account a rather carefully worked-out theory concerning the mechanics of karma and rebirth, which is made available to the non-philosopher through appeal to the model of rice-farming. (Potter 1983: 248)

While acknowledging that metaphors are a fundamental way to construct and apprehend abstract ideas, I disagree with Potter's assessment of the model of rice-farming as a 'dumbing-down' of philosophy for laypersons. As I have argued, metaphors are not ornamental, nor in this case for the purpose of simplifying or conveying information, but are rather integral to soteriology in this period. The basis of such metaphors was, most likely, experiential.

In the north-western areas (such as Kashmir and Gandhara), the earliest crops grown were wheat and barley, whereas rice-farming was established early in the Central Gangetic Plain (correlating partly to Greater Magadha), the Bengal Delta regions and South India (Pejros and Shnirelman 1998: 384–5).[51] Indeed, the north-eastern region – with its coastal belt, river valleys and deltas – provided ideal conditions for growing rice (Sattar et al. 2010: 225–6).[52] And, as Chakrabarti and others have noted, the Gangetic Valley had a uniquely 'fertile alluvium', which was especially suitable for the wetland and irrigation methods required by rice-farming in this period (Chakrabarti 1995: 169).[53]

Since rice-farming first thrived in the Gangetic Plain, it may indicate that this was a relevant 'live' or 'creative' context in which the rice-grain metaphor was used to conceptualize a mental seed in relation to action (*karman*) and affliction (*kleśa*). This would support Bronkhorst's thesis of Greater Magadha as a location for the cultural emergence of karmic theory (Bronkhorst 2007). Although the first major urban centres (during the Second Urbanization) included the regions of the Central Gangetic Plain and the Northwestern Borderlands, the largest early urban centre was in the Gangetic Plain (Allchin 1995). Such growth of urban centres may have been a result of surplus rice production (Sattar et al. 2010: 231), which facilitated the stability and prosperity that economically fuelled the new political states and cities (Gombrich 1988: 37). To sum up: the Gangetic Plain was potentially the earliest location of both rice-farming and large urban centres during the Second Urbanization. There is also evidence of the north-west as a location for thriving rice-farming. This establishes two possible generative and geographical contexts for rice-seed metaphors in *bhāvanā*, both of which were sites of fertile religious cultures in the so-called classical period – Gandhara and Kashmir as key centres of Buddhism and the Gangetic Plain as associated with the Upaniṣads and *śramaṇa* movements.

We find many technical descriptions of rice-farming in relation to meditation in the texts that we are examining. For example, the *Abhidharmakośabhāṣya* explains that the elimination of affliction (*kleśa*) in the mind is like the process of burning rice seed by fire,[54] using the example of *vrīhi*, a particular type of rice grain.

> So when the substratum has come to be without the seeds of afflictions, like rice that has been burnt by fire, someone is called 'one who has abandoned defilements' – or when [the substratum has] seeds that have been damaged by the ordinary path. (AKBh 2.36)[55]

The text also refers to the *śāli* form of the rice seed when the Sautrāntikas recount their ontological concept of the 'state' of the seed (*bījabhāva*) (discussed in Chapter 2):

> By 'seed' one should understand a certain capacity to reproduce the *kleśa*, a power belonging to the person engendered by the previous *kleśa*. In this same way, there exists in a certain person the capacity of producing a certain consciousness of memory, a capacity engendered by a consciousness of perception; in this same way, the capacity to produce rice, which belongs to the plant, the shoot, the stalk, etc. is engendered by the rice seed. (AKBh 5.1: trans. Pruden 1988, 3: 770)[56]

Indeed, such is the prevalence of rice-seed imagery in the *Abhidharmakośabhāṣya* that the concept of affliction (*kleśa*) is introduced almost entirely in these terms. In the chapter on the latent seeds of afflictions (*anuśaya*s), affliction is described as accomplishing ten actions to ensure its longevity, which include making its own roots solid to prevent them from becoming broken, reproducing itself, adapting to the field conditions, engendering its own offspring, causing misrecognition of what it fundamentally is, bending the mind (down) towards the wrong object or towards rebirth, causing a falling away of the good and becoming a bond in itself (AKBh 5.1). I suggest that these are all qualities that are mapped from the domain of the wild rice species, the very enemy of the cultivation of the 'tame' or 'good' rice species (see below). As we will see in the next chapter, the *Pātañjalayogaśāstra*, too, contains many references to the seed of affliction (*kleśabīja*) as a rice seed, including the elaborate description of the irrigation of rice paddies in relation to causality (PYŚ 4.3). This passage describes contemporaneous techniques for irrigating the land and removing common weeds to preserve rice cultivation. In order to understand the conceptual significance of these technical accounts of rice-farming in relation to meditation in both the *Abhidharmakośabhāṣya* and the *Pātañjalayogaśāstra*, let us now turn to some further historical material detail.

Techniques of rice cultivation and their relevance to soteriology

The cultivated Asian rice species is called *Oryza sativa* or *O. sativa* (Sharma 2010: 1). Rice itself comes in many variant forms. The husk can be fawn, yellow, golden or purple; the grain type can be short and round or long and slender; the colour can be white, chalky, red or black; some plants mature in 70 days and some in 180 days (Sharma 2010: 2). Such details become significant when considering the descriptions in our texts, which contain accounts of how long rice takes to mature (as an analogy of how karma matures), how a grain of rice can be dehusked to render it non-fertile (in relation to rendering the afflictions, or *kleśa*s, impotent) and how a rice seed is parched to destroy its potency (again, in relation to destroying the afflictions). Since the properties of the domain of rice-farming were mapped to techniques of spiritual cultivation, we can only improve our semantic decoding by getting to grips with the original creative context in which such metaphors were generated.

For example, if we fundamentally misunderstand what is meant by 'scorching a rice-seed', both the method and its significance, we may miss a vital detail in what is meant by scorching the seed of affliction (*kleśa*) to attain liberation. When translators choose how to render technical rice-farming terms in the *Pātañjalayogaśastra*, it is important to know that *tandula* is dehusked rice (Sattar et al. 2010: 231), that *śāli* is usually a late maturing or transplanted plant, while *vrīhi* is an early maturing variety (Sattar et al. 2010: 233). Such technical distinctions have semantic bearing on the theories that are put forward about *kleśa* and karma. For example, a dehusked grain is one that has less chances of self-reproducing. See, for instance, this technical elaboration of the three primary afflictions (greed, aversion and delusion; or *lobha*, *dveṣa* and *moha*) in the *Aṅguttara Nikāya*:

> It is monks, as with seeds that are undamaged, not rotten, unspoiled by wind and sun, capable of sprouting and well embedded: if a man were to burn them in fire and reduce them to ashes, then winnow the ashes in a strong wind or let them be carried away by a swiftly flowing stream, then those seeds would have been radically destroyed, fully eliminated, made unable to sprout and would not be liable to arise in the future. Similarly, it is, monks with actions done in non-greed, non-hatred and non-delusion. Once greed, hatred and delusion have vanished, these actions are thus abandoned, cut off at the root, made barren like palm-tree stumps, obliterated so that they are no more subject to arise in the future. (AN 1.135; Nyanoponika and Bodhi, 1999: 50)

Additionally, technical rice terms and descriptions may also provide some hints about the geographical contexts for our texts; for example, there was a special type of *mahāśāli* rice (a large grained variety) that was only available in Magadha (Sattar et al. 2010: 234).

Wild rice and cultivated rice

We have already noted that the cultivated form of rice in India is called *O. sativa*. However, there was also a wild rice, *O. nivara*,[57] which was the likely progenitor of rice in South Asia. It is my contention that differences in how these two types of rice were perceived are reflected in the soteriology of cultivation (*bhāvanā*) in the early Common Era.

Sharma notes the key properties of the wild rice called *O. nivara*: it acquired an 'annual habit, self-pollination, gregarious habit, synchronous flowering and seed setting, higher seed productivity and bolder seeds' than cultivated rice (Sharma 2010: 5). Wild rice was therefore difficult to control and was regarded as a weed (Armpong-Nyarko and De Datta 1991: 101). If one assesses the growth pattern of wild rice as 'habitual', 'self-producing' and 'bold', these are all qualities used to characterize the negative patterns of the mind, or *kleśa*. Furthermore, wild rice's pattern of simultaneous 'flowering' and 'seeding' is characteristic of the cycle of karma as containing the seed of future action in the present action. Thus, wild rice was a plant that was especially bold and self-sufficient in its reproduction and was a direct threat to cultivated rice. The wild rice seed provided a useful metaphor through which to express anxiety about the uncontrolled growth of negative habit in the human personality. In the agricultural field, the contrast between cultivated order and wild divergence from such order was visibly stark: 'When rice is seeded or transplanted in rows, it is easy to differentiate wild rice growing between the rows' (Armpong-Nyarko and De Datta 1991: 101).

Understanding growth patterns of rice is useful for decoding the soteriological notion of how *kleśa*s thrive automatically. Even amongst desirable rice plants, there were two growth periods: vegetative growth (stems and leaves), followed by generative (reproductive) growth (Matsubayashi et al. 1968: 34). A key feature of wild rice (*O. nivara*) is that its seeds are highly dormant; they are 'adapted to the environment of cultivated rice, are competitive, and have grains that are highly dormant and shatter easily' (Armpong-Nyarko and De Datta 1991: 101). The seed dormancy of wild rice means that it can lie undetected for a long time and then suddenly spring up. Furthermore, since the grain husk breaks easily, the grain inside is rapidly freed and, because it contains its own seed, it can quickly propagate again. Therefore, the farmer has to continuously eliminate wild rice seed in favour of cultivated seed. After the rice harvests, there were various techniques to kill wild rice seeds, such as burning or flooding the field, to prevent germination (Armpong-Nyarko and De Datta 1991: 101). While cultivated rice plants have to be deliberately germinated with various fertilization techniques, wild rice is self-germinating.

However, even in cultivated rice plants, reproductive growth has a negative aspect after the harvesting period. Thus when rice was harvested, the grain had to be 'parched' or 'scorched' in order to remove its germination potential. This ensured that the lifespan of stored rice was extended and the food supply was preserved. The higher the moisture content in rice, the greater the perishability (Matsubayashi et al. 1968: 65). The method of scorching is as follows. Rice must be dried, usually in the sun. Subsequently, it is smoked, parched (slow roasted) or scorched in a container over fire. This destroys the inner germ or seed and stops the seed from sprouting or germinating during storage (conjuring up the Buddhist image of *ālayavijñāna* as the 'store' or 'storehouse' consciousness). The chaff (hull or husk) is threshed (loosened) and then winnowed (falls off). The sterile hard rice kernel is what remains.

I have explored these technical dimensions of how wild rice growth threatens cultivation because similar features may be identified in the way in which affliction (*kleśa*) is theorized in the *Pātañjalayogaśāstra* and the *Abhidharmakośabhāṣya*. In its latent form, *kleśa* is a dormant seed, is self-propagating, is described as having a root system, and the seed of *kleśa* must be eliminated by scorching. In spiritual practice, eliminating affliction is the raison d'être of *bhāvanā*, just as in rice-farming, eliminating wild rice is the very basis of rice cultivation. Therefore, in the metaphor 'seed of *kleśa*' (*kleśabīja*) the domain-mapping employs not just any seed as the source but specifically the rice seed.

This consideration of rice cultivation methods in the early Common Era highlights that in agricultural terms there was an existential anxiety about taming wild patterns in nature, preventing self-germination of weeds and maximizing the lifespan of food harvests. Indeed, as Schmithausen points out, in the *Manobhūmi* of the *Yogācārabhūmiśāstra*, *dauṣṭhulya* (badness or evil) is characterized as the seed or plant that is beyond cultivation: *dauṣṭhulya* is 'unwieldy' and has a 'lack of controllability'. It can be 'permeating' (*-anugata*), 'infesting' (*-upagata*) or 'sticking in' (*sannviṣta*) the basis of personal existence (Schmithausen 1987: 66–7).[58] As we will see in Chapter 2, the dormancy and the self-propagation of the seed of *kleśa* are central problems in both the *Abhidharmakośabhāṣya* and the *Pātañjalayogaśāstra*. The struggle that we witness in the metaphoric depiction of meditation during the classical period reflects a wider struggle between 'nature' and 'culture', between the attempt to bring wild areas of land under control for cultivation, and thus to harness the means to create an agricultural surplus, a necessary condition for urbanization.

I suggest that this is the generative context in which the metaphorical complex of *bhāvanā* was created. Thus, the existential anxiety about food supply was transferred to the domain of the inner self and reproduced as an existential anxiety about cultivating the inner mind and impulses to ensure the survival, or liberation, of the 'self' (in a range of doctrinal contexts).

Labour: A basis for the metaphor of *bhāvanā*?

As Lakoff and Johnson put it, there is an 'inseparability of metaphors from their experiential bases' (Lakoff and Johnson 1980: 19). In this section, I argue that there is an inherent logic to using cultivation as a metaphor to describe the spiritual path, which is reflected in the prevalence of *bhāvanā* as a religious paradigm in the early Common Era. Although the theory of karma was integrally constructed using metaphors of cultivation (seeds and fruits), there were also other dominant metaphors for the mechanisms of karma: for example, the wheel of *saṃsāra* as a cyclical force or the metaphor of liberation as the crossing of an ocean with, or without, a boat or raft.[59]

Let us briefly examine one of these metaphors: that of the wheel. The wheel metaphor, in fact, refers to a complex of related metaphors used to conceptualize karma. For example, the wheel of existence (*bhavacakka*) is associated with the twelve links of dependent origination (as its spokes) and is referred to in the *Visuddhimagga* as having 'no known beginning'.

> Becoming's Wheel reveals no known beginning;
> No maker, no experiencer there;
> Void with a twelvefold voidness, and nowhere
> It ever halts; forever it is spinning.
>
> (Vism. 18; trans. Ñāṇamoli 2010: 598)[60]

A near-synonym to *bhavacakka* is *saṃsāracakka*, the wheel of rebirth, which is also constructed conceptually by mapping qualities from the domain of the chariot wheel, such as the spoke, axle, hub and rim. In this passage, again from the *Visuddhimagga*, the process of domain-mapping is visible in the syntactic structures. Only the Buddha can smash the spokes of this wheel:

> Now, this wheel of the round of rebirths with its hub made of ignorance and of craving for becoming, with its spokes consisting of formations of merit and the rest, with its rim of ageing and death, which is joined to the chariot of the triple becoming by piercing it with the axle made of the origins of cankers (see M I 55),

> has been revolving throughout time that has no beginning. All of this wheel's spokes (*ara*) were destroyed (*hata*) by him at the Place of Enlightenment, as he stood firm with the feet of energy on the ground of virtue, wielding with the hand of faith the axe of knowledge that destroys kamma – because the spokes are thus destroyed he is accomplished (*arahanta*) also. (Vism. 8; trans. Ñāṇamoli 2010: 188–9)[61]

Similarly, one allegorical etymology of the noble one (*arahant*) is the 'breaker of the spokes of the wheel of transmigration', *saṃsāracakkassa arānaṁ hatattā* (Pd; Hardy 1901: 106, 1–2). Another important context for the wheel metaphor is the wheel of power or sovereignty, such as *dhammacakka* (the wheel of dharma), *cakkavatti* (the turner of the wheel, or sovereign earthly ruler) and *Brahmacakka* (the doctrine of the Buddha).[62]

From the preceding examples, the primary generative context for the wheel metaphor in relation to karma appears to be that of the chariot or carriage: *rathacakka*.[63] See, for example,

> Just as a chariot wheel, when it is rolling, rolls [that is, touches the ground] only on one point of [the circumference of] its tire, and, when it is at rest, rests only on one point, so too, the life of living beings lasts only for a single conscious moment. (Vism. 8; trans. Ñāṇamoli 2010: 233)[64]

In this context, the carriage or chariot appears to be associated with harmonious movement, stability and balance, although the quality that is most often stressed is that of continuous rotation. However, there is another less common generative context for the wheel metaphor in which *cakra* appears to be associated with machinery. So, for example, in the compound *yantacakka*, a *yanta* (Skt. *yantra*) is a formation – in this instance a mechanical formation – and the *cakka* is the wheel that drives it. In the *Jātaka*s, we encounter a description of the Buddha's piety as being like the tremendous force of the wheel of an oil mill (P. *telayantacakka*; Skt. *tailayantracakra*) or a sugar mill (P. *ucchuyanta*; Skt. *ikṣuyantra*).

> These are all the conditions in the world that bring Buddhaship
> to perfection;
> Beyond these are no others, therein do thou stand fast.
> While he grasped these conditions natural and intrinsic,
> By the power of his piety the earth of ten thousand worlds quaked.
> The earth sways and thunders like a sugar mill at work,
> Like the wheel of an oil-mill so shakes the earth.
>
> (Ja i.25, 339; trans. Rhys Davids 2000: 26)[65]

In this description of a mill, the rotating wheel of the mill produces an earth-shaking thunderous force, altogether different to the chariot wheel and far more deadly.[66] Another example of a mill wheel that features in this period is the wheel that raises water (*jalayantracakra*). These mechanical metaphors express the idea of a giant rotating force that is harmful and can potentially crush one. Underpinning this notion is the category of the fetters (*saṃyojana*) that bind one to the wheel of transmigration (*saṃsāracakra*).[67] These fetters vary in number but suggest an unpleasant fate whereby one is crushed under the force of a rotating wheel.[68] In this context, the 'cessation' of liberative attainment can only be the cessation of the unrelenting turning wheel.[69] There is further research to be done on identifying how the material context of these mills – oil, sugar, water – and the prevalence of related metaphors in literature can indicate approximate geographical locations for the production of specific texts. However, central though the wheel of *saṃsāra* and the raft of liberation were to religious thought, they were not used as the basis to elaborate an entire soteriology technically in the way that *bhāvanā* was. What, then, were the specific factors that initiated the dominance of the botanical cultivation metaphor in this period?

Despite the Second Urbanization (Thapar 2003; Olivelle 2004), agriculture was still at the centre of daily experience for the majority of the population in South Asia in the early Common Era. A primary feature of crop cultivation that was mapped to spiritual cultivation was that of 'work': arduous striving and hard labour. Success in both endeavours, farming and spiritual practice, require 'labour': labour in the fields and the labour of ascetic efforts. The association of spiritual practice with labour may be rooted in the lifestyles and living conditions of the early renouncer (*śramaṇa)* communities. The inception of these ascetic communities in the north-eastern region is widely understood as a reaction against the beginning of the Second Urbanization. The *śramaṇa*s adopted remote rural environments and engaged in extreme bodily practices. This combination of bodily mortification and punishing natural environments meant that religious existence was certainly 'hard work' in the sense of corporeal 'labour'. This is reflected in the meaning of the word *śramaṇa* itself, which denotes 'striver'. Forest-dwelling and mendicancy, which relied on hunter-gatherer techniques and alms-seeking for food, would surely have been a lifestyle replete with anxiety about food supply (whatever the doctrinal teachings to the contrary).

There were also manifold early Buddhist examples of the metaphor of botanical cultivation[70] in a positive context.[71] In the *Petavatthu*, we are told, 'like fields are the *Arhata*; the givers are like farmers. The gift is like the seed, (and) from this arises the fruit' (Pv 1.1; trans. Collins 1982: 219). Elsewhere, for laypersons, 'doing good deeds, which bring rebirth, what is given to the monkhood is rich in fruit' (SN i 233; AN iv, 292; trans. Collins 1982: 219).[72] The *Saṃyutta Nikāya* states, 'Gifts to those who in this world are worthy of gifts [i.e. monks] bring great fruit, just like seeds sown in a good field' (SN i, 233; trans. Collins 1982: 219).[73] As Collins outlines, the image of an 'unsurpassable field of merit' (*anuttara puññakhetta*) is used to describe the Buddha, advanced monks and the institution of monkhood as a whole.[74] Religious striving is said to depend on morality (*śīla*) just as seeds and plants depend on the earth (*Milindapañha* 75–6). Elsewhere, this teaching is framed as the seed of faith, the root of morality and the shoot of meditation and insight (SN i 172f; Sn 12f; SN-a i 250; Sn-a 144). In one particularly striking image, monkhood is a field in which the seed of the Dharma is planted. Thus, monks are like seedlings that require nurturing; and if they do not see the Buddha, they wither away for lack of water (MN 1.457; SN 3.91–92 and 4.314).[75] These are all positive early accounts of the function of the seed and, as Collins observes, appear to situate monasticism and the religious life in relation to the secular toil of agriculture (Collins 1982: 219). There may therefore have been a cultural impetus to metaphorically endorse the value of monkhood in the terms of secular agricultural life.

However, other early Buddhist contexts portray the labour of cultivation as a negative phenomenon. One passage suggests that monkhood might offer a pleasurable escape from the endless labour of toiling the soil. In a conversation in which two young men discuss becoming monks, they describe the household life as an endless cycle of sowing, irrigating, ploughing, tending, harvesting and so on (Vin ii 180–181). This attitude reflects the lure of newly emerging urban and mendicant life in contrast to the traditional and fixed conditions of rural dwelling. It also hints at a paradox that although spiritual progress is represented by the paradigm of botanical cultivation, it is the very cyclical rounds of cultivation that represent the type of existence from which the religious aspirant seeks to escape. As Collins spells out, '*saṃsāra* is a life of constant agriculture, planting seeds and reaping their fruit, while *nirvāṇa* is the abandonment of such a life' (Collins 1982: 220). This is reflected in the urban metaphor of liberation as the 'city of nirvāna'.[76] For some monks, the escape from *saṃsāra* was viewed as an escape to the urban centre, away from the hard toil of the fields in which cultivation was not symbolic but literal.[77]

The question then arises: why did Buddhist thinkers not simply characterize religious striving in the terms of urban experience, if it was a more privileged or newly emerging type of social dwelling? There are several possible answers to this question. First, we have to consider the hypothesis that *bhāvanā* was an earlier śramaṇic metaphor that effectively became a 'dead' metaphor in the strands of Buddhism that thrived in urban centres. Nonetheless, the paradigm of *bhāvanā* still served as an explanatory tool to recruit new converts to Buddhism, because of continuous social migration between rural areas and towns or cities. Another hypothesis is that, in the interests of social order, there may have been a need to 'justify' the work of monks in secular terms so as to retain a valid social and ethical basis for the value and output of monastic 'labour' – without the paradigm of *bhāvanā*, it may have been difficult to account for ascetic monks' material and economic 'non-productivity' in society, relatively speaking. This latter theory seems relevant when we read in the Buddhist canon the story of a layman who complains that while he works hard in the fields, the Buddha does nothing.[78] In response to their complaints, the Buddha explains:

> My seed is faith, austerity the rain; insight is my yoke and plough, my pole modesty, mind the strap; mindfulness my plough-share and goad; … energy is for me the ox which bears the yoke, drawing on towards rest from work. (*Saṃyutta Nikāya* 1.172f and *Sutta Nipāta* 12f; cited in and trans. Collins 1982: 221)

In the religious context then, the value of communal labour was transposed to the realm of the individual body; the external domain of the tended field was internalized to the 'field' of the mind.[79] This was partly due to the everyday visceral experiences of agriculture as a generative context for *bhāvanā*, but may also have been due to a more strategic need to justify monastic (non-)production in secular economic terms.

The tension between cultivating and stopping growth

A fundamental paradox in the elaboration of the *bhāvanā* paradigm in the classical era is that although in society growth was good (growth = harvest; rural surplus leads to urban expansion), in the yogic meditation practices discussed in our texts the emphasis is on stopping growth: Patañjali's maxim of cessation (*cittavṛttinirodha*, YS 1.2) or his paradigms of non-cognitive concentration (*asaṃprajñāta samādhi*) and seedless concentration (*nirbīja samādhi*), the Abhidharma techniques for cessation of affliction (*kleśanirodha*), Buddhist tranquility practices (*śamatha*) or the higher attainment of cessation (*nirodhasamāpatti*) or *nirvāṇa* itself. Why then is *bhāvanā*, a paradigm that purports to be about cultivated growth, so preoccupied with non-growth? I have already accounted for this paradox, in part, by highlighting the agricultural tension between wild and cultivated rice growth in order to argue that there was a material anxiety about uncontrollable proliferation in a new ascendance of culture over nature. But the tension between growth and non-growth is also related to meditation itself.

A primary orientation of meditation in the texts that we are surveying is towards cessation. Cessation in these texts is presented metaphorically as the cessation of growth – stopping the flourishing of the seed or cutting the roots of a plant. Specifically, this checking of undesirable growth pertains to the afflictions (*kleśas*) and karma.[80] Textual prescriptions of meditation also share a common metaphoric tension between the image of the ground (where seed and roots reside in the substratum) and the image of the sky (where the liberating *dharmamegha*, the cloud of dharma, resides). The phenomenon of growth is identified as occurring at ground level and is generally depicted as a spiritual hindrance. In contrast, liberation occurs at the sky level, whereby the unboundedness of the sky represents freedom from limits and weight, as well as freedom from growth (i.e. change) itself. In our texts, the seed (*bīja*) metaphors often denote states of spiritual captivity, and *dharmamegha* denotes an atemporal state of spiritual liberation. In short, meditation can be both cessative and aspirational at the same time – at some point, mundane mental activity must be ceased to facilitate a 'higher' goal. Cultivation itself is a paradigm that references both growth and non-growth in equal measure and therefore provides logically substantiated reasoning to construct a conceptual scheme, an orientational metaphor, of spiritual cultivation.

Conclusions

Metaphors are integral to conceptuality, and since soteriological thinking is inherently conceptual, it cannot happen without metaphors. In the sharing of conceptual metaphors, different religious groups can scaffold an experiential field, such as 'meditation', with identical metaphors (drawn, for example, from agrarian cultivation). However, it is not necessary to reproduce the semantic value of that metaphor because selective editing (of the qualities) in domain-mapping can facilitate different semantic values, while retaining logical integrity. This means that Pātañjala yoga, Sautrāntika and Sarvāstivāda Abhidharma can all use the metaphor of *bhāvanā* to conceptualize the process and outcomes of meditation, even though the content of that meditative experience is described differently by each school – and so they can shuttle between theories of growth and non-growth, between theories of meditation as productive and non-productive.

The investigation of a material context for the metaphor of *bhāvanā* has shown that the reasons for the employment of the metaphor of cultivation to conceptualize spiritual practices and attainments were many and complex. I hope to have demonstrated that the semantic and structural dimensions of the metaphor of *bhāvanā* extend beyond the experiential to social and economic aspects. In the elaborate metaphorical system of *bhāvanā*, there was a transference of qualities from the domain of botanical cultivation to soteriological acts, so that forms of religious striving through meditation and asceticism were framed in the terms of labour. During the historical period under investigation, religious success was primarily measured using the markers of sustenance and longevity, that is food production. Sautrāntika and Pātañjala authors and proponents may have coexisted in a geographically proximate or similar environment in which there was anxiety about food supply – relating to rice cultivation being overrun by wild rice, to a shortage of water supplies or to the maintenance of expanding urban centres. At a basic level in the fourth to fifth century CE, there was, then, a conceptual link between soteriology (religious 'survival') and food production (existential survival).

In the religious paradigm of *bhāvanā*, growth can take two forms: either wild proliferation that is difficult to control and is potentially dangerous or controlled cultivation that yields the right fruits. Yet they are both forms of cultivation, one negative that requires eliminating the wrong growth and one positive that nurtures the right growth. *Bhāvanā* then is not paradoxical, but adequately expresses and encompasses both of these growth forms in one paradigm. This is why *bhāvanā* was so successful conceptually: it could 'contain' the two the dominant soteriological approaches to liberation in the so-called classical period, 'the cessative' and the 'aspirational'.[81]

2

Seeds of bondage and freedom: Eliminating the afflictions (*kleśa*s) in the *Pātañjalayogaśāstra* and the *Abhidharmakośabhāṣya*

Introduction

There are several ways in which the *Pātañjalayogaśāstra* shares its discourse of liberation with a particular strand of Buddhist Sarvāstivāda Abhidharma: namely, the Sautrāntika positions recorded in Vasubandhu's *Abhidharmakośabhāṣya*.[1] Specifically, the botanical image of the seed (*bīja*) and its seedbed (*āśraya*) is used to explain the concept of mental affliction (*kleśa*) within a wider theory of retributive action, or karma. A set of intertextual passages from PYŚ 2.4 and AKBh 5.1 demonstrate the shared use of conceptual metaphor.

The *Pātañjalayogaśāstra* foregrounds the negation of all afflictions as a fundamental criterion for the attainment of spiritual liberation. This is done by constructing a particular conceptual metaphor: seed of affliction (*kleśabīja*) or AFFLICTION HAS A SEED.[2] Many qualities contained in Patañjali's metaphor are those we find in the Buddhist *Abhidharmakośabhāṣya*, notably, (1) the seed can only be destroyed by scorching it to destroy its germination potential and (2) the seed is a potent form that resides in a seedbed or substratum. The specificity of the domain-mapping that occurs in the botanical metaphor of affliction points to significant conceptual interaction between the Pātañjala and concurrent Buddhist soteriologies. In the following sections, I explore how this is expressed in a metaphorical scheme centred on forms of contemplative reflection (*prasaṃkhyāna* and *pratisaṃkhyā* – both defined further along), affliction (*kleśa*), seed of affliction (*kleśabīja*) and mental substratum (*āśraya*), which is comprised of the seeds of affliction.

Sarvāstivāda Abhidharma

The Abhidharma tradition of Buddhism was part of the Mainstream (Śrāvakayāna) school and was a scholastic approach that sought to systematize the teachings (the Dharma) of the early Buddhist *sūtras*.[3] Abhidharma, which emerged in the centuries after the Buddha's life, developed highly technical terminology and schemes to present the Buddhist teachings in a more comprehensive and objective way. It reflects an analytical style of doctrinal exegesis and innovated complex taxonomies to classify the constituents or factors of reality (*dharmas*). The textual tradition of Abhidharma is called the Abhidharmapiṭaka,[4] and it highlights in detail the components of soteriology and the stages on the path (*mārga*) to attain the goal of enlightenment.[5] The Sarvāstivāda Abhidharmapiṭaka contains seven texts that were compiled in Kashmir around the second century CE,[6] and the commentarial tradition consists of three commentaries, collectively called the *Vibhāṣā*. The longest and most famous of them is the *Mahāvibhāṣā*,[7] which establishes the orthodox doctrinal positions for the Sarvāstivāda school that came to be known as Kashmiri Vaibhāṣika. The label Vaibhāṣika (denoting those who follow the *Vibhāṣā*) was used interchangeably with the label Sarvāstivāda (Kritzer 2005: xxi).

Within the Sarvāstivāda textual tradition, Vasubandhu's[8] *Abhidharmakośabhāṣya* sits as a late work and is perhaps the culmination of the Abhidharma comprehensive summaries.[9] The *Abhidharmakośabhāṣya* consists of two parts: the *Abhidharmakośakārikā*, presented in verse form, and the longer auto-commentary or *bhāṣya*.[10] The text presents the orthodox Vaibhāṣika doctrines, but situates them in a debate with a rival group called the Sautrāntikas, who were apt to win most of the arguments.[11] The discourse of this text is less obviously intermingled with the *Pātañjalayogaśāstra* than the *Yogācārabhūmiśāstra* (see Chapters 3 and 4) in that the *Abhidharmakośabhāṣya* does not declare itself to be a text about yoga. However, like the *Pātañjalayogaśāstra*, the *Abhidharmakośabhāṣya* is concerned with the path to liberation and the graded levels of meditative attainment and is therefore of interest to this study.[12]

Vasubandhu and the *Abhidharmkośabhāṣya*

Vasubandhu is dated to the fourth to fifth centuries, when he produced an extensive literary output of some twenty works.[13] His identity is bound up with the traditional identities of schools of Buddhism. Nineteenth- and twentieth-century scholarship drew clear lines of division between Sarvāstivāda,

Sautrāntika and Yogācāra. This meant that the oeuvre of Vasubandhu, which seemed to span all three schools, appeared to be philosophically inconsistent.[14] Tradition accounted for this discrepancy in Vasubandhu's output with a standard story: Vasubandhu trained in the Vaibhāṣika tradition and composed the *Abhidharmakośakārikā* (AKK) as a treatise of what he learned, but after some time, in which Vasubandhu's doctrinal views changed, he composed an auto-commentary (the *bhāṣya*), which criticized aspects of that Vaibhāṣika system.[15] Another story proposes that Vasubandhu converted to Mahāyāna because it was his brother Asaṅga's dying wish. Gold argues that these 'doxographic identities' of Vasubandhu (first Sarvastivāda, then Sautrāntika, then Yogācāra) are, in fact, later inventions (Gold 2015: 19).[16] On the whole, contemporary scholarship now accepts that there was one Vasubandhu who produced a philosophically and doctrinally varied output over time.[17] A further issue has been the question of Vasubandhu's relationship to Asaṅga, which has bearing on the textual interrelationship of their two flagship texts, the *Abhidharmakośabhāṣya* and the *Yogācārabhūmiśāstra*. Kritzer has demonstrated a strong interrelation between the *Abhidharmakośabhāṣya* and the *Yogācārabhūmiśāstra* by offering the first systematic comparison of passages between the two texts (Kritzer 2005).

The Sautrāntikas

The Sautrāntikas were a group loosely affiliated to the Sarvāstivāda Abhidharma Buddhist community, but distinguished by their doctrines.[18] Their literary works (such as the *Sautrāntikavibhāṣā*) have been lost, and we have only the representations of them that exist in other texts, particularly from the debate in the *Abhidharmakośabhāṣya*. Because many of the Sautrāntika positions in the *Abhidharmakośabhāṣya* concur with the later Yogācāra positions, some scholars have characterized Sautrāntika as 'a kind of bridge between Hīnayāna Sarvāstivāda and Mahāyāna Yogācāra' (Kritzer 2005: xxvii). The Sautrāntikas defined themselves in opposition to the Vaibhāṣikas,[19] and claimed to adhere to an earlier textual tradition, that of the Buddhist *sūtras* (P. *suttas*), which they believed more accurately represented the Buddha's teachings.[20] There is a great deal about the identity and beliefs of the Sautrāntikas that remains unknown,[21] and the first reliable reference to them as a distinct group occurs in the *Abhidharmakośabhāṣya* (Cox 1995: 38).[22] The founder of Sautrāntika is taken to be Śrīlāta,[23] who is said to have composed the *Sautrāntikavibhāṣā*, a lost work that has been partly reconstructed from the *Nyāyānusāra*, a commentary by Kashmiri Sarvāstivāda scholar Saṅghabhadra *c.*420–80 CE.[24]

Notably, there is a long-standing debate as to whether the Sautrāntikas were identical to the Dārṣṭāntikas, another outlying group. The literal meaning of Dārṣṭāntika is 'user of simile[25]/examples', an appellation that is relevant to our discussion of metaphors. The confusion between the two groups was already there in the early period. In one Chinese source, Dārṣṭāntika is the name for a Sautrāntika teacher, while elsewhere the label indicates a dissident group within Sautrāntika (Kritzer 2005: xxvi). Cox suggests that Dārṣṭāntika may have been a pejorative name for the Sautrāntikas (Cox 1995: 37–41). Most scholars now see the two groups as connected, if not the same.[26] For Deleanu, the Sautrāntika/Dārṣṭāntika designation simply signals a divergent position from the orthodox Vaibhāṣika one, and although the authors and redactors of the *Śrāvakabhūmi* expressed such divergent views, they were still (Mūla-)Sarvāstivādins (Deleanu 2006, 1: 159). Deleanu casts the Sautrāntika/Dārṣṭāntika position as a set of 'scholastic views' or an 'interpretive pattern' that represented 'hermeneutical freedom' (Deleanu 2006, 1: 159–60). For the purposes of this study, it is sufficient to note that the *Abhidharmakośabhāṣya* seems to treat the two names almost synonymously; there are nineteen positions attributed to the Sautrāntikas, all of which Vasubandhu agrees with (Kritzer 2005: xxvi–xxvii),[27] and only two positions to Dārṣṭāntika, with which Vasubandhu disagrees (Cox 1995: 39).[28] By observing that the Sautrāntikas appear to win most of the debates in the *Abhidharmakośabhāṣya*, many scholars now characterize Vasubandhu as a Sautrāntika (or at least assert that he agreed with the philosophical positions of the Sautrāntikas).[29] The reasons for the lack of concordance between the *kārikās* and *bhāṣya* continues to be the subject of speculation.[30]

The metaphor of affliction

The Sanskrit word *kleśa* (P. *kilesa*) – derived from the root verb √*kliś*, which means 'to distress' (Whitney 1895: 27) – indicates a negative mental state (such as anger or ignorance). The term appears widely in the *Pātañjalayogaśāstra*, the *Abhidharmakośabhāṣya*, and the *Yogācārabhūmiśāstra* to denote a set of factors that must be eliminated in order for an adept to make spiritual progress. The afflictions are also a driving force in the theory of karma, for they are reinforced through past actions and must be eradicated in order to achieve liberation from the cycle of rebirth. In line with most scholars of Pātañjala yoga, I have chosen to translate *kleśa* as 'affliction', which sticks closely to its etymological roots, but other common translations are 'defilement', 'taint', 'passion', 'contaminant' and 'blemish'.[31] From its core semantic field of bodily 'distress', 'injury' or 'pain', we can deduce that the original context of *kleśa* was medical discourse. *Kleśa* is an important and recurring term in the *Pātañjalayogaśāstra*. Even from PYŚ 1.1 the *kleśa*s are situated in the initial outline of the soteriological path.

> But when the mind is one-pointed, that [concentration; *samādhi*] which illuminates an existing (real) object, destroys the afflictions [and] loosens the bonds of karma; it conduces towards cessation. That cognitive [concentration] is called yoga.[32]

In the opening chapter, we are told that the mental modifications (*vṛttis*) can be both afflicted and unafflicted (*kliṣṭākliṣṭāḥ*) (YS 1.5).[33] Patañjali later characterizes the five afflictions as erroneous cognitions (*viparyayā*) (PYŚ 2.3). In order to evaluate the significance of Patañjali's concept of *kleśa*, I will now sketch the role of this term in early Buddhist and Brahmanical sources in order to demonstrate that the primary discursive context was Buddhist.

In canonical and classical Buddhism, the afflictions (*kleśa*s) are frequently formulated through two metaphors: AFFLICTIONS ARE UNWHOLESOME ROOTS and AFFLICTIONS ARE POISONS. The three primary afflictions are called the three roots (*trimūla*) or the three poisons (*triviṣa*), and the standard formula is attachment (*rāga/lobha*), aversion (*dveṣa*) and delusion (*moha*). These three unwholesome roots (*akuśalamūla*) have counterparts in the wholesome roots (*kuśalamūla*): non-attachment (*alobha*), non-aversion (*adveṣa*) and non-delusion (*amoha*). The unwholesome roots are to be countered with respective contemplations on non-beauty (*aśubha*), compassion (*maitrī*) and wisdom (*prajñā*). In AFFLICTIONS ARE UNWHOLESOME ROOTS, the qualities of roots are domain-mapped to afflictions; hence the *kleśa*s are conceived as difficult to remove, penetrating the soil at depth, unseen, produced over a period of time from a seed or bulb and so on. In the canonical sources, a common technique for elimination of the afflictions is that of 'cutting off' the roots (e.g. AN 3.404).[34] Although the generative context for the metaphor of roots is botanical, the context for poisons is less clear.[35] In the metaphor AFFLICTIONS ARE POISONS, the qualities of poisons are domain-mapped to afflictions, so that *kleśa*s are injurious, dangerous, potentially fatal, require an antidote and so on.

Indeed, there is a third metaphor related to the afflictions that would appear to provide a missing link between these metaphors of roots and poisons: that of 'fault' or 'defect' (*doṣa*). In early āyurvedic texts, the three faults are the principal causes of disease in the body: wind (*vāta*), bile (*pitta*) and phlegm (*śleṣman*). This āyurvedic model is also taken up in classical Buddhist medical texts such as Dharmakṣema's *Sutra of Golden Light* (*Suvarṇabhāsottamasūtra*).[36] As Salguero states, in the *Suvarṇabhāsottamasūtra* there is a clear mapping of the three faults (*doṣas*)[37] onto the three afflictions (*kleśas*): 'There is … a frequent connection made between the physical *doṣa* and the three mental and emotional poisons (*vāta* being equated to greed, *pitta* to hatred, and *śleṣman* to ignorance)' (Salguero 2017: 30). Sharfe (1999) offers a comprehensive analysis of the *doṣas* in early Brahmanical and Buddhist medical sources and suggests a close correspondence between *doṣa* and *viṣa* in some sources, for example, the formulation of the three *doṣas* as 'bile, poison, and wind (*pitta-viṣa-māruta*)' (*Caraka Saṃhitā* Sūtra-sthāna 26.43.1; cited in Scharfe 1999: 620) rather than the standard bile, phlegm and wind. To sum up, the conceptual blend from *doṣa* to *kleśa* is relatively straightforward to trace,[38] but the blend that occurs between *kleśa* and *viṣa* is more difficult to identify; one can speculate that since 'poison' (*viṣa*) is closely connected with 'defect' (*doṣa*) in the medical discourse, when the *doṣas* were conceptually overlaid onto the *kleśas*, the *doṣas* carried with them a blended metaphor of *viṣa*. This eventually created a new hyperblend of the three concepts fault-poison-affliction (*doṣa-viṣa-kleśa*), all gradually compacted within the term *kleśa*. It may also be the case that the confusing slide between these three terms is partly a product of semantic slippage or extension in translation. Salguero notes that while *doṣa* was often translated using Chinese terms for 'fault' or 'defect' (thus accurately representing the āyurvedic context), 'poison' was also strategically chosen as an effective translation for cultural transference, being more resonant for Chinese audiences (Salguero 2014: 58–9). We encounter a similar slipperiness in the translation of *kleśa* in modern-day English-language scholarship. For example, Groner, the translator of Hirakawa (1990), and Gombrich both translate '*tridoṣa*' as 'three poisons' (Hirakawa 1990: 204, 306; Gombrich 1996: 66–7), and Salguero translates *kleśas* as 'poisons' (Salguero 2017: 30). Therefore, when scholars choose 'three poisons' to translate the 'great afflictions' (*mahākleśas*) or the three poisons (*tridoṣa*), there can occur both semantic slippage and metaphorical blending of the accidental and deliberate varieties.

Gombrich argues that these two common metaphors for afflictions (roots and poisons) are not the earliest. The *kleśas* are also represented in Buddhism as the three fires. Since fire in Buddhism is presented negatively to explain the condition of suffering, *nirvāṇa* is the extinguishing of the fires of the passions (*āsravas*), of which *kleśas* are a subgroup.[39] This metaphor is AFFLICTION IS FIRE or the closely related AFFLICTION IS FUEL FOR FIRE. When the *kleśas* no longer provide fuel to the fire of suffering, it goes out and liberation is attained. Over time, this original metaphoric context of *nirvāṇa* (as quenching fire) was forgotten. In this forgetting, the three fiery *kleśa*s were reconceptualized as 'the three poisons'[40] while *nirvāṇa* itself was largely replaced by the metaphor of awakening (*bodhi*) (Gombrich 1996: 66–7).[41] Gombrich also proposes that because the primary afflictions in Buddhism number three, this corresponds to the three fires of the Brahmin householder (the eastern, western and southern fires) (Gombrich 1988: 17–20). Thus, the emancipatory concept of *nirvāṇa* was constructed in opposition to the central concept of Brahmanism, the ritual fire. The soteriological basis of Buddhism renders the literal sacred fires of Brahmanism into dangerous fires of delusion, greed and desire, which must be extinguished. Against such an intense dialectical backdrop, we cannot view the theory of affliction (*kleśa*) in the *Pātañjalayogaśāstra* as merely incidental.

One variation on AFFLICTION IS A ROOT is AFFLICTION IS/HAS A SEED. The metaphor of *kleśa* as a bad seed is developed at length from early Buddhist sources onwards.[42] The *Aṅguttara Nikāya* specifies that bad actions are those informed by greed, aversion and delusion – the three primary afflictions. This is accompanied by two images that are relevant. The first image is that the seeds of affliction are like those planted in fertile soil with abundant rain, and the second is that only by burning and throwing away the seeds of *kleśa* can the bad fruits be stopped (AN 1.134–135, cited in Collins 1982: 298 fn. 6). Arguably, the underlying root metaphor[43] for AFFLICTION IS A SEED is THE LIFE CYCLE IS A PLANT CYCLE (e.g. a child is a 'young sprout', a pregnant woman is 'in full bloom', someone in old age 'withers away').

Entailment and contradiction

The metaphors that I have outlined here – AFFLICTION IS A ROOT/POISON/SEED/FIRE – are not all compatible. While AFFLICTION IS/HAS A ROOT and AFFLICTION IS/HAS A SEED map qualities from the same domain (botanical cultivation), AFFLICTION IS A POISON and AFFLICTION IS A FIRE map different, contradictory qualities. However, as Lakoff and Johnson state, multiple metaphors for the same concept can either be part of the same image-schema (root and seed are part of a larger botanical image-schema) or they can offer alternative ways of conceptualization, as long as they share one or more entailments. While the metaphors AFFLICTION IS A POISON and AFFLICTION IS A FIRE share the entailment 'affliction is dangerous', AFFLICTION IS A (BAD) SEED and AFFLICTION IS A (STUBBORN) ROOT share a different set of entailments, most obviously 'affliction is unseen' (beneath the surface) and 'affliction is unwanted growth'. However, all of these conceptual metaphors share at least one entailment: that affliction (*kleśa*) is an undesirable factor that must be eliminated.[44]

In contrast to the proliferation of technical discussions of *kleśa* in Buddhist soteriology, the presence of the term *kleśa* in Brahmanic soteriology is relatively sparse. While the concept appears briefly in *Śvetāśvatara Upaniṣad*[45] and is employed generically in the *Bhagavad Gītā*,[46] we find the term used more frequently in the 'Śānti Parvan' of the *Mahābhārata*, where it is used to denote four primary *kleśa*s of greed (*lobha*), anger (*krodha*), attachment (*rāga*) and aversion (*dveṣa*).[47] These are clearly counterparts to the Buddhist trio discussed above. However, in none of these contexts is affliction (*kleśa*) presented in relation to the seed (*bīja*) and its substratum (*āśraya*). Furthermore, we do not encounter the term *kleśa* in the *Sāṃkhyakārikā* (SKK), although it does contain a similar idea of a threefold causal basis of suffering (internal, external and supernatural causes). The opening lines of the *Sāṃkhyakārikā* declare that the goal of the Sāṃkhya method is to remove the three inflictions of suffering: *duḥkhatrayābhighātā* (SKK 1). This Sāṃkhya notion of 'infliction' or 'injury' (*abhighātā*) is closely related to the idea of *kleśa* as 'affliction', 'distress' or 'harm'. Indeed, Patañjali reproduces Sāṃkhya's account of forms of suffering related to delusion.

Both the *Sāṃkhyakārikā* and the *Pātañjalayogaśāstra* list five forms of delusion (*tamas*, *moha*, *mahāmoha*, *tāmisra* and *andhatāmisra*), but only Patañjali's text equates them to the five afflictions (*kleśa*s).[48] Broadly speaking, the concept of affliction (*kleśa*) is not prevalent in Brahmanic discourse in the way that it is in Buddhist soteriology. More common in Brahmanism is the related concept of fault (*doṣa*) in the sense of physical or mental defect within āyurvedic medical discourse (discussed above).[49] Yet since they both literally denote bodily distress, *kleśa* and *doṣa* appear to have been generated in medical discourse and were only later blended with the botanical metaphor.

Pratisaṃkhyā and *prasaṃkhyāna*

In order to provide a full context for my discussion of soteriological metaphors, it is necessary to firstly elucidate some detail on how *kleśa*s fit in to the soteriologies of the *Pātañjalayogaśāstra* and the *Abhidharmakośabhāṣya*. Here, I discuss two closely related terms: Vasubandhu's *pratisaṃkhyā* ('contemplative disjunction', also called *pratisaṃkhyāna*) and Patañjali's *prasaṃkhyāna* ('contemplative discernment').

Pratisaṃkhyā: Contemplative disjunction in the *Abhidharmakośabhāṣya*

While the *Abhidharmakośabhāṣya* does not identify an entity or practice called 'yoga' in its discussion of the unconditioned factors of existence (*asaṃskṛta dharmas*), it posits a technique called disjunction (*visaṃyoga*)[50] that entails cessation via analysis[51] (*pratisaṃkhyānirodha*).[52] This contemplative technique generates insight (*prajñā*)[53] and is equivalent to cessative liberation (*nirvāṇa*). Specifically, *visaṃyoga* indicates the disjunction of the afflictions (*kleśa*s) from the mind (*citta*)[54] (AKBh 1.6; Pradhan 1975: 4, 7–8). The three primary afflictions of attachment (*rāga*), aversion (*dveṣa*) and delusion (*moha*) form part of the set of impure factors (*sāsrava dharma*s), which belong to the conditioned state.[55] Therefore to attain an unconditioned state, one must be free of the *kleśa*s. Depending on whether one takes the Vaibhāṣika or the Sautrāntika position, disjunction (*visaṃyoga*) can respectively result in mere cessation of the *kleśa*s or total elimination thereof including any latent forms (*anuśaya*s). Within Buddhist literature, this function of destroying the *kleśa*s by disconnecting from them is consistent and long-standing. Cox notes the primacy of destroying the *kleśa*s in late Sarvāstivāda soteriology:

> Later Sarvāstivādin texts do not present either the practice of concentration or the acquisition of knowledge as the ultimate religious goal, but rather as means for abandoning and preventing the future arising of defilements. (Cox 1992: 66)[56]

The next question then is, in practice, what exactly is disjunction (*visaṃyoga*), or cessation via analysis (*pratisaṃkhyānirodha*)?[57] It entails an act of understanding by reviewing the content of the four noble truths (AKBh 1.5; Pradhan 1975: 4, 1).[58] The disjunction that is produced by such analysis not only leads to a cessation/elimination of the afflictions, but is also prerequisite for the state of *nirvāṇa*, or cessative liberation:[59] 'He who takes refuge in the dharma takes refuge in *nirvāṇa*, or cessation via analysis' (AKBh 4.32).[60] Indeed, *nirvāṇa* is defined as the cessation of the afflictions and of suffering.[61]

According to the Vaibhāṣikas, disjunction (*visaṃyoga*) takes place not just once, but repeatedly. Thus disjunction/cessation via analysis must take place separately for each *kleśa*: 'The acquisition of disjunction from them occurs many times' (AKBh 5.62).[62] There are as many cessations as there are afflictions to be abandoned. The condition in which afflictions are perpetuated makes cessation via analysis non-absolute, but rather a provisional, continuous and repeated process – in short, a contemplative practice. In contrast, for the Sautrāntikas, cessation via analysis (*pratisaṃkhyānirodha*) is the extinction of the latent forms of affliction (*anuśaya*) and the extinction of any future arising of life (*janman*) (AKBh 2). For them, there is an additional quality of permanence to the extinction of the latent form – once it is eliminated, it will not arise again.[63] According to the Sautrāntikas, only the higher paths represent the result of disjunction (*visaṃyogaphala*) and indicate *nirvāṇa* without remnant (*nirupadhiśeṣanirvāṇa*).[64] And what is this remnant? It is the trace of past karma that contains the seed of future karma – only *pratisaṃkhyānirodha* (= *visaṃyogaphalam*) marks the attainment of this seedless state.

We should, at this point, have a clear sense of how privileged and important a term *pratisaṃkhyā* is in the *Abhidharmakośa*'s discourse of liberation.[65] It is situated within a network of equivalences (*visaṃyoga* = *pratisaṃkhyānirodha* = *prajñā* = *nirvāṇa*). It refers to a contemplation that entails reflecting on enumerated content in sequence, such as the four noble truths. For the Sautrāntikas, it permanently eliminates the afflictions and their seed.

Prasaṃkhyāna: Contemplative discernment in the *Pātañjalayogaśāstra*

In the *Pātañjalayogaśāstra*, Patañjali uses the term *prasaṃkhyāna* – analytical or discerning contemplation – to denote a form of contemplation that relates to the afflictions,[66] and the way in which he employs the term *prasaṃkhyāna* resembles the Sautrāntika soteriology of Vasubandhu's text. Let us first trace the conceptual link between *prasaṃkhyāna* and the afflictions in Patañjali's text. Pātañjala yoga also posits a theory of *kleśa*. The five afflictions are nescience, egoity, attachment, animosity and clinging to life (***avidyāsmitārāgadveṣābhiniveśāḥ kleśāḥ***, YS 2.3), although they are also defined using a threefold formula of greed, anger and delusion (*lobhakrodhamoha*; YS 2.34). In the fivefold model, nescience is a field (*kṣetra*), which is the propagative ground (*prasavabhūmi*) of the other four afflictions. In total, there are five states in which the afflictions may exist, and they are all explained via the idea of plant propagation: (1) dormant (*prasupta*), (2) attenuated (*tanu*), (3) cut (*vicchinna*), (4) sustained (*udāra*) and (5) burnt (*dagdha*), the last of which is the ideal state (PYŚ 2.4). Even though the metaphysical framework is different, Pātañjala yoga, like the contemporaneous Buddhist soteriology, also describes a meditative technique to cut off from the *kleśas*: cognitive concentration (*saṃprajñāta samādhi*).[67] Furthermore, diminishing the *kleśas* is one of the two stated goals of the yoga of action (*kriyā yoga*), one of the main path structures of the *Pātañjalayogaśāstra*.[68] The growth of concentration (*samādhi*) is proportional to the non-growth of the afflictions. As long as the roots of *kleśas* exist, the seeds will mature in the form of birth, duration of life and experience (YS 2.13). Destroying the afflictions produces cessation (*nirodha*), which leads not to cessative liberation (*nirvāṇa*) in this case but to the epistemological and ontological isolation (*kaivalya*) of pure consciousness (*puruṣa*) from materiality (*prakṛti*), the central teaching of Sāṃkhya.

In the *Pātañjalayogaśāstra*, one of the chief means of tackling the afflictions is a mental process called *prasaṃkhyāna*. This is a specific form of absorption (*dhyāna*) (PYŚ 2.11) and is also called the absorption of the cloud of dharma (*dharmameghadhyāna*):

> When that very [purity] is established in its own form, without the least measure of dynamism, being merely the cognition of the distinction between purity and pure consciousness, it is conducive to the absorption of the cloud of dharma. Those versed in absorption call this [*dharmameghadhyāna*] '*prasaṃkhyāna*'. (PYŚ 1.2)[69]

As a form of absorption, *prasaṃkhyāna* is a higher practice that is pursued after the goals of action (*kriyā yoga*) have been attained: *kriyā yoga* can attenuate the afflictions, but the practice of *prasaṃkhyāna* will be required to render them impotent (PYŚ 2.2, 2.11). In the final stage, however, the technique of *prasaṃkhyāna* must also be abandoned, and, as long as the presence of discriminating discernment (*vivekakhyāti*) remains unwavering, the *samādhi* that conduces to the cloud of dharma (*dharmamegha samādhi*) will arise (YS 4.29). This is the final liberation.

To summarize, *prasaṃkhyāna* is a form of object-centred meditation that can lead to cognitive concentration (*saṃprajñāta samādhi*).[70] It is an act of contemplation that eradicates the afflictions and produces the ultimate form of discriminating discernment (*vivekakhyāti*) – discerning the difference between *prakṛti* and *puruṣa*.[71] We have established, then, that in the *Pātañjalayogaśāstra*, analytical contemplation or *prasaṃkhyāna* is a key soteriological technique that destroys the afflictions.

Prasaṃkhyāna and *pratisaṃkhyā* as related soteriological terms

Patañjali's *prasaṃkhyāna* and Vasubandhu's *pratisaṃkhyā* are related and belong to the same semantic and conceptual family.[72] These terms broadly refer to a contemplative act of reviewing distinct principles with analytical or discriminative application in order to gain understanding (knowledge).[73] Although the content of the contemplative act differs in Brahmanical and Buddhist traditions, the approach or vehicle of meditation is comparable. Equally, the structural function of this contemplation (its role and placement within a broader soteriological scheme of karma theory) is also resonant. There is an enumerative aspect to an act of *pratisaṃkhyā* or *prasaṃkhyāna*, which is inextricably part of the analytical act. *Pratisaṃkhyā* and *prasaṃkhyāna* indicate both seeing and counting at the same time (either the four noble truths, or *prakṛti* and *puruṣa*) and are structured by the primary metaphor KNOWING IS SEEING. However, *pratisaṃkhyā* carries a specific sense of the sequential consideration of a group of factors (the four noble truths), which is not conveyed by *prasaṃkhyāna*. Additionally, while the doctrinal content of both forms of contemplation is, of course, different, they share the goal of destroying the *kleśa*s.

Stcherbatsky speculated that the *pratisaṃkhyā* of the *Abhidharmakośabhāṣya* is identical with the *prasaṃkhyāna* of the *Yogasūtra*. Although reductive, his argument is worth considering in that he asserts that only the prefix *prati-* expresses an orthodox Sarvāstivāda doctrinal point – that each disjunction from *kleśa* must occur individually on a separate basis (Stcherbatsky 1991: 51 fn. 1). However, it is not clear that a singular approach to each *kleśa* is necessarily excluded from Patañjali's *prasaṃkhyāna*. Although the *Pātañjalayogaśāstra* does not state explicitly that the *kleśa*s must each be treated singly, we are told that their nature is to arise one at a time (PYŚ 2.4; Angot 2012: 381, 9–11), and therefore, presumably, they must be dealt with in similar fashion. Furthermore, in the *Pātañjalayogaśāstra* the phrase '*vivekadarśana-abhyāsa*' (PYŚ 1.12; Maas 2006: 40, 6–7) indicates a practice (*abhyāsa*) of discriminating discernment (*vivekakhyāti*), and thus implies the repeated application of the technique of *prasaṃkhyāna* to achieve this state.[74] Such repeated application also implies that *kleśa*s must be addressed individually. Additionally, the *prasaṃkhyāna* of the *Pātañjalayogaśāstra* appears to entail not the provisional *kleśanirodha* adhered to by the Vaibhāṣikas but rather the permanent destruction of the *kleśa*s adhered to by the Sautrāntikas; in the *Pātañjalayogaśāstra*, the *kleśa*s must be utterly 'destroyed' (*hata*) (PYŚ 4.30; Angot 2012: 723).

To sum up: Vasubandhu's *pratisaṃkhyā* and Patañjali's *prasaṃkhyāna* both produce disjunction from the *kleśa*s by reflecting on enumerated content during contemplation so as to correctly perceive reality. In the way that *pratisaṃkhyā* produces cessation (*nirodha)*, so is *vivekakhyāti* a form of ultimate *nirodha* in that it produces the cessation of false identification with, and therefore disjunction from, materiality.[75] The doctrinal or methodical significance of the two prefixes '*prati-*' and '*pra-*' is not entirely clear. However, the *Abhidharmakośa*'s soteriological continuum from *pratisaṃkhyā* to *nirvāṇa* shares semantic and structural form with the Pātañjala yoga continuum from *prasaṃkhyāna* to *kaivalya* – they both entail the destruction of the *kleśa*s. It is only by reading the *Pātañjalayogaśāstra* intertextually that we glean these insights of the semantic and technical framework of the term *prasaṃkhyāna* in Pātañjala yoga. Unless we read this term, and others, through the Buddhist context, we simply miss out on dense layers of meaning.

The visceral action of removing unwanted roots and seeds from soil is used to structure the idea that a *kleśa* in the mind is difficult to uproot and that, even when it appears to be removed, a persistent root or seed may regrow and have to be pulled up again. Equally, seeds and roots that are embedded in soil are unseen and difficult to find. The sensorimotor experiences of cultivating the soil are used to construct a conceptual system of spiritual cultivation in which cultivation is understood as repetitive and hard work (e.g. pulling up roots or finding and destroying bad seeds). This specific conceptual metaphor of *kleśa* as a botanical plant/seed/root is of course part of the scheme of karma. In karma theory, the proposition that each action has a consequence is structured via the metaphor that the end product of a plant (e.g. its fruit or flower) is directly concomitant to the conditions of growth – that is, intensive cultivation produces a high yield and non-intensive cultivation produce a low yield. The metaphors of *kleśa*, then, are part of the wider orientational metaphor of karma theory, which also governs cultivation (*bhāvanā*).

The seed of *kleśa*

The general karmic metaphor that you reap what you sow (that the seed matches the fruit) is of course common to all early Indic philosophical thought.[76] Nonetheless, it is important to differentiate some distinct contexts: namely seed growth as a positive phenomenon[77] contrasted with seed growth as a negative phenomenon.[78] Furthermore, I wish to distinguish between a general karmic theory of seed and a particular and detailed theory of seed in relation to *kleśa*, that of the Sautrāntikas.[79] Moreover, we see that the elaboration of the seed of *kleśa* (*kleśabīja*) in Buddhist sources is more prolific and technical than in Brahmanical.[80] Here I argue that *kleśabīja* is a uniquely Sautrāntika metaphorical elaboration within Sarvāstivāda Buddhism and that Patañjali co-opts this image from the Sautrāntika discursive sphere.

The metaphorical power of *prasaṃkhyāna* in the *Pātañjalayogaśāstra* is not restricted to the image of 'discriminating vision'. It is also explained using the metaphor of fire. We are told that the fire of *prasaṃkhyāna* sterilizes the diminished *kleśa*s 'like fire, during the process of roasting sterilizes seeds'.[81] By observing the shared image of fire between *tapas* (asceticism) and *prasaṃkhyāna*, Endo associates *prasaṃkhyāna* with the *tapas* of *kriyā yoga* (Endo 2000: 78).[82] However, as we have noted, *prasaṃkhyāna* is not part of *kriyā yoga* but is rather an advanced practice beyond *kriyā yoga* (PYŚ 2.2, 2.11), which is only suitable for the practitioner whose mind is still in an active state (PYŚ 2.1). Where Endo's analysis falls short is in focusing solely on the image of fire and not on the image of the seed. Thus, he conflates the heat of *tapas* with the fire of burning the seed, an image attached to *prasaṃkhyāna*. Indeed, *prasaṃkhyāna* contains two different metaphors of sterilization: one is purificatory (sterilizing impurity) and the other is non-propagative (sterilizing potency).[83] The non-propagative status of the seed is, in many ways, more significant than the image of purificatory fire.

This image of the seed of *kleśa* is crucial in the intertextual discourse of classical yoga in the fourth to fifth centuries. As we have noted, in the *Abhidharmakośabhāṣya*, the Sautrāntika account of liberation insists that *pratisaṃkhyānirodha* (= *visaṃyoga*) is not just the cessation of the *kleśa*s but also the destruction of the latent form of *kleśa*, the *anuśaya*, which stops the production of all future seed (*bīja*) of affliction.[84] As in Patañjali's text (see above), the image of the burnt seed[85] of *kleśa* that cannot sprout (*na prarohasamartha*) also appears in the *Abhidharmakośabhāṣya*:

> For the substratum of the Noble Ones is thus transformed due to the capacity of the paths of seeing and cultivation, such that there is no recurrence of the germination potential of the *kleśa*s to be abandoned by those [two paths]. So when the substratum has come to be without the seeds of afflictions, like rice that has been burnt by fire, someone is called 'one who has abandoned defilements' – or when [the substratum has] seeds that have been damaged

> by the ordinary path. In other circumstances, someone is one who has not abandoned the *kleśa*s (AKBh 2.36c–d).[86]

Both the Pātañjala and Sautrāntika soteriologies, then, rely on a seedless state of *kleśa*. And both refer to a technique of burning the seed of *kleśa* in order to sterilize its potency.

The seedless state

In Sautrāntika discourse, the destruction of the *anuśaya* (the latent form or seed of *kleśa*) is due to the presence of insight, *prajñā*. Patañjali's *nirbīja samādhi* (presented in the first chapter of the *Pātañjalayogaśāstra*) also requires the presence of *prajñā* to achieve the seedless state. This *prajñā* – specifically, truth-bearing insight (*ṛtaṃbharā prajñā*)[87] – eventually leads to the destruction of all latent imprints of *karma*, which are called *saṃskāras*.[88]

> **When that [special *saṃskāra*] is ceased, as a result of everything being ceased, the *samādhi* is without seed.** (YS 1.51)[89]

For this line of enquiry, it is essential to render *nirbīja* literally (at YS 1.51) as meaning 'without seed', rather than translate it as 'without object', as some scholars have done.[90] Those who render *nirbīja* metaphorically to mean 'without object' do so in order to make the state of *nirbīja samādhi* correspond to the other paradigms in the first *pāda* of the *Pātañjalayogaśāstra* – in particular to correlate it to non-cognitive or objectless concentration (*asaṃprajñāta samādhi*).[91] While I must concur that seedless concentration (*nirbīja samādhi*) is a non-cognitive state in which the practitioner no longer engages in objective cognition, this does not account for the technical meaning or function of the seed within this process.[92]

The overall semantic range of seed (*bīja*) in the *Pātañjalayogaśāstra* is 'seed of *kleśa*' rather than 'seed of cognition', or 'object' (e.g. PYŚ 2.2, 2.4, 2.11, 2.13).[93] Thus the primary meaning of seedless (*nirbīja*) in *sūtra* 1.51 refers not to the absence of an object in concentration but to the concentration that contains no seed, that concentration which is devoid of any future generative seed of affliction and the resulting karma, as the later commentator Śaṅkara explains.[94] The *bhāṣya* makes this point clear by explaining how the karmic imprints (*saṃskāras*) are prevented from future arising. The end of the material function of mental operation (*adhikāra*) can occur only after the generation of the mental imprints of isolation (*kaivalya)*, which have the effect of sublating all other imprints (*saṃskāras*):

> Due to this, when its function[95] comes to an end, the mind ceases together with those imprints that are conducive to isolation (*kaivalya*). (PYŚ 1.51)[96]

Eventually, these *kaivalya*-inducing imprints will also cease to exist because they contain no seed.[97] There is a parallel here with the Sautrāntika theory that, in order for disjunction (= cessation) (*visaṃyoga)* to occur, the latent form of affliction (i.e. the *anuśaya*, which contains the seed) must also be eliminated.

The dormant seed

Hwang argues that the Sautrāntikas made a unique innovation to the Buddhist theory of the two *nirvāṇas* (enlightenment and final liberation at death)[98] in order to elaborate their theory of causality (Hwang 2006: 90–7).[99] The Sautrāntikas highlighted a distinction between *nirvāṇa* with remainder of karmic deposit and of life (*janman*) (*sopadhiśeṣanirvāṇadhātu*) and *nirvāṇa* that is devoid of remnant of karmic deposit and of arising of future life (*nirupadhiśeṣanirvāṇadhātu*) (Hwang 2006: 92).[100] To explain the idea of karmic deposit, the early Dārṣṭāntika-Sautrāntikas shifted the emphasis from affliction to a latent form of affliction (a dormant seed), which they called *anuśaya* and which became their doctrinal cornerstone (Park 2014: 464–9; Hwang 2006: 90–7).[101] As Park has noted in his study of the seed in relation to karmic theory in early Buddhism,

> this sequential model of causation based on the botanical imagery of seed growth is a characteristic marker by which to discern the Dārṣṭāntika-Sautrāntika affiliation. (Park 2014: 311)

At this point, *anuśaya* was not a common term in the Buddhist canon, and as Hwang states, 'this small terminological shift seems to be the key to understanding how nirvana was explained in the Sautrāntika system' (Hwang 2006: 92). The metaphor model used by the Sautrāntikas to anchor these doctrinal distinctions was that of the seed (Hwang 2006: 93), and it was typical of later Sarvāstivādin Abhidharma texts to engage in 'heated sectarian controversy' over 'the possibility of a distinction between latent and active defilements' (Cox 1992: 69). In the *Abhidharmakośabhāṣya*, this argument plays out between the Vaibhāṣikas, who deny that there are any latent afflictions, and the Sautrāntikas, who maintain a dual distinction between the manifest affliction (*paryavasthāna*) and the latent affliction (*anuśaya*).[102] Thus Patañjali's discussion of concentration as being with seed and without seed (*sabīja* and *nirbīja samādhi)* is particularly resonant of the specific debates happening in Sautrāntika circles during the fourth to fifth centuries.

The argument for such resonance is supported by comparing the two following passages, which define the seed state of affliction. Patañjali claims that dormancy (*prasupta*) is when the *kleśa* remains in a seed state (*bījabhāva*) and is not awakened (*prabodha*). In the *Abhidharmakośabhāṣya*, the Sautrāntikas define the dormant affliction as a seed in similar terms (see Table 2.1).

The passages seem to echo each other, and although I am wary of asserting a direction of influence, it is worth noting that the metaphor of the seed in Buddhist soteriology was technically employed even before the *Abhidharmakośabhāṣya*.[103] The *Mahāvibhāṣaśāstra* (first to second century CE, and of which the

Table 2.1 *Pātañjalayogaśāstra* 2.4 and *Abhidharmakośabhāṣya* 5.1

Pātañjalayogaśāstra	***Abhidharmakośabhāṣya***
tatra kā prasuptiḥ? cetasi śaktimātrapratiṣṭhānāṃ bījabhāvopagamaḥ. tasya prabodha ālambane saṃmukhībhāvaḥ (PYŚ 2.4; Angot 2012: 381, 2–3)	*prasupto hi kleśo 'nuśaya ucyate / prabuddhaḥ paryavasthānam / kā ca tasya prasuptiḥ / asaṃmukhībhūtasya bījabhāvānubandhaḥ / kaḥ prabodhaḥ / saṃmukhībhāvaḥ / ko 'yaṃ bījabhāvo nāma. ātmabhāvasya kleśajā kleśopādanaśaktiḥ* (AKBh 5.1; Pradhan 1975: 278, 20–4)
Of these [modes of existence], what is dormancy? It is having the seed state (*bījabhāva*) of those [*kleśa*s] that remain in the mind in potential-form only (*śaktimātra*). Its awakening means that it is becoming present (face-to-face)* with regard to an object.	The dormant *kleśa* is called *anuśaya*. The opposite is [the *kleśa* in] an awakened state. And what is its dormancy? It is a series of seed states (*bījabhāvānubandha*) of [an affliction] that has not become present. What is awakening? The becoming present (face-to face). And what is it that is called the seed state (*bījabhāva*)? The capacity of *kleśa* to be productive in one whose self is generated by *kleśa*.

* What is being emphasized is the notion of contact with an object: becoming present here is the condition of contact that creates the awakening. It should be noted that *saṃmukhībhūta* or *-bhāva* is a technical term in Buddhist meditation for a face-to-face meeting with the Buddha, e.g. in this passage from the *Bodhisattvabhūmi: yad bodhisattvaḥ tathāgata-kāyaṃ vā tathāgata-caityam vā saṃmukhībhūtam adhyakṣaṃ pūjayati. iyam asya saṃmukha-pūjety ucyate* (BoBoh 1.16; Wogihara 1930–6: 231, lines 13–15). 'Regarding this [topic], the act of worship that a bodhisattva performs while standing face-to-face before a tathāgata's body or a tathāgata shrine, and while [either of them] is perceptible to his or her own senses, is called "face-to-face" worship' (trans. Engle 2016: 388).

Abhidharmakośabhāṣya is a summary)[104] records that the Vibhajyavādins reject the possibility of retrogression for an *arhat*:[105]

> The Vibhajyavādins further say that *anuśaya* is the *bīja* of *paryavasthāna*. The *anuśaya* is *cittaviprayukta* in its intrinsic nature. The *paryavasthāna* is *cittasaṃprayukta* in its intrinsic nature. *Paryavasthāna* arises from *anuśaya*. Retrogression results from the manifestation (*saṃmukhībhāva*) of *paryavasthāna*. The *arhat*-s have already abandoned the *anuśaya*-s; the *paryavasthāna*-s not arising, how can an *arhat* retrogress? Hence they (the Vibhajyavādins) assert that it is logical that there is no retrogression. (MVŚ 313a; trans. Dhammajoti 2009: 340)[106]

This *Mahāvibhāṣa* passage is one that gives rise to the *Abhidharmakośabhāṣya*'s later discussion of the seeds of *kleśa* and how they manifest.[107] A similar passage also appears in one of the supplementary sections of the fourth-century *Yogācārabhūmiśāstra*, the *Viniścayasaṃgrahaṇī*:[108]

> There the active (**samudācarita*) and manifest (**saṃmukhībhūta*) *kleśa* is called *paryavasthāna*. Its seed, which has not been abandoned (**aprahiṇā*) or destroyed (**asamudghātita*), is called *anuśaya* or *dauṣṭhulya*. Since it is [in a] dormant [state] (*aprabuddha*-[*avasthā*]), it is *anuśaya*, and since it is in the awakened state (**prabuddhāvasthā*), it is **paryavasthāna*. (trans. Park 2014: 436)[109]

It seems that this particular elaboration of the seed of *kleśa* as having latent and manifest forms is a Buddhist one and that Patañjali is drawing on such descriptions – if not on the text of the *Abhidharmakośabhāṣya* itself. Both texts assert that a *kleśa* has latent and manifest states and map these properties from a botanical domain. The properties 'latency' and 'manifestation' are then logically extended to propose that seeds can be 'dormant' and 'awake'. The domain-mapping in this metaphor is so specific that it points towards one author utilizing the words of the other.

Destroying the power of the seed by burning it

In the above comparison of PYŚ 2.4 and AKBh 5.1, there is one other technical term that merits consideration. The above passage from the *Pātañjalayogaśāstra* includes the term *śaktimātra* ('by power/capacity alone') in relation to the seed. The term *śakti* is also used in the Sautrāntika theory of the seed as a synonym for *sāmarthya*, which indicates the potential of the seed. These terms are central in explaining the ontology and causality of Sautrāntika. Interestingly, the PYŚ also refers to this highly technical concept of the potential of the seed (*bījasāmarthya*). This passage occurs in a description of dormant *kleśa*s as seeds and how they are rendered impotent (see Table 2.2).[110]

In Sautrāntika, the *śakti* or *sāmarthya* of the seed refers to the capacity or potential of the seed to produce future afflictions in an individual existence (*ātmabhāva*) (AKBh 5.2). The *śakti* or *sāmarthya* is intricately bound up with the concept of *bījabhāva* (which features in both the compared passages here: PYŚ 2.4 and AKBh 5.1).[111] This 'capacity' or 'potential' of the seed forms a key doctrinal point in the Sautrāntika theory of causality within the doctrine of momentariness.[112] For the Sautrāntikas,

> this seed-state itself arises from another, previous defilement and contains the power to produce a subsequent defilement, thereby forming a series (*bījabhāvānubandha*) that belongs to the material basis (*ātmabhāva, āśraya*) of a sentient being. (Cox 1992: 73)

Park points out that *bījabhāva* was a technical Sautrāntika definition of *anuśaya* and that Vasubandhu uses it to emphasize 'the agency or ontological basis of these seeds' in relation to the notion of *āśraya*, as the ontological basis of mind (AKBh 2.36) (Park 2014: 452–3).[113] The seed with its connotations of potential and contiguous states allows the Sautrāntika concept of karma and retribution to be different to the Vaibhāṣika concept.[114] Using these technical concepts of the power and potential of the seed, the Sautrāntikas rejected the Vaibhāṣika notion that the action continues to exist at the same time as the effect (the 'three times' theory).

We have observed that *kleśa-bīja-anuśaya-āśraya* emerges as a metaphorical scheme through which the Sautrāntika discourse of liberation is constructed.[115] This scheme is also present in the *Pātañjalayogaśāstra*, albeit in a condensed form (as befits the *sūtra* genre). Such is the dominance of 'seed of affliction' (*kleśabīja*) in the discourse of the *Pātañjalayogaśāstra*, that, at points, the text defines yoga as the destruction of the afflictions and its seeds: it is the light of yoga that destroys the darkness of the afflictions (PYŚ 3.51),[116] and isolation (*kaivalya*) is achieved by one in whom the seeds of affliction have been burnt (PYŚ 3.55).[117] As discussed, the image of the burnt seed is a recurrent one in Pātañjala yoga and is the only way to destroy the capacity (*sāmarthya*) of the seed to reproduce across time. Now that we have enriched our understanding of how the metaphor of *kleśabīja* works in Pātañjala yoga, we can return to analytical contemplation or *prasaṃkhyāna*: if *prasaṃkhyāna* destroys the seed, it must lead to the *samādhi* that is seedless

Table 2.2 *Pātañjalayogaśāstra* 2.4 and *Abhidharmakośābhāṣya* 2.36

Pātañjalayogaśāstra	***Abhidharmakośabhāṣya***
satāṃ kleśānāṃ tadā bījasāmarthyaṃ dagdham iti viṣayasya saṃmukhībhāve 'pi sati na bhavaty eṣāṃ prabodha ity uktā prasuptir dagdhabījānām aprarohaś ca (PYŚ 2.4; Angot 2012: 381, 6–7).	*āśrayo hi sa āryāṇāṃ darśanabhāvanāmārgasāmarthyāt tathā parāvṛtto bhavati, yathā na punas tatpraheyāṇāṃ kleśānāṃ prarohasamartho bhavati / ato 'gnidagdhavrīhivad abījībhūte āśraye kleśānāṃ prahīṇakleśa ity ucyate / upahatabījabhāve vā laukikena mārgeṇa / viparyayād aprahīṇakleśaḥ* (AKBh 2.36 c–d; Pradhan 1975: 63, 20–1)
Since the potential of the seeds (*bījasāmarthyam*) is then burnt up in those remaining (*satām*) *kleśa*s, even though there is direct (face-to-face) encounter with the object, they [the *kleśa*s] do not awaken – thus is described dormancy and the non-germination of the burnt seed.	For the substratum (*āśraya*)* of the Noble Ones is thus transformed (*parāvṛtti*) due to the capacity of the paths of seeing and cultivation, such that there is no recurrence of the germination potential of the *kleśa*s to be abandoned by those [two paths]. So when the substratum has come to be without seeds of *kleśa*s, like rice has been burnt by fire, someone is called 'one who has abandoned *kleśa*s' – or when [the substratum has] seeds that have been damaged by the ordinary path. In other circumstances, someone is one who has not abandoned *kleśa*s.

*Yamabe translates *āśraya* in this passage as 'body' and 'our personal existence centred on the body' (Yamabe 1997: 198).

(*nirbīja samādhi*).[118] In addition to a specific association of *kleśa* with *bīja* and the use of a specific contemplative technique to eradicate such seeds (*prasaṃkhyāna*), Patañjali's text has recourse to a range of other related technical concepts that appear in Sautrāntika:

1. the distinction between latent and manifest affliction (*kleśa*) with the blended concept of dormant and awake seeds (*prasupti* and *prabodha*),
2. the potency of the seed (*bījasāmarthya*; *śakti*),
3. the state of the seed (*bījabhāva*) in sequence that forms the ontological basis of mind (*āśraya*) and
4. the necessity of burning the seed (*dagdhabīja*) to make it non-germinating (*apraroha*).

There can be little doubt that the discourse surrounding *kleśa* in Patañjali's and Vasubandhu's texts is an integrated one. While the conceptual metaphor of *bīja* within karma theory is not unique to Sautrāntika, they had a particular elaboration that was distinct, even within Buddhist discourse.[119] Thus, the technical metaphors that we see in the *Pātañjalayogaśāstra* around *kleśabīja* are closer to Sautrāntika than anything we encounter in Brahmanical sources. On this basis, I conclude that Patañjali was aware of and drawing on Sautrāntika metaphorical discourse and in particular had access to or knowledge of the *Abhidharmakośabhāṣya*.[120]

Mental substratum (*āśraya*) as seedbed of *kleśa*

There is one final point to explore in relation to the seed of *kleśa*: the Sautrāntika theory of seed also relates to the idea of a psychophysical substratum (*āśraya*), a concept that Patañjali develops in a way that is concordant with the Sautrāntika position.

In the *Abhidharmakośabhāṣya*, both *āśraya* and *āśaya* are key concepts, respectively denoting 'mental basis/substratum' and 'intention/disposition'. According to the Sautrāntikas, when the *kleśa*s are eliminated, the mental basis, the *āśraya*, also disappears. This is because there is a semantic continuum between the term for latent affliction, *anuśaya*, and the term for the basis, the *āśraya*.[121] Let us look more closely at the semantics. Although *āśraya* and *āśaya* are derived differently in Sanskrit,[122] the two terms are semantically related.[123] Furthermore, as Edgerton points out, in Buddhist-Hybrid Sanskrit, *āśaya* (disposition) and *anuśaya* (latent affliction) are near-synonyms. *Anuśaya*[124] is glossed in Abhidharma by the term *bīja*. Indeed, the very quality of latency (*anuśaya*) is an attribution of the seed form.[125] Collectively then, the *anuśayas*, which are in fact seeds, form the substratum (mental basis; *āśraya*) and cause afflictions.[126] The substratum is therefore a seedbed.[127] This semantic continuum between *anuśaya-āśaya-āśraya* in the *Abhidharmakośabhāṣya* means that the terms are sometimes used interchangeably.[128]

In the discourse of the *Pātañjalayogaśāstra*, the terms *āśraya* and *āśaya* are also significant, although *āśaya* is by far the more prominent term.[129] *Anuśaya* appears in a limited context in the *Pātañjalayogaśāstra* (and only in relation to the *kleśa*s),[130] but it is possible that *āśaya*, a near-synonym, stands in for it because, as Edgerton states, occurrences of *anuśaya* in Sanskrit are rare, making it 'essentially a Buddhist word'.[131] As in the Buddhist literature, there is also a degree of semantic fuzziness between the terms *āśaya* and *āśraya* in the Buddhist-inflected discourse of the *Pātañjalayogaśāstra*.[132] In the *Pātañjalayogaśāstra*, *āśaya* appears most often in the compound *karmāśaya* and is a term that is conceptually resonant with the Sautrāntika *āśraya* as the 'karmic substratum' or 'mental basis'. *Karmāśaya* is the substratum of karmic deposits, and *āśaya* is stated as the cause of *kleśa*:

> The afflicted [*vṛttis*], having *kleśas* as their cause, are the fields of operation in respect to the accumulation of karmic deposits (*karmāśaya*). (PYŚ 1.5)[133]

In the way that *āśraya* in the *Abhidharmakośabhāṣya* indicates the latent ontological basis of mind (*citta*) that gives rise to affliction, *āśaya* in the *Pātañjalayogaśāstra* is used to indicate the substratum of mind (*citta*) in which the latent form of affliction dwells and thus the seed of future action. In this respect, Patañjali's text seems to be in dialogue with a proto-Yogācāra notion of *āśraya*[134] that had already been put forward in the *Saṃdhinirmocanasūtra* (third century CE) as the storehouse consciousness (*ālayavijñāna*).[135] Additionally, like the Sautrāntikas, the *Pātañjalayogaśāstra* posits the complete destruction of the substratum as necessary for liberation:

> From attaining that (cloud of dharma), the afflictions of nescience, etc. are cut by root and branch and the karmic deposits, good and bad, are destroyed utterly. (PYŚ 4.30)[136]

It is not only *āśaya* that is discussed in the *Pātañjalayogaśāstra* but also *āśraya*, which denotes 'basis' in relation to the karmic trace (*vāsanā*). *Vāsanā* is a 'subtle effect', 'trace' or 'perfuming' within the substratum and is also a key term in the *Pātañjalayogaśāstra*, particularly in its fourth chapter:[137]

> On the other hand, a mind with its activity is the substratum (*āśraya*) of traces (*vāsanās*). For in a mind whose activity has come to an end, the traces, having no basis [*nirāśraya*], cannot remain. (PYŚ 4.11)[138]

Again, this reinforces that, in concord with the Sautrāntikas, Pātañjala yoga entails the elimination of the basis (*āśraya*).[139] While the *Abhidharmakośabhāṣya* focuses on the seed (*bīja*) and its power (*sāmarthya*) to account for karma, the predominant images of the *Yogācārabhūmiśāstra* are the basis (*āśraya*)[140] and the trace (*vāsanā*) (Park 2014: 377).[141] Thus Patañjali's discourse appears to be aware not only of the core seed metaphor of the *Abhidharmakośabhāṣya* but also of the predominant trace (*vāsanā*) metaphor of the *Yogācārabhūmiśāstra*[142] and with the *anuśaya-āśaya-āśraya* semantic continuum of both Buddhist texts.[143]

Divergent Jain metaphors: Resin, ladder, door

The metaphorical overlaps of the Sautrāntika and yoga discourses are not merely generic but, rather, are specific. To underline this point, it is worth highlighting that in the same period the Jains employ a different metaphoric treatment of the *kleśa*s in relation to liberation. Patañjali and the Sautrāntikas envisaged the afflictions as functioning like seeds that grow, but Umasvāti's *Tattvārthasūtra*, a *c.* fifth-century treatise on Jain soteriology, also has a theory of the 'passions' (*kaṣāya*). In classical Jainism, there are four varieties of *kaṣāya*: anger, pride, deceit and greed (*krodha*, *māna*, *māyā* and *lobha*, TvS 8.10) (Zyndenbos 1983: 14) – closely mirroring the primary faults (*doṣa*s) and afflictions (*kleśa*s) of Brahmanic yoga and Buddhism. *Kaṣāya* is usually translated by Jain scholars as the 'passions', but it literally means 'resin'. Thus, the source domain of the Jain passions is not that of 'seed in a field' but rather of a sticky plant resin that entraps.[144] Zyndenbos elucidates that the term *kaṣāya* is utilized metaphorically to mean 'that by which karma is stuck to the soul' (Zyndenbos 1983: 15). *Kaṣāya* is primarily associated with delusion (*moha*), which is a kind of 'master-karma' that binds other karmas (Zyndenbos 1983: 15).[145] One is reminded here of the 'master role' of nescience (*avidyā*) in Pātañjala yoga and Buddhism as the field (*kṣetra*) of all others. The *kaṣāya* combines with 'yoga' (the attracting capacity of the soul) to produce karmic influxes (*āsrava*), and these produce a state of spiritual bondage (*saṃsāra*) (Zyndenbos 1983: 15). This metaphorical mapping of the domain of 'resin' and its quality of 'stickiness' to explain the workings of the passions is quite different to the seed domain that we have examined.

In relation to *dhyāna*, the Jain theory of liberation also contains metaphors of vision and ascendancy via a ladder. There are obscuring actions (*āvaraṇīya-karmans*) that are associated with the sense organs, and which are explained as factors that obstruct the vision and progress of meditation (*dhyāna*). The Jain canon[146] classifies *dhyāna* itself as a ladder to liberation: there are four types (*ārta*, *raudra*, *dharma* and *śukla*), which are each further divided into four to create sixteen steps.[147] The twelfth step of the stages of virtue (*guṇa-sthāna*) on this 'ladder' is the destruction of the passions (*kṣīna-kaṣāya*).[148] Beyond the *kaśaya*s, there are other metaphors of liberation in Jainism such as liberation as a doorway. This image is found in the *Aṇuogaddārāiṃ*, a Prakrit text from *c.* fourth century CE, which conceptualizes liberation as attained by scriptural knowledge (*śrūtajñāna*) (Petrocchi 2016: 236). As the title of the work indicates, its purpose is to elucidate the doors of investigation (*aṇuyoga* in Sanskrit) (Petrocchi 2016: 237).[149] This metaphor of liberation – going through a door that takes you to a better place – is one that we do not, for example, encounter in our yoga schemes and is much less prominent in Buddhist soteriology.[150] The divergence of Jain soteriological metaphors in this period strengthens the argument of proximal development between Pātañjala yoga and Sautrāntika.

Overall, the Sautrāntika and the Pātañjala discourses of liberation share the following structural components:

1. a disjunction of mind (*citta*) from the afflictions (*kleśa*s),
2. cessation due to analysis/discriminative reflection (*pratisaṃkhyā* or *prasaṃkhyāna*),
3. cessation of the latent form of affliction (i.e. the dormant seed),
4. the transformative function of and eventual abandonment of wisdom (*prajñā*),
5. the permanence of disjunction and cessation from the afflictions,
6. the disappearance of the mental basis/substratum when the afflictions are eliminated,
7. the centrality of the image of the seed, and its power, to understanding *kleśa* and *karma* and
8. access to an unconditioned and liberated state (*nirvāṇa* or *kaivalya*).

In particular, the metaphor of the seed rests on the mapping of a specific set of key technical qualities from the domain of agriculture, which I have argued pertain to rice cultivation specifically (see Chapter 1):

1. *kleśa*s are self-germinating (self-propelling) and so contain their own seeds,
2. dormant seeds, which are *kleśa*s in latent form, are dangerous,
3. the way to eliminate the seed is to destroy its potential by scorching it.[151]

It would, of course, be reductive to claim that the soteriological systems presented in the *Abhidharmakośabhāṣya* and the *Pātañjalayogaśāstra* are identical because, clearly, they are not. There are profound differences in the philosophy and orientation of the two texts.[152] Neither am I claiming to be able to identify a definitive direction of influence in the dialogic resonance, although my suggestion is that Patañjali's text is reflecting the Sautrāntika discourse. The redactor Patañjali was, it seems, deeply engaged with the notion of destruction of the *kleśa*s (*kleśanirodha*) via analysis, a distinctly Buddhist approach to liberation. We should be in no doubt as to the unique elaboration of the role of *kleśas* within Buddhist Abhidharma soteriology and of *kleśabīja* in Sautrāntika thought.[153] In comparison, there is no such developed theory of *kleśa* and its seed in the classical Brahmanical sources on yoga.

It is thus time to shine a spotlight on Patañjali's path of *kriyā yoga* with its theory of *kleśabīja* – which has been overshadowed historically by disproportionate scholarly, religious and popular emphasis on the *aṣṭāṅga* path structure – and to highlight *kriyā yoga*'s[154] centrality to liberation as well as its integral relationship to Buddhist discourse.

Conclusions

As this chapter has illustrated, within a dialogic context of soteriology, conceptual metaphor was more easily transferable between traditions than doctrine. In one sense, metaphors were used to 'smuggle' in doctrines and philosophical positions from other schools. The intertextual examples that I have examined between the *Pātañjalayogaśāstra* and the *Abhidharmakośabhāṣya* demonstrate that the majority of the technical discussions of the seed of affliction take place in Patañjali's second chapter (*pāda*), leading to the conclusion that this portion of the text has a particular basis for interaction with the Sarvāstivāda and Sautrāntika sphere. My suggestion is that the early section of Patañjali's second *pāda* (dealing with *kriyā yoga*) was either an independent text incorporated into the *Pātañjalayogaśāstra* or exists as a specific point-by-point response to a Buddhist orator such as Vasubandhu or to a text such as his *Abhidharmakośabhāṣya*.

In shifting the focus to a *discourse* labelled 'classical yoga' we must view beyond doctrines and texts to wider conceptual and metaphoric frames (often interlocking intricately). A practice does not have to be explicitly labelled 'yoga' for it to share the same discourse or episteme as the *Pātañjalayogaśāstra*. In exploring the discourse of 'classical yoga', it is useful to think about soteriological path structures rather than an overall 'entity' called yoga; this can aid us in identifying subtle but structural interconnections between distinct religious traditions. This chapter has presented a few examples of the many shared metaphors and paradigms in the *Pātañjalayogaśāstra* and the *Abhidharmakośabhāṣya*. The *Abhidharmakośabhāṣya* presents a soteriology that it does *not* call yoga and the *Pātañjalayogaśāstra* presents a discursively similar soteriology that it *does* call yoga. Next, I will examine how these two texts share an overlapping discourse with the *Yogācārabhūmiśāstra*.

3

The 'other' yoga *śāstra*: The *Yogācārabhūmiśāstra*

Introduction

This chapter argues that since the *Pātañjalayogaśāstra* and Asaṅga's *Yogācārabhūmiśāstra* have their final redaction *c.* the fourth century CE and are self-labelled *śāstra*s (treatises) about yoga, we have two 'classical' *yogaśāstra*s. Furthermore, historical contextualization shows that the earliest layers of the *Yogācārabhūmiśāstra* most likely predate the *Pātañjalayogaśāstra* and contain systematized accounts of yogācāra (yoga discipline). Therefore, we can study detailed, non-Brahmanical accounts of yoga that precede Pātañjala yoga.

By tracing the historical textual formation of the *Yogācārabhūmiśāstra*, we can consider what was meant by the label 'yogācāra' in its earliest context. Scholars now draw a distinction between yogācāra (early and ascetic) and Yogācāra (later and systematized philosophy). Deleanu, for example, differentiates between the early stages of yogācāra around the beginning of the Common Era, in which ideas and practices were emerging, and a later philosophical school of Yogācāra which by the time of the fifth to sixth century was formalized around a set of doctrines (Deleanu 2006).[1] In the fourth to fifth centuries, then,

> there is strong reason to doubt that the term 'Yogācāra' had its later, doxographic meaning – referring to a particular philosophical school. (Gold 2015: 3)

As Lusthaus points out, most of the distinctively Yogācāra ideas had already appeared in the *Saṃdhinirmocanasūtra* (discussed below) around a century before Asaṅga and Vasubandhu lived. He concludes that the standard claim that the two brothers are the founders of Yogācāra is a 'fictitious' one (Lusthaus 2002: 7). Although the *Yogācārabhūmiśāstra* has been categorized as a quintessentially Mahāyāna text, the majority of the content of the *Yogācārabhūmiśāstra* is, in fact, Śrāvakayāna with nascent strands of Mahāyāna (Deleanu 2006; Kragh 2013a).

By drawing on contemporary research in Buddhist studies, we can map out a richer and more granular picture of yoga discipline in the early Common Era that extends beyond the *Pātañjalayogaśāstra*.

Historical textual formation of the *Yogācārabhūmiśāstra*

The *Yogācārabhūmiśāstra* is a complex text, both in its constitution and in its formation. By establishing a chronology for this text in relation to the *Pātañjalayogaśāstra*, it can be argued that Patañjali may have been aware of the prior textual tradition of yogācāra.

Structure of the *Yogācārabhūmiśāstra*

The *Yogācārabhūmiśāstra* consists of two parts (see Appendix 3): 'The Basic Section' (*Maulī Bhūmi*) and the 'The Supplementary Section' (*Saṃgrahaṇī*).[2] The 'The Basic Section' contains fourteen 'books' that describe seventeen stages/foundations (*bhūmis*) of yoga discipline (*yogācāra*). Each book is divided into sections titled 'topic of yoga' (*yogasthāna*).[3] 'The Supplementary Section' contains four parts that comment on the books, as well as on other topics, and includes an independent work called the *Saṃdhinirmocanasūtra*. One of the four sections of the *Saṃgrahaṇī*, the *Viniścayasaṃgrahaṇī*, contains additional materials on the books of 'The Basic Section.[4] The three further supplementary sections are the *Vastusaṃgrahaṇī* (which explains the content of the Tripiṭaka), the *Paryāyasaṃgrahaṇī* (which classifies and explains synonyms found in the Buddhist *sūtras*) and the *Vivaraṇasaṃgrahaṇī* (which describes the principles for interpreting scripture). 'The Basic Section' is partially extant in Sanskrit, while the majority of 'The Supplementary Section' is extant only in Chinese and Tibetan.

Dating of the *Yogācārabhūmiśāstra*

The dating of the *Yogācārabhūmiśāstra* is not straightforward, given that the text is so extensive. As a treatise, or *śāstra*, it typically collates different units of knowledge into a coherent whole. The prevailing view now among scholars is that the *Yogācārabhūmiśāstra* was compiled over a substantial period of time. The organization of the material and the absence of a self-conscious frame or map that lays out the contents is 'evidence that the work was not compiled on the basis of a unitary plan but grew gradually from separate textual units and materials' (Deleanu 2006: 155).[5] Most scholars date the final redaction of the *Yogācārabhūmiśāstra* to the fourth century CE (e.g. Kragh 2013b: 26).[6] This locates the final text to approximately the same period as the *Pātañjalayogaśāstra*, which Maas dates between 325 and 425 CE (Maas 2013) – and he has recently suggested that *c.* 400 CE might be the more likely date in that range (Maas 2018). Yet parts of the *Yogācārabhūmiśāstra* most likely predate the *Pātañjalayogaśāstra*. The earliest two layers of the *Yogācārabhūmiśāstra* are the books titled *Śrāvakabhūmi* and *Bodhisattvabhūmi*,[7] which are from the third century CE if not before,[8] while another early layer is the *Saṃdhinirmocanasūtra*.[9] Given that the *Śrāvakabhūmi* and the *Bodhisattvabhūmi* present systems of yoga discipline, I argue that the earlier systematization of yoga discipline appears not in the *Pātañjalayogaśāstra* but in the *Yogācārabhūmiśāstra*.[10] In this discussion of what comprises a 'system' of yoga discipline, I am not addressing the early proto-systems such as those we see in the *Bhagavad Gītā*, the *Sānti Pārvan* and parts of the *Upaniṣads*, since those have been discussed extensively. Rather, I am defining a 'system' as labelled stages of practice arranged into a coherent whole that offers a discrete and sequential path structure to liberation. In the Brahmanic sources, this would include the six-auxiliary yoga or *ṣaḍaṅga yoga*[11] of the *Maitrī Upaniṣad* (MU 6.18), generally dated to the start of the Common Era. However, this *ṣaḍaṅga* system – although an important template for Patañjali's later *aṣṭāṅga yoga* – contains only a skeletal frame without any details. As we will see, the early layers of the *Yogācārabhūmiśāstra* contain systems of yoga discipline that are expounded in considerable detail.

The proto-layers of the *Yogācārabhūmi*

In tracing the early development of the *Yogācārabhūmiśāstra*, we encounter two meditation treatises that are extant only in Chinese but which appear to have been translated from, or modelled on, a Sanskrit work called the **Yogācārabhūmi*.[12] This work, now lost, is thought to have been an early forerunner of the *Yogācārabhūmiśāstra*. Scholars refer to it as **Yogācārabhūmi* to distinguish it from the later and much longer śāstric redaction of the fourth century.[13] In fact, if the **Yogācārabhūmi* can be said to contain an earlier part of the *Yogācārabhūmiśāstra*, it relates to the two books that I have highlighted: the *Śrāvakabhūmi* and the *Bodhisattvabhūmi*.

The two Chinese meditation manuals that were based on a work called the **Yogācārabhūmi* are the *Xiuxing dao di jing* (*Yogācārabhūmi* of Saṅgharakṣa)[14] and the *Damoduoluo chan jing* (*The Meditation* (dhyāna) *Scripture [Taught] by Dharmatrāta)* (Demiéville 1951).[15] The earliest of these two works, the *Xiuxing dao di jing*, is based on the work of Saṅgharakṣa, a Sarvāstivādin patriarch who lived around the end of the first and the beginning of the second centuries CE (Demiéville 1951: 343–7; Deleanu 2006: 157) and appears to contain one of the earliest instances of the term *yogācāra* (Deleanu 2006: 195). An Shigao partly translated this text into Chinese in the second century (*Dao di jing*), and Dharmarakṣa made a fuller Chinese translation in 284 CE (*Xiuxing dao di jing*).[16] This meditation treatise is a Sarvāstivādin text, which contains 'a Mahāyānist fragment' that 'appears to be an appendix added to the original text of the **Yogācārabhūmi* in China' (Deleanu 2006: 157). The other meditation treatise, the later *Damoduoluo chan jing*, was authored by the Sarvāstivādin Buddhasena (but based on the teachings of Dharmatrāta),[17] who is usually described in Chinese sources as 'one of the most famous Buddhist meditation masters active in Kashmir around the end of the 4th and beginning of the 5th century' (Deleanu 2006: 158).[18] Buddhasena's treatise was translated into Chinese by Buddhasena's disciple, Buddhabhadra, in 413 CE, as the *Damoduoluo chan jing*. The existence of these two texts (*Xiuxing dao di jing* and *Damoduoluo chan jing*), each containing an early prototype layer of the *Yogācārabhūmiśāstra*, demonstrates that a tradition of Buddhist meditation called yogācāra had been established in South Asia by the early second century CE.

In this early period, the proto-*Yogācārabhūmi* (**Yogācārabhūmi*) was not the only text that was outlining systems of yogācara. The content of the *Damoduoluo chan jing* partly correlates with that of the *Saddharmasmṛtyupasthānasūtra* (*Saddhsu*), a *c.* second to fourth century CE yogācāra meditation treatise that was a Sarvāstivāda text with Mahāyāna leanings (Stuart 2015, 1: 264).[19] As Stuart sees it, the *Damoduoluo chan jing* partly draws on the material preserved in the *Saddhsu*. The *Damoduoluo* contains references to the fulfilment of the *bhūmi*s in conjunction with the ten levels of meditative practice, which can be connected to texts such as the *Daśabhūmikasūtra* or the *Mahāvastu* (Stuart 2015, 1: 265).[20] Furthermore, Saṅghabhadra transmitted to China the legends of four early Kashmiri yoga practitioners, Sarvāstivādin masters who lived between the first and third centuries CE – Vasumitra, Maitreyaśrī, Saṅgharakṣa and Dharmatrāta.[21] Besides the two Chinese yogācāra meditation treatises, these other transmissions illustrate that a strand of soteriological thought called yogācāra was established in Indian Buddhism by the second century. Therefore, systematized yogācāra meditation treatises were in circulation up to two centuries before the final redaction of the *Pātañjalayogaśāstra* in the fourth century. As Deleanu puts it,

> since Saṅgharakṣa appears to have been active around the end of the 1st century and the beginning of the 2nd century ... and his **Yogācārabhūmi* (compiled ca. 100) reflects an already developed stage in the codification of the yogic theory and practice, it would seem that the ascetic tradition crystallised in this work had already existed for at least one century. It is not excluded, however, that the roots of the Sarvastivādin yogic tradition might go even further back in time. (Deleanu 2006: 243 fn. 261)

Therefore, it is reasonable to assert that Patañjali may have been aware of a prior text or tradition of meditation called yogācāra. Furthermore, given that the *Pātañjalayogaśāstra* appears to textually revise certain passages from the *Abhidharmakośabhāṣya* (as I discussed in Chapter 2) and that the *Abhidharmakośabhāṣya* revises passages from the *Yogācārabhūmiśāstra*,[22] Patañjali may also have been aware of the *Yogācārabhūmiśāstra*. Moreover, as the **Yogācārabhūmi* was composed in Sarvāstivādin circles, this suggests a line of Sarvāstivādin influence that is shared between the *Yogācārabhūmiśāstra*, the *Abhidharmakośabhāṣya* and the *Pātañjalayogaśāstra* in relation to yogic soteriology.

Early yogācāra

In this section, I assert that yogācāra is not simply a generic term for any or all spiritual practice in Buddhism but pertains to a specific identity and set of techniques. I then highlight the relationship between Sarvāstivāda Abhidharma and yogācāra. Finally, I consider what we know about the technical details of the discipline of yogācāra.

What does yogācāra mean?

The nuanced meaning of the term *yogācāra* is still under debate. In contrast to the later doxographical use of Yogācāra to refer to a philosophical school, the early uses of this term are more shadowy. The key questions in the debate are whether the term is generic, whether it can be associated with any specific concepts of 'yoga' and whether it refers to 'practice' or 'practitioner'. While Silk argued that yogācāra was a generic word for spiritual practice (Silk 2000: 303), there is a growing consensus that yogācāra had a more specific meaning. It is, of course, possible to acknowledge that some connotations of yogācāra were not fixed without resorting to the extreme position that the term meant nothing in particular. Buescher underscores this point:

> At some time, the notion of yogācāra referred very generally to anyone practicing any stage of a non-visionary path; later, in a different context, it designated an expert in visualization techniques; at one place it is restricted to refer to a Śrāvakayāna monk; in another milieu, a *yogācāra* is *the* bodhisattva per se, etc. (Buescher 2008: 13 fn. 3)

For Davidson the earliest meaning of yogācāra was, quite simply, 'yogin' (Davidson 1985: 127). Kragh follows this line of reasoning: depending on context, *yogācāra* means '*yoga* practitioner' and secondarily means '*yoga* practice' (Kragh 2013b: 30). He even goes so far as to define the fourth-century usage of the term in the *Yogācārabhūmiśāstra* as 'School of Yoga Practitioners' (Kragh 2013b: 23). For Deleanu, 'yoga' in the compound yogācāra carries not just the generic meaning of 'application' or 'purpose' but reflects that the *Yogācārabhūmiśāstra* was closely connected to a 'yogic milieu' which denoted Buddhist groups that practised specialist spiritual cultivation (Deleanu 2006, 1: 158–9). In the *Saddharmasmṛtyupasthānasūtra* (*Saddhsu*), the narrative framing of the text[23] means that the *sūtra* 'can be read as a text detailing the making of a yogācāra' (Stuart 2015, 1: 109). In the *Saddhsu*, yogācāra communities referred to themselves as having a practice of 'yoga': a yogācāra monk is described as *yogam āsthitaḥ*, established in the practice of yoga (*Saddhsu* 7.12.7; trans. Stuart 2015, 1: 176).[24]

Stuart traces the evolution of 'the common term yogācāra … as a Sanskritized form of the canonical Middle Indic term yoggācariya' (Stuart 2015, 1: 227). In the Pāli canon the term *yoggācariya*[25] denoted animal trainer or horse charioteer (Stuart 2015, 1; 229), a familiar image that we have also encountered in the Brahmanic literature (discussed in Chapter 1). Although in the early Pāli canon the use of *yoggācariya* seems to be 'a master of training' (Stuart 2015, 1: 232), the term comes to mean not just practitioner of yoga but also master of yoga.[26] Rejecting Silk's assessment of yogācāra as a generic term, Stuart posits that the *Saddhsu* demonstrates the use of the term yogācāra, 'in a precise way, to refer to a specific type of meditation practitioner, with a specific set of practices and a mastery of karma' (Stuart 2015, 1: 226). Given that the ideal subject of the *Saddhsu* is a yogācāra, the identification of this subject as a yogin reinforces the connection between the two terms:[27]

> He who, not taken up with unwholesome action,
> constantly delights in wholesome action,

> is one who delights in purity, [which is like the cool] rays of the moon.
> Such a person is a practitioner [*yogī*].[28]
> (trans. Stuart 2015, 1: 377)

This book assumes a working definition of yogācāra as 'one who practises a discipline of yoga'. *Yogācāra* in the *Yogācārabhūmiśāstra*, then, appears to have been a general appellation for Buddhist practitioners of yoga in the way that yogin was a general label for those practising in Brahmanic circles. Deleanu, for one, wants to keep the terms yogin and yogācāra separate and proposes that yogin should denote a Brahmanic yogin and yogācāra a Buddhist ascetic (Deleanu 2006: 35 fn. 4). In the interest of clarity and consistency, I will follow this convention.[29]

Sarvāstivāda yogācāra

The **Yogācārabhūmi* was first composed in Śrāvakayāna[30] circles, specifically Sarvāstivāda,[31] even though the *Yogācārabhūmiśāstra* was later designated as part of Mahāyāna tradition.[32] Centuries before Yogācāra was identified as a distinct approach of philosophy (in the fifth to sixth centuries), there were already yogācāra communities in the Sarvāstivāda Abhidharma stream of Śrāvakayāna Buddhism. Deleanu argues that the early yogācāra scribes of the *Śrāvakabhūmi* were straightforward adherents of Sarvāstivāda doctrines (Deleanu 2006: 169). Indeed, the very title of the *Śrāvakabhūmi* reflects its Śrāvakayāna affiliation. It is evident, then, that yogācāra, as a strand of Buddhist meditative practice, emerged within the Sarvāstivāda tradition.

> Already in the 1st century CE, a tradition of Sarvāstivāda *yogācāras*, with its own theoretical and praxis-related peculiarities, commences to be active in the production of meditation treatises and manuals. (Deleanu 2006: 161–2)[33]

Yamabe also supports this argument, noting that the close connections between the **Yogācārabhūmi* of Saṅgharakṣa (*Xiuxing dao di jing*), An Shigao's *Dao di jing* and Asaṅga's *Yogācārabhūmiśāstra* suggest that '*yogācāra* meditators were forming their own, somewhat distinct circle within the general Sarvāstivāda community' (Yamabe 2013: 601). Later on, these Sarvāstivāda yogācāras became influenced by the *bodhisattva* path or the *Saṃdhinirmocanasūtra* (Deleanu 2006: 170).[34] Although yogācāra communities emerged within Sarvāstivāda, an enhanced focus on yoga discipline became a key marker by which Mahāyāna sought to distinguish itself from Śrāvakayāna Buddhism (Kragh 2013b: 25).

In summary, it is an overstatement to characterize the *Yogācārabhūmiśāstra* as a Mahāyāna text. Early yogācāra practice was liminal, existing at the threshold of Śrāvakayāna and Mahāyāna.[35] The fourth-century *Yogācārabhūmiśāstra* contains not just one model of yoga but rather at least two: one indebted to Sarvāstivāda Abhidharma scholasticism and one intent on forging an innovated and applied concept of yoga discipline, yogācāra. This characterization of yogācāra as partly Sarvāstivādin in origin is relevant to our consideration of the *Pātañjalayogaśāstra*. As I argued in Chapter 2, there are overlaps and interactions between the *Pātañjalayogaśāstra* and the Sarvāstivādin *Abhidharmakośabhāṣya*. All this points to a strong role for the Sarvāstivāda school of Śrāvakayāna Buddhism in the formation of early yoga. To put it another way, we might argue that at least some of the roots of 'classical yoga' are firmly planted in the Sarvāstivāda tradition and its inherently scholastic and doctrinal character.

Early yogācāra was affiliated with the north-west region of India, and the legendary yogācāra masters are described as hailing from Kashmir (Demiéville 1951: 364–6). Given the association of early yogācāra with Sarvāstivāda thought, this is no surprise; the Kashmir Valley also formed the central region for the Sarvāstivāda-Vaibhāṣika tradition that produced the *Abhidharmakośabhāṣya* (Buescher 2008: 11 fn. 3).[36] Indeed, the second-century *Abhidharmamahāvibhāṣaśāstra* refers to Sarvāstivāda meditation practitioners[37] – yogācāra or yogācārya – on some 140 occasions (Deleanu 2006: 213 fn. 61).[38]

> Though not a school apart, the *yogācāras* seem to have constituted a distinct group or groups, and the scholastic masters (*vaibhāṣika*) usually mention their views with much respect. (Deleanu 2006: 158)

Furthermore, in terms of the emergence of Mahāyāna, Demiéville argues that there were yogācāra Maitreya cults in the north-west region in the early centuries of the Common Era (Demiéville 1951). Of course, we must be prepared to think beyond an exclusive association with the north-west because the *Abhidharmamahāvibhāṣaśāstra* also mentions 'Northern yogācāras', 'Southern yogācāras' and 'yogācāras everywhere'.[39] Deleanu's assessment is that these regional groups were not doctrinally different, but rather 'the difference between these groups refers to a gloss of a linguistic nature' (Deleanu 2006: 213 fn. 62). Generally, however, we can assert that Kashmiri Sarvāstivāda yogācāras played a major role in the formation of the early *Śrāvakabhūmi* and *Bodhisattvabhūmi* and that early yogācāra developed in the north-west.

What was early yogācāra practice?

We have established that early yogācāras were adherents of the Sarvāstivāda tradition. Let us now try to understand who they might have been and what they practised. What did the 'yoga discipline' in the *Yogācārabhūmiśāstra* entail?

Yogācāra primarily denoted systems of meditation. This is evident in the general yogācāra literature of the period and specifically in the *Yogācārabhūmiśāstra*. In his translation of the *Saddharmasmṛtyupasthānasūtra* (*Saddhsu)*, a Sarvāstivāda meditation sūtra, Stuart renders yogācāra as not only 'meditation practitioner' (Stuart 2015, 1: 6) but more specifically 'master of yoga' (Stuart 2015, 1: 37). Yogācāra denoted 'a master practitioner whose spiritual presence can be interpreted as an instantiation of the power of the Buddha in the world' (Stuart 2015, 1: 30–1). In the *Saddhsu*, yogācāra is a meditative practice of discernment (*prajñā*), specifically in relation to the laws of karma, with one gaining a level of omniscience comparable to the Buddha's (Stuart 2015, 1: 227). Furthermore, the yogācāras are depicted as a unique group with elevated status: not only does the Buddha state that he does not see anyone other than his yogācāra disciples (*yogācāo macchrāvakaḥ*) (Stuart 2015, 1: 61), but the Buddha himself was originally a part of this community (Stuart 2015, 1: 235). Buescher proposes that there was a distinctive visionary quality to the practices called yogācāra that developed in north-west India (greater Kashmir, Gandhara, Afghanistan, Gilgit) (Buescher 2008). This point was also previously made by Schlingloff, who provided a summary of the visionary experiences of the yogācāras described in the 'Kyzyl Yoga Fragment'. Found in Central Asia and dated to *c.* fifth century CE,[40] this text may originally have come from Kashmir (Schlinghoff 1964: 28–56). It describes visual meditative exercises related to the four elements (*dhātu-prayoga*), repulsion towards the physical (*aśubha-prayoga*), the aggregates (*skandhaparīkṣā*), aspects of the dependent co-arising model (*pratītyasamutpāda*), the four immeasurables (*apramāṇās*), as well as contemplations (*anusmṛti*) of the Buddha, the dharma and so on.[41]

The *Yogācārabhūmiśāstra* refers to the existence of exclusive communities of yogācāras who were not just ordinary meditation practitioners but rather an advanced or elite class of 'rigorous meditators, whose commitment to *yoga* practice was extraordinary and incessant' (Kragh 2013: 31).[42] At the outset of the **Yogācārabhūmi* of Saṅgharakṣa (first to second century CE), we are provided with definitions of both *yogācāra* and *yogācārabhūmi*:

> Definition of *yogācāra*: the practice of cultivation and the exercises.
>
> Definition of *yogācārabhūmi*: one who is practicing the practice, this is the ground of practising. (SYCB 182 b29–182c14)[43]

Here we have an instance in which yogācāra refers not to a practitioner but to the practice itself. Specifically, the **Yogācārabhūmi* of Saṅgharakṣa supports these definitions with two prescriptions of what one should refrain from (anger, lust, etc.) and what one should cultivate (kindness, chastity, etc.). In practice, there are two steps of meditation: tranquillity (*śamatha*) is contemplation of impurity (*aśubha*) and controlled breathing techniques, and insight (*vipaśyana*) is contemplation of emptiness (Demiéville 1951: 399).

In terms of lifestyle, many yogācāras were ordained.[44] Yogācāra often appears in the phrase '*yogācāra bhikṣu*', which Kragh translates as 'yoga practitioner monk'. This suggests not only that many such meditation adepts were ordained but also that the intended audience of the *Yogācārabhūmiśāstra* were monks and nuns who formed 'a circle of meditation savants' (Kragh 2013b: 31). Kragh asserts that the monastic component of the yogācāra's identity may in fact be a central feature in the *Yogācārabhūmiśāstra*, irrespective of whether yogācāras in the earlier periods were so inclined (Kragh 2013b: 31).

The section on general meditative objects in the *Śrāvakabhūmi* ends by explaining how a monk who is a yoga practitioner should practise the next set of foci. He is referred to using the common epithet '*bhikṣur yogī yogācāraḥ*', a label that combines three states of monk, yogin and practitioner of yoga. Buescher points out that *bhikṣur yogī yogācāraḥ* is a 'standing phrase' in works such as the *Revatasūtra*, which is quoted in the *Śrāvakabhūmi* (Buescher 2008: 11).[45] All three nouns appear in the nominative case and are apposite, indicating that *bhikṣu*, *yogin* and *yogācāra* were three distinct categories. Silk suggests that, in this phrase, *yogin* is a synonym for *yogācāra bhikṣu* (Silk 2000: 302–3). However, I concur with Stuart, who plausibly translates the phrase as 'meditator monk, a yoga practitioner' (Stuart 2015, 1: 281). We can suggest that a *bhikṣur yogī* was a gloss for *yogācāra*. Thus, a yogācāra was conventionally a monk-yogin.

There are competing theories as to how Mahāyāna ideology arose within Buddhism. One disputed argument is that Mahāyāna emerged as an orthodox response among ascetic forest monks to restore what they saw as a purer form of Buddhism.[46] This locates the roots of Mahāyāna yoga in forest-dwelling monastic asceticism. Whatever the outcome of the larger debates regarding Mahāyāna, the meditation manuals depict the yogācāra as a forest-dweller – which refers to any isolated place, not necessarily a forest as such (Harrison 2003; Stuart 2015, 1: 227).

This feature of isolation is a basic condition of asceticism. The **Yogācārabhūmi* of Saṅgharakṣa describes the yogācāra as engaging in solitary meditation in his hermitage under a tree (SYCB 24. 219a-b; Demiéville 1951: 419) and, in another chapter, in his hermitage or in an isolated place (SYCB 7.190, 12-16c; Demiéville 1951: 401). In its account of the practice of cultivation (*bhāvanā*), the *Bhāvanāmayī Bhūmiḥ* explains how adverse conditions arise in different types of practitioners: householders (*āgārika*), renunciants or ordained persons (*pravrajita*) and those who have entered into solitude to practise yoga.[47] This very statement implies that yoga is not practised by a householder, a renunciate or a monastic – but that yoga discipline is reserved for a different or special class of practitioner, one who operates in solitude. The *Bhāvanāmayī Bhūmiḥ* also describes how the yogācāra enters deep seclusion with tranquility practices and attains mastery through devotion to ascetic austerity. These higher stages of isolated ascetic austerity indicate that the most advanced levels of yogācāra were uniquely demanding and not conducive to the social life of the householder or even a monk in a monastery. The *Śrāvakabhūmi* extols the *arhat* Revata (ŚBh 2.8b.4–5c; Wayman 1960: 86), who was declared by the Buddha to be 'foremost among the forest-dwellers' (*araññakānaṃ*) (*Aṅguttara Nikāya* i.24) and who delighted in solitude, sitting cross-legged (Malalasekera 1938 II: 753–4). The conditions for yoga discipline in the *Śrāvakabhūmi* are a state of retreat, isolation in a desolate place, sitting all day in seated posture, cultivating one-pointedness of mind (*cittaikāgratā*) and attaining *samādhi*, which is a stream of mind characterized by bliss whose focus is an object of constant mindfulness. Again, it is clear that this level of isolated meditation practice is not compatible with social living and relies on intensely continuous cultivation and an ascetic lifestyle in a remote setting. This point is underlined in the *Saddharmasmṛtyupasthānasūtra* in which a yogācāra is a forest-dwelling ascetic monk who practises sense control. However, asceticism in itself is not the goal but rather the lifestyle that facilitates the practice of pure meditation:

> He whose mind delights in
> abodes of groves and forests,
> or in beds of grass in the charnel ground,
> such a person is a [true] monk.
>
> (*Saddhsu* 5.2.12.9; trans. Stuart 2015, 1: 461)[48]

The opposite state of yogācāra meditation, here, is indolence (*kausīdya*), hinting at the role of austerity in this lifestyle:

Skillful in the practice of meditation,
far removed from indolence,
he who practices for the benefit of beings
is known as a forest monk.

(*Saddhsu* 5.2.12.17; trans. Stuart 2015, 1: 463)[49]

To sum up: another defining feature of yogācāra was isolated asceticism away from the daily activities and routines of the monastery setting.

In assessing the identity of the subject and audience of the *Yogācārabhūmiśāstra*, we must not overlook the frame of the text itself. Who produced the voluminous *Yogācārabhūmiśāstra* (now that we have put to one side the notion of a single author)? Hakamaya argues that the *Yogācārabhūmiśāstra* must have been compiled by monks who were scholars as well as meditators (Hakamaya 2013). Stuart depicts the yogācāras as a 'textual community' that was involved in the production and transmission of texts (Stuart 2015, 1: 227). Scholarly credentials would certainly have been required, given the erudite nature of the Sarvāstivāda content of much of the *Yogācārabhūmiśāstra*. Indeed, Kragh points out that the *Yogācārabhūmiśāstra* appropriated the authoritative prestige of the large Abhidharma treatises 'by imitating their literary guise' (Kragh 2013b: 46). Such learned scribes were perhaps one and the same as the forest meditators. In short, we should not assume that yogācāras were 'mere' practitioners of yoga, devoid of philosophical speculation. Deleanu asserts that, whenever necessary, yogācāras could become 'part-time Ābhidharmikas' to discuss their own doctrines (Deleanu 2006: 217 fn. 91).

The Sarvāstivāda *Abhidharmakośabhāṣya* also contains references to *pūrvayoga*, which is generally taken as referring to 'ancient yoga' (Hirakawa 1963: 241) and also to *pūrvacārya*s, the 'old masters'.[50] There has been much written on the identity of the *pūrvācārya*s and to the likelihood that some of the references are to yogācāras.[51] Deleanu posits that in the *Abhidharmakośabhāṣya* the *pūrvācārya*s, or 'masters of yore', refers specifically to the Sautrāntikas and that some positions attributed to the Sautrāntikas in the *Abhidharmakośabhāṣya* also appear in the *Yogācārabhūmiśāstra*. Indeed, there is a body of scholarship on the likely doctrinal influence of the Sautrāntikas on the philosophical orientation of the *Śrāvakabhūmi* (Deleanu 2006: 159). Nishi, for example, proposed that individual groups of yogācāras identified their philosophical views as belonging to Sautrāntika/Dārṣṭāntika (Nishi 1975). In his commentary on the *Abhidharmakośabhāṣya*, Yaśomitra (commenting on AKBh 3.15c) equates the two terms and refers to '*pūrvācāryā yogācārā āryāsaṅgaprabhṛtayaḥ*', which means '[the expression] "earlier masters" [refers to] the Yogācārās, starting with the noble Asaṅga and so forth' (trans. Skilling 2013: 773 fn. 3).[52]

The distinct, or perhaps elite, status of yogācāras as advanced practitioners may also point to initiation and secrecy. Arguing that the *Bodhisattvabhūmi* distinctly reworks Nāgārjuna's two truths for a new audience, Aramaki suggests that 'a bodhisattva yogācāra is an expert in the secrets of mind, conception, and consciousness' (Aramaki 2013: 420). Being an expert in 'supreme truth' allows the yogācāra to teach on the mundane or conventional truth of *citta*, *manas* and *vijñāna*. What qualifies the yogācāra to access supreme truth is initiation, which then enables him/her to teach to uninitiated *bodhisattvas* (Aramaki 2013: 421). Yogācāras were also granted special status due to their supernatural powers. A passage from the *Mahāvastu* warns bodhisattvas of being distracted on the path by yogācāras who constantly dwell in meditation (Senart 1882–97: 1.120). Stuart suggests that this association with supernatural powers was also a defining feature of early yogācāras and set them apart: 'certain folks were threatened by yogācāras precisely because they were practitioners with supernormal status' (Stuart 2015, 1: 304). This is evidenced by a passage from Buddhasena's *Yogācārabhūmi*:

> [From] one lofty state to another, he gradually controls the mind. Flying and transforming as he likes, unhindered, he is called a yogācāra due to the strength of his subtle and wondrous powers. (Bybh CBETA, T15, no. 618, p. 319a 25–7; cited in and trans. Stuart 2015, 1: 304)

Therefore, the elite ranking of yogācāras may have reflected not only their mastery of techniques, their privileged association with the Buddha and their learned status, but also the fact that some were initiated and were perceived to have supernatural capacities.

To sum up: the early yogācāras were conventionally monks, but they were not everyday monks. They appear to have been a distinct group of advanced practitioners who spent extended periods in meditation in austere conditions of isolated retreat. They were focused on cultivating wisdom (*prajñā*) and their meditative practices sometimes had a visionary quality. These yogācāras were also connected to a learned and philosophical community that recorded and systematized these practices of advanced meditation in texts, primarily reflecting Sarvāstivāda thought. They may have undergone special initiation and were perceived to hold secret teachings and to possess extraordinary powers. Finally, they appear to have been concentrated in the north-west regions, particularly Kashmir. Doctrine aside, in this profile of the yogācāra, the main distinguishing features from the yogin of Patañjali's *yogaśāstra* are that a yogācāra was a monastic and may have emphasized techniques of visualization. While Patañjali's yogin was a Brahmin (addressed as such in PYŚ 2.30–2.33), the other features of yogācāra identity (asceticism, isolation, scholasticism, mastery of meditation, possessing supernatural powers, residing in the northwest, etc.) can be regarded as shared aspects of ascetic identity.

Path systems of yogācāra in the *Yogācārabhūmiśāstra*

It is beyond the scope of this book to provide an in-depth analysis of the entirety of 'The Basic Section' (*Maulī Bhūmi*) or 'The Supplementary Section' (*Saṃgrahaṇī*) of the *Yogācārabhūmiśāstra*.[53] Rather this study engages selectively with three books of the *Yogācārabhūmiśāstra* that are available in Sanskrit and which discuss the topic of yoga in ways that prove most relevant for an intertextual analysis with the *Pātañjalayogaśāstra*. In particular, I focus on the earliest two books of the *Yogācārabhūmiśāstra*, the *Śrāvakabhūmi* and the *Bodhisattvabhūmi*, since their presentations of yogācāra most likely predate the *Pātañjalayogaśāstra*. Additionally, I consider the *Bhāvanāmayī Bhūmiḥ*, not only because of its intertextuality with the *Śrāvakabhūmi* but also because, as a manual on meditative cultivation, it details a precise and unique discipline that is pertinent to Pātañjala yoga. Lastly, I highlight aspects of the *Saṃdhinirmocanasūtra* (embedded in 'The Supplementary Section'), which also contains key discussions of yogācāra. Since each of these books or parts of the *Yogācārabhūmiśāstra* started out as an independent meditation treatise, each textual unit contains its own system of yogācāra, or yoga discipline.

Śrāvakabhūmi

The *Śrāvakabhūmi* is the second largest book in 'The Basic Section' (*Maulī Bhūmi*); only the *Bodhisattvabhūmi* is longer. Regarded as the oldest layer of the *Yogācārabhūmiśāstra* (Sugawara 2013: 847; von Rospatt 2013: 854), it is a key book in assessing the early formation of yogācāra. Versions of the *Śrāvakabhūmi* were in circulation independently before being incorporated into the *Yogācārabhūmiśāstra*.[54] The contents of the *Śrāvakabhūmi* and the *Bodhisattvabhūmi* are interlinked, with the latter generally thought to be dependent on the former. Along with the *Pratyekabuddhabhūmi* and the *Bodhisattvabhūmi*, the *Śrāvakabhūmi* forms one text in a sequential trio that describes the 'vehicles' of Buddhism. As we have noted, the *Yogācārabhūmiśāstra* is not a Mahāyāna text in the majority of its content, and so, contrary to expectation, the *śrāvaka* and *pratyekabuddha* paths of practice are given just as much space, context and importance as the distinctly Mahāyāna *bodhisattva* path, which is nonetheless the ideal path.[55] In these texts combined, then, we encounter a particular strand of yogic ascetic thought from the early centuries CE.

As the name suggests, the *Śrāvakabhūmi* is a work dedicated to the Śrāvakayāna spiritual path, and the ideal is the attainment of arhatship (in contrast to the *pratyekabuddha* or *bodhisattva* ideal). The *Śrāvakabhūmi* is a technical book that explains the requisites (*saṃbhāra*s) for practice in great detail. It contains two parallel paths, the mundane path (*laukika mārga*) and the supramundane path (*lokottara mārga*). The mundane path consists of eight attainments (*samāpatti*s), and the supramundane path is comprised of contemplation of the four noble truths and knowing them as they are in reality (*yathābhūtaṁ prajānāti*).[56]

The second *yogasthāna* opens with a series of questions about yogācāra:

> What is the instruction (*śikṣā*)? What are the natures consistent with the instruction? What is the breakdown of *yoga*? What are the *yoga*s? What is the mental orientation (*manaskāra*)? How many are the practitioners of yoga (*yogācāra*)? What is the business of yoga? What is the intense contemplation of yoga (*yogabhāvanā*)? What is the fruit of intense contemplation? (trans. Wayman 1960: 83)[57]

The *yogasthāna* then goes on to answer these questions in turn, providing technical definitions and an overall definition of yoga as consisting of four elements: (1) faith (*śraddhā*) (2) aspiration (*chandas*) (3) perseverance (*vīrya*) and (4) application of spiritual methods (*upāya*: *tatra yogaḥ katamaḥ / āha / caturvidho yogaḥ / tadyathā śraddhā chando vīrye upāyaś ca*) (Śbh 9B.7-7b; Wayman 1960: 92). It also describes three different kinds of yoga practitioners who make up the seven steps of the path of contemplation (*manaskāra*). The first is the beginner (*ādikarmiko yogācāraḥ*) who has not yet achieved one-pointedness and is practising the lowest level of contemplation, *manaskāra*. The second is the adept (*kṛtaparicaya*), who is more developed and practises the second to sixth levels of *manaskāra*. The third is one who has transcended *manaskāra* (*atikrāntamanaskāra*) and has reached the seventh level or fruit of the practice. The final goal of *śrāvaka* meditation is a twofold process: the old basis of existence ends (*āśrayanirodha*) and a transformed one replaces it (*āśrayaparivarta*). As I discussed in Chapter 2, this process of the destruction of the ontological substratum (*āśraya*) is also central to the process of mental liberation in the *Pātañjalayogaśāstra*.

Bodhisattvabhūmi

The *Bodhisattvabhūmi* (BoBh) is the culmination of the three books that deal with the types of practitioners from the three vehicles or *triyāna*: *śrāvaka*s, *pratyekabuddha*s and *bodhisattva*s (with the *bodhisattva* belonging to the Mahāyāna vehicle). Together with the *Śrāvakabhūmi*, this is one of the oldest parts of the *Yogācārabhūmiśāstra*, and it is the longest book. The goal of *yogācāra* for the *bodhisattva* is personal liberation while alive, in which one remains embodied in order to work tirelessly for the liberation of all sentient beings, achieved through teaching. This yoga is crystallized in the practising of the six perfections of generosity (*dāna*), moral conduct (*śīla*), patience (*kṣānti*), vigour (*vīrya*), meditation (*dhyāna*) and wisdom (*prajñā*).[58]

The *Bodhisattvabhūmi* contains a sevenfold path of stages (*bhūmi*s), which is offset against thirteen abodes (*vihāra*s) (Kragh 2013: 211–12). The seven *bhūmi*s are:

1. stage of innate potential (*gotrabhūmi*),
2. stage of firm conviction (*adhimuktacaryābhūmi*),
3. stage of superior aspiration (*śuddhādhyāśayabhūmi*),
4. stage of correct practice (*caryāprattipattibhūmi*),
5. stage of certainty (*niyatabhūmi*),
6. stage of determined practice (*niyatacaryābhūmi*) and
7. stage of arrival at the ultimate (*niṣṭhāgamanabhūmi*).

This progressive path is correlated to a better-known system of *bhūmi*s, the ten *bhūmi*s (*daśabhūmi*), which also appear in the *Daśabhūmikasūtra*. In this correlation, the seventh stage in the above path, *niṣṭhāgamanabhūmi*, is understood to correspond to the tenth stage of the *daśabhūmi*s, also called the stage of the cloud of dharma (*dharmameghabhūmi*), which represents the apex of attainment and enlightenment itself. However, scholars regard the two soteriological systems in the *Bodhisattvabhūmi* (the sevenfold *bhūmi*s and the tenfold *bhūmi*s) as independently co-evolved.

Bhāvanāmayī Bhūmiḥ

The *Bhāvanāmayī Bhūmiḥ* (BhāvBh) is book nine of the *Yogācārabhūmiśāstra*. Sections of the *Bhāvanāmayī Bhūmiḥ* are based on the content of the

Śrāvakabhūmiḥ and both books recount a path of seven stages of contemplation (*manaskāra*). The *Bhāvanāmayī Bhūmiḥ* may originally have been an independent work that was revised to fit in with the *Śrāvakabhūmi* and the *Bodhisattvabhūmi*, after being joined to them (Sugawara 2013: 849). Like the *Śrāvakabhūmi* (and most of the *Yogācārabhūmiśāstra*), the orientation of the *Bhāvanāmayī Bhūmiḥ* is Śrāvakayāna.[59] Whereas the *Śrāvakabhūmi* presents the seven stages of contemplation more doctrinally, the *Bhāvanāmayī Bhūmiḥ* is concerned with the practical details (von Rospatt 2013: 854). Within the structure of the *Yogācārabhūmiśāstra*, the *Bhāvanāmayī Bhūmiḥ* is grouped with two other books and occupies the last place in a threefold exposition: the *Śrutamayī Bhūmiḥ*, the *Cintāmayī Bhūmiḥ* and the *Bhāvanāmayī Bhūmiḥ*. Together, the three texts reflect a path structure of listening, reflecting and practice – representing a continuum from absorbing teachings to implementing them correctly.

As its title suggests, the *Bhāvanāmayī Bhūmiḥ* explains the foundation (*bhūmi*) of meditative cultivation (*bhāvanā*), which is defined as yoga.[60] The *Bhāvanāmayī Bhūmiḥ* foregrounds the obstacles to meditation and the appropriate counterstate (*pratipakṣa)* for each case. Yoga is defined as the cultivation of the counterstates to the obstacles (*pratipakṣabhāvanā*). The *Bhāvanāmayī Bhūmiḥ* presents four sequential stages of the cultivation of yoga (*yogabhāvanā*): the conditions for cultivating yoga (*yogabhāvanāpada*), the foundation for the cultivation of yoga (*yogabhāvanopaniṣat*), the cultivation of yoga (*yogabhāvanā*) and the result of cultivation (*bhāvanāphala*). This fourth stage bifurcates into two paths, worldly purification and supramundane purification. The worldly and supramundane outcomes mirror the two pathas (*mārgas*) of the *Śrāvakabhūmi* – the *laukikamārga* and the *lokottaramārga* – but the *Śrāvakabhūmi* is a more comprehensive treatise. In the *Bhāvanāmayī Bhūmiḥ*, the four stages of *yogabhāvanā* are mapped within a wider structure of seven book segments.[61] The four stages are as follows (Sugawara 2013):

1. Yogabhāvanāpada

The initial conditions for cultivation (*yogabhāvanāpada)* are tenfold.[62] Each of these ten conditions is itself a counterstate for a converse condition (i.e. finding a good teacher is the counterstate to not having a good teacher), but also, specifically, the condition of the five obstructive acts or obstacles (*pañcāntarāyaṇi karmāṇi)* is remedied by the perfection of being free of the obstacles of karma (*karmānāvaraṇa-saṃpat*).[63]

2. *Yogabhāvanopaniṣat*

The basis of the cultivation of practice (*yogabhāvanopaniṣat*) is described in three auxiliaries (*aṅgas*), which deal with listening to the genuine Dharma, the benefits of listening and the proper absorption of the teaching via listening.[64]

3. *Yogabhāvanā*

The next topic of yoga (*yogasthāna*) deals with the ensuing cultivation of practice (*yogabhāvanā*). This section recounts the ten obstacles (*vipakṣa*)[65] to *yogabhāvanā* and their counterstates (*pratipakṣa*).[66] These obstacles apply to three different classes of practitioner: two obstacles apply to the householder (*āgarikāvasthā*), four obstacles apply to the ascetic (*pravrajitāvasthā*) and four obstacles apply to the solitary disciple who cultivates in seclusion (*praviviktasya pratisaṃlayanayogabhāvanāvasthā*). As the entire section on countering obstacles is titled *yogabhāvanā*, we can propose that the cultivation of yoga *is* the countering of obstacles.[67] In short, *yogabhāvanā* is *pratipakṣabhāvanā*.[68]

4. *Bhāvanāphala*

The next and final phase of practice yields the fruit of cultivation (*bhāvanāphala*). As with the *Śrāvakabhūmi* (ŚBh), there is a bifurcation of the outcomes into purification at the mundane level (*laukika*) and purification at the supramundane level (*lokottara*). At the mundane level, the focus is on concentration (*samādhi*), which is broken down into three steps: the acquisition of *samādhi* (*samādhilābha*), the fulfilment of *samādhi* (*samādhiparipūri*) and the mastery of samādhi (*samādhivaśitā*). At the supramundane level, the four noble truths are realized via a reflective process called *abhisamaya* (*satyābhisamaya*).[69] The mind must be suitably frightened or flurried (*cittasaṃvigna*) and steadied (*cittasthiti*), with all obstacles countered and all *anuśaya* (seeds of *kleśa*) eliminated. Then ensues final liberation.

Saṃdhinirmocanasūtra

The *Saṃdhinirmocanasūtra* (SNS) is an independent text that is quoted in its entirety (bar its prologue and colophons) in the supplementary section of the *Viniścayasaṃgrahaṇī* that discusses the *Bodhisattvabhūmi*. The *Saṃdhinirmocanasūtra* is seen as pivotal in the advent of Mahāyāna thought in that it announces itself as the third 'turning of the wheel of dharma' and elaborates the core doctrines of store consciousness (*ālayavijñāna*), the three aspects (*trisvabhāva*) and appearance-only (*vijñāptimātratā*). This short work[70] is extant only in Chinese and Tibetan.[71] This text has a chapter dedicated to yoga and shares the tenfold path system of yogācāra that we find in the *Bodhisattvabhūmi* (with an eleventh stage added, the *tathāgatabhūmi*). It posits its yoga path as superior to all to other yogas in polemical fashion.

Conclusions

In this chapter, we have reviewed recent research in Buddhist studies to trace both the historical emergence of yogācāra as a distinct strand of Buddhist meditative practice and the formation of its core text, the *Yogācārabhūmiśāstra*. This enables us to think about Asaṅga's treatise as a significant *yogaśāstra* in its own right, alongside the *Pātañjalayogaśāstra*.

If we follow Maas's dating for the *Pātañjalayogaśāstra* (325–425 CE),[72] then, the *Śrāvakabhūmi*, the *Bodhisattvabhūmi* and *Saṃdhinirmocanasūtra* were all significantly earlier meditation treatises that contain the first systematized accounts of yogācāra, or yoga discipline. What do these proto-systems and systems look like? The *Śrāvakabhūmi*, the *Bodhisattvabhūmi* and the *Bhāvanāmayī Bhūmiḥ* map out a systematic frame of ten counterstates (*pratipakṣas*) to corresponding obstacles and, in the case of the *Śrāvakabhūmi* and the *Bhāvanāmayī Bhūmiḥ*, correlate this tenfold frame to a sevenfold path.[73] In the *Bodhisattvabhūmi* and the *Saṃdhinirmocanasūtra*, the tenfold path is itself constituted by a counterstate (*pratipakṣa*) to remove an affliction (*kleśa*). Among these four texts (all sections of the *Yogācārabhūmiśāstra*), the most detailed presentation of yoga as the cultivation of the counterstate (*pratipakṣabhāvanā*) in the *Yogācārabhūmiśāstra* occurs in the *Bhāvanāmayī Bhūmiḥ*. In the next chapter, we will consider how these structures of Buddhist yoga discipline intersect with conceptual schemes of practice in the *Pātañjalayogaśāstra*.

4

Pātañjala yoga and yogācāra: The cultivation of the counterstate

Introduction

Let us now bring Patañjali's *yogaśāstra* back into focus in order to demonstrate the presence of shared conceptual metaphors in the systems of yogācāra and yoga. The *Pātañjalayogaśāstra* and the *Yogācārabhūmiśāstra* present a definition of yoga as 'the cultivation of the counterstate' (*pratipakṣabhāvanā*).[1] Both the *Pātañjalayogaśāstra* and the *Yogācārabhūmiśāstra* employ the notion of the counterstate as that which removes factors that impede liberation. This counterstate is designated as the *pratipakṣa* or *vipakṣa*, which both mean 'opposite'. *Pratipakṣabhāvanā*, then, is the systematic application of a counterstate in order to negate an unwanted factor, and each sequential application (of the counterstate) marks a stage on the path. Since *pratipakṣabhāvanā* is not a common paradigm in Brahmanic thought and is a key soteriological paradigm in both the *Pātañjalayogaśāstra* and the *Yogācārabhūmiśāstra*, I propose that Patañjali's inclusion of this term is drawing on Buddhist sources.

The cultivation of the counterstate (*pratipakṣabhāvanā*)

Pratipakṣabhāvanā explains the elimination of affliction (*kleśa*), not by using the seed model (as in burning the seed of *kleśa* to eliminate germination potential) but rather using the binary model of factor/counterfactor or state/counterstate. Within this conceptual frame, there are three distinct structural metaphors that appear in both the *Pātañjalayogaśāstra* and the *Yogācārabhūmiśāstra*:

YOGA IS AN ANTIDOTE (= *KLEŚA* IS A POISON)
YOGA IS A PATH (= *KLEŚA* IS AN OBSTACLE)

YOGA IS CLEAR VISION (= *KLEŚA* IS AN OBSCURATION)[2]

Scholars of Buddhism frequently translate the term *pratipakṣa* by using a medical term – that of the 'antidote',[3] 'remedy' or 'cure'. However, I argue that, in relation to all of our texts, such blanket usage of the term 'antidote' for *pratipakṣa* (or *vipakṣa*, a common synonym) is unsuitable because it foregrounds the medical paradigm of disease/remedy (YOGA IS AN ANTIDOTE) at the expense of two other structural metaphors (YOGA IS A PATH, YOGA IS CLEAR VISION) that also govern the topic of 'unwanted states and how to remove them'.[4] Instead, I propose that *pratipakṣabhāvanā* may be best translated by examining the metaphoric context of each use. These structural metaphors are combined to create the conceptual scheme of *pratipakṣabhāvanā*, which is, in turn, a constituent part of the larger and more complex orientational metaphor of mental/spiritual cultivation (*bhāvanā*). As I discussed in Chapter 1, cultivation is an orientational metaphor that centres on the agricultural image-schema of cultivating the soil. In this section, I narrow my analysis of *bhāvanā* to examine systematic accounts of *pratipakṣabhāvanā* as the yogic means to liberation. In the soteriologies under review in this book, affliction (*kleśa*) is the key factor that opposes spiritual liberation. An affliction must be overcome using a technique of systematically applying the appropriate counterfactor or counterstate, generally known as the *pratipakṣa*.

Pratipakṣabhāvanā in Pātañjala yoga

When we turn to the soteriology of Pātañjala yoga, we find that the concept of the counterstate (*pratipakṣa*) is vital. In Patañjali's path of *kriyā yoga* (the goal of which is to reduce the afflictions), the overcoming of the afflictions (*kleśas*)[5] is, by definition, the application of positive counterstates to eradicate negative states.[6] Patañjali foregrounds *pratipakṣabhāvanā* as a technique for success:[7]

> When, for [the yogin], the contrary ideas that are to be abandoned become of sterile quality, as a result of *pratipakṣabhāvanā* of the cause, then there arises for the yogin power caused by that, and it is an indication of success (PYŚ 2.35).[8]

This explanation weaves in the notion of sterility and non-propagation (*aprasava*) as the purpose of *pratipakṣabhāvanā*, reflecting that the obstacles are forms of the afflictions, the seeds of which must be destroyed to succeed in yoga. In this example, Patañjali's elaboration of the counterstate is another expression of the theory of the elimination of the seed, and we are returned, again, to the notion of dialogue with the Sautrāntikas. The path of *kriyā yoga* – the path that exterminates the afflictions by countering them – is often overlooked in scholarship on Pātañjala yoga. I argue that it has as important a place in Patañjali's exposition of yoga as does the well-known *aṣṭāṅga* system[9] and therefore merits greater analysis.[10] It is in the exposition of *kriyā yoga* that cultivation of the counterstate is most clearly explained as a means to eliminate the afflictions:

> The afflictions become diminished when they are damaged by the cultivation of a counterstate (*pratipakṣabhāvana*). This is the definition of diminishment (PYŚ 2.4).[11]

The outcome of *pratipakṣabhāvanā* is cessation.[12] The importance of the paradigm of state and counterstate in Patañjali's text is also evident in a more subtle way in the nine obstacles (*antarāyas*), each of which is neutralized with a counterstate (discussed below).[13] In order to better understand this context of *pratipakṣabhāvanā* in the *Pātañjalayogaśāstra*, we benefit from turning to the Buddhist sources of the period.

Pratipakṣabhāvanā in the *Yogācārabhūmiśāstra*

The technique of *pratipakṣa* is widely employed in the *Yogācārabhūmiśāstra*.[14] In the *Bodhisattvabhūmi*, for example, there is a fivefold scheme in which each affliction can be removed by a specific oppositional contemplation designed to negate it (see Table 4.1). In the *Bhāvanāmayī Bhūmiḥ*, cultivation of the counterstate is the very definition of yoga. The *Bhāvanāmayī Bhūmiḥ* puts forward four stages of yoga and defines the third stage, the cultivation of yoga (*yogabhāvanā*), as the cultivation of the counterstate (*pratipakṣabhāvanā*). In this sense, the text presents yoga as a set of techniques (solutions) to overcome obstacles (problems). *Pratipakṣabhāvanā* also forms the core practice of the *Śrāvakabhūmi*, in which the four classes of meditative objects are presented as counterstates to the obstacles (*āvaraṇa*):

> How many types of purifying the obstacles are there? It is said that there are four causes which, when correctly applied to the obstacles by the yogin, purifies his own *citta*: perception of his own form, the 12 interdependent links (*nidāna*), perception of danger (*ādīnava*) and cultivation of the counterstate[15] (*pratipakṣa*).[16]

Table 4.1 The *kleśas* and their counterstates in *Bodhisattvabhūmi* 1.12

Affliction (*kleśa*)	Opposing contemplation (*pratipakṣa*)*
Passion (*rāga*)	Cultivation of the unattractive (*aśubhabhāvanā*)
Animosity (*dveṣa*) or malice (*vyāpāda*)	On the *brahmavihāra* of *maitrī* (compassion)
Delusion (*moha*)	On *pratītyasamutpāda* (twelvefold chain of dependent origination)
Discursive thought (*vitarka*)	Mindfulness of breathing (*ānāpānasmṛti*)
Ego (*asmimāna*)	On the eighteen sense fields (*dhātus*)

Note: See BoBh 1.12.21–27 (Wogihara 1930–6: 204–5). For the conceptual symmetry between *vipakṣa* and *pratipakṣa*, see also BoBh 1.8 (Wogihara 1930–6: 98 line 17–21).

* It is also worth noting that of the Buddhist *pratipakṣas* listed here, the *Pātañjalayogaśāstra* also advocates the counterstates of friendliness *maitrī* (YS 1.33) and *prāṇāyāma* (PYŚ 1.34, 2.52).

Both the *Śrāvakabhūmi* and the *Bhāvanāmayī Bhūmiḥ* contain a list of ten *vipakṣas*,[17] which are opposed with counterstates (*pratipakṣas*).[18] These are all ideational cultivations (*saṃjñābhāvanā*) or contemplations:

1. contemplating the unattractive (*aśubhasaṃjñā*),
2. contemplating impermanence (*anityasaṃjñā*),
3. contemplating the suffering in what is impermanent (*anitye duḥkhasaṃjñā*),
4. contemplating selflessness regarding suffering (*dukhe 'anātmasaṃjñā*),
5. contemplating disagreeability to food (*āhāre pratikūlasaṃjñā*),
6. contemplating indifference to anything worldly (*sarvaloke anabhiratisaṃjñā*),
7. contemplating light (*ālokasaṃjñā*),
8. contemplating detachment (*virāgasaṃjñā*),
9. contemplating cessation (*nirodhasaṃjñā*) and
10. contemplating death (*maraṇasaṃjñā*).[19]

Each *pratipakṣa* governs not just one obstacle but groups and subgroups of obstacles. Therefore, there are more obstacles than *pratipakṣas*. For example, there is the *vipakṣa* called 'obstacle to expertise in yogic contemplation' (*yoga manasikārākuśalatā*), which is the lack of expertise in yogic contemplation that occurs when one is not eager to listen and thus not inquisitive (BhāvBh

142b5-a1; von Rospatt 2013: 858).[20] This is countered by cultivation of unattractive images (*aśubhasaṃjñābhāvanā*). Another obstacle is laziness and indolence (*ālasyakausīdya*) in applying oneself to the constant cultivation of wholesome dharmas (*kuśaladharmabhāvanāsātatyābhiyoga*) (BhāvBh 142a3; von Rospatt 2013: 858). This obstacle has as its counterstate the contemplation that regards the impermanent as entailing suffering (*anitya duḥkhasaṃjñābh āvanā*). From this range of examples in the *Yogācārabhūmiśāstra*, we can see that cultivation of the counterstate (*pratipakṣabhāvanā*) is a central technique to liberation.

The conceptual metaphors of *pratipakṣabhāvanā*

Let us now examine the three structural metaphors of *pratipakṣabhāvanā* to demonstrate conceptual sharing between the *Pātañjalayogaśāstra* and the *Yogācārabhūmiśāstra*. *Pratipakṣa* has a general meaning of 'opposing side',[21] and this semantic breadth allows it to be a 'container' for different structural metaphors. Each metaphor develops the basic idea that every state has a counterstate (or every force has a counterforce). In this way, '*yoga*' and '*kleśa*' mirror each other as opposing states or forces.

YOGA IS AN ANTIDOTE (= *KLEŚA* IS A POISON)
YOGA IS A PATH (= *KLEŚA* IS AN OBSTACLE)
YOGA IS CLEAR VISION (= *KLEŚA* IS AN OBSCURATION)

Each structural metaphor has an underlying root metaphor.[22]

YOGA IS AN ANTIDOTE relies on BAD FEELINGS ARE POISONS.
YOGA IS A PATH relies on LIFE IS A JOURNEY and DIFFICULTIES ARE IMPEDIMENTS.
YOGA IS CLEAR VISION relies on KNOWING IS SEEING.

Each of these structural metaphors demonstrates the process of domain-mapping: a counterstate can be conceived of as the remedial force of an antidote to a poison (YOGA IS AN ANTIDOTE), or the physical force that moves a material obstacle out of the way (YOGA IS A PATH), or the physical force that moves a material obscurant out of the field of vision (YOGA IS CLEAR VISION). In each of these cases, the basic idea is that a physical object or substance must be removed: a poison from the body, an obstacle from the path or an obscurant from the field of vision. Indeed, *Pātañjalayogaśāstra* 1.30 is striking in that it appears to acknowledge the prevailing choices of metaphors available in conceptualizing yoga as a counterstate. It offers three ways of understanding the obstacles (problems) to yoga: impurities of yoga (*yogamala*), opposites of yoga (*yogapratipakṣa*) and impediments to yoga (*yogāntarāya*).

1. Yoga is an antidote: Ethical precepts as cures

The conceptual metaphor YOGA IS AN ANTIDOTE rests on the root metaphor that BAD FEELINGS ARE POISONS. In literal terms, negative psychological states are not poisons, of course, but their metaphorical designation as such is reflected in everyday utterances such as the English phrases 'he was poisoned by jealousy' or 'love is the cure'. In our Sanskrit texts, yoga is understood as a remedy or cure for negative psychological, emotional or ethical states. As an example, I will now look at how ethical precepts are understood as antidotes in *pratipakṣabhāvanā*.

In Patañjali's preparatory stages of *aṣṭāṅga yoga*, the ethical precepts of the restraints (*yama*s) and observances (*niyama*s) are presented as positive counterstates to neutralize unwanted behaviours.[23] Because these ten ethical precepts are only understood in relation to the violations or transgressions that they counter, I propose that the *yama*s and *niyama*s are presented within the paradigm of state/counterstate.[24] Indeed, Patañjali presents the ethical precepts as *pratipakṣabhāvanā*. When the five *yama*s are introduced at YS 2.32, they are defined as counterstates to their obstacles.

> On this it is said: and then for one who has mastered turning the thoughts inwards, the obstacles (*antarāya*) cease to exist.
>
> Of these *yama*s and *niyama*s:
>
> **When there is obstruction by discursive thought, [there should be] cultivation of the counterstate *(pratipakṣabhāvana)*** (PYŚ 2.31-32).[25]

The commentary to YS 2.33 then gives instruction on how a Brahmin should practice cultivation of the counterstate – it is the practice of the restraints (*yama*s). For example, in the case of harm (*hiṃsā*), yoga offers a meditation to access its counterstate (*ahiṃsā*):

> Thus, being harassed by the intensely blazing affliction that opposes and that is the decline out of the path, one should cultivate the counterstate of that: 'Being roasted on the terrible embers of *saṃsāra*, I have attained refuge. *Yogadharma* arises by means of bestowing safety to all beings.' One should cultivate: 'However, having abandoned the contrary ideas (*vitarka*),[26] I accept (*ādadāna*) similar

ones again, by means of acting like a dog.[27] In the way that a dog licks up its own vomit, so do I again take up [those contrary ideas] (PYŚ 2.33).'[28]

The implication here is that one keeps regurgitating and redigesting foul things/substances until they are countered with an antidote. The next instruction is to repeat the above *pratipakṣa* meditation technique for the remainder of the *yama*s and *niyamas*.[29] The example given is a person who has contemplated murder; his cultivation of the opposite (*pratipakṣabhāvanā*) should be the contemplation of his own death, so that his waking hours become a living hell. In all of these examples, *pratipakṣabhāvanā* is suffused with images of physical suffering or affliction: such as burning in fire, reconsuming vomit or contemplating one's own death. These images of pain, distress and disease in the body point to the generative context for the metaphors of *pratipakṣabhāvānā*: the medical domain of affliction and cure.[30]

The nature of the counterstate in Patañjali's examples – visualizing oneself in degrading and foul terms – is not dissimilar to the Buddhist practice of visualizing the human body as unpleasant or frightening (*aśubhabhāvanā*).[31] *Aśubha* was a practice that focused on contemplation of various bodily states as unattractive, disagreeable, impure or in various stages of decomposition – what Deleanu refers to as 'vividly imaged samsāric horror' (Deleanu 2006 1: 21).[32] In the Sarvāstivāda tradition, *aśubha* is often prescribed as the counterstate for sensual craving and for the character type in whom greed predominates (Chan 2013: 102).[33] The practice of contemplating the unattractive is a central meditation technique in the *Śrāvakabhūmi* in its account of *yogabhāvanā*, where it is prescribed for those afflicted by passion (*rāga*) (ŚBh 9B.9-1a; Wayman 1960: 96). In the *Bhāvanāmayī Bhūmiḥ*, *pratipakṣabhāvanā* is employed to frighten the mind so that the practitioner will see that saṃsāra is terrible and that nirvāṇa is sublime.[34]

To sum up: in Pātañjala yoga and yogācāra one can visualize an unpleasant image of the body in order to obtain a 'remedy' or 'antidote' for ethical disease in the body-mind complex. This structural metaphor maps qualities from the domain of medicine to ethics, so that yoga is understood as curative or healing.

2. Yoga is a path: The *bhūmi*s and the *mārga*

Spiritual progress is often conceived of as a journey, not just any type of journey but a specific route with a purpose, goal and a clearly defined end destination. The conceptual metaphor YOGA IS A PATH is based on LIFE IS A JOURNEY, which in turn is derived from the image-schema SOURCE-PATH-GOAL (based on embodied or visceral experience).[35]

The conceptual metaphor SPIRITUAL PROGRESS IS A PATH is also one that we encounter in Brahmanism. Here, the 'Śānti Parvan' identifies the connection between yoga and the path of liberation (*mokṣamārga*):

> For one who is established in yoga there is attainment of the *mokṣamārga*. (MB 12.319.006a; Belvalkar 1954, 16: 1802)[36]

However, in Brahmanic asceticism, although the wandering ascetic follows a path with a destination (*mokṣa*), it is not always rigidly defined in the way that Buddhist paths typically are. Buddhist soteriology (particularly Sarvāstivāda Abhidharma) is often precisely mapped out and definitively signposted at every step and stage. Gethin points out that in the Nikāyas, 'Buddhist thought is about the Buddhist path' and that there is an inextricability between the concept of path (*mārga*) and the concept of spiritual development as *bhāvanā* or *yoga* (Gethin 2007: 18).[37] The best-known metaphor used to describe Pātañjala yoga is not that of the path but that of *aṅga* or limb, for example, *aṣṭāṅga yoga*.[38] This draws on a different root metaphor THE WHOLE IS A BODY (as in 'body of thought', 'body of work', 'body of the state' or 'body of knowledge') and is expressed in *Maitrī Upaniṣad*'s outline of *ṣaḍaṅga yoga*. The logical drive of the *aṅga* metaphor is different to that of the stage/foundation and the path (*bhūmi* and *mārga*): whereas the end goal of the *aṅga* metaphor is to express the relationship of a part to whole, *bhūmis* presuppose the structure of a path and a journey to a destination. The *aṅga* metaphor conceptualizes 'a sum total' while the *bhūmi* infers 'an ultimate destination'. These metaphors cannot be said to be overlapping because they do not share the same entailments. And yet, since we find both metaphors in the *Pātañjalayogaśāstra*, the text can be regarded as an integration of different conceptual systems.

Patañjali's *aṣṭāṅga yoga* appears to be drawing on older conceptual systems in the Vedas and *Upaniṣads* that rely on THE WHOLE IS A BODY: such as the cosmic dismemberment of a primordial body as a positive, generative process, as in the 'Puruṣa Sūkta' of the *Ṛg Veda* (RV 10.90); or the correlations of one's body (part) to the cosmic body (whole) in the *Upaniṣads* – expressed not only in connections (*bandhus*) but ultimately in the *ātman-brahman* correspondence. Such is the predominant interpretation of *aṅga* as the key metaphor in Patañjali's system of yoga, however, that scholars have overlooked how Patañjali also uses the conceptual metaphors of *bhūmi* and *mārga* to construct an understanding of yoga as cultivation (*bhāvanā*). If we look beyond *aṣṭāṅga yoga*, we see that the issue of what constitutes the system of Pātañjala yoga is considerably more complex. *Kriyā yoga* is, for example, in some details and in structure close to the Buddhist Sarvāstivāda and yogācāra systems of *mārga*. Next, I highlight how Patañjali's conceptual metaphor YOGA IS A PATH intersects with the Buddhist equivalent YOGĀCĀRA IS A PATH.

The very title of the *Yogācārabhūmiśāstra* itself expresses the idea that yogācāra is a path. *Bhūmi* literally means 'ground', 'soil' or 'foundation', and the qualities of this domain are mapped to soteriological practice to convey the concept of 'stage' or 'step' in a progressive sense. The *bhūmis*, then, are the stages or steps that make up the path of practice, the *mārga*. In both Mahāyāna and Sarvāstivāda Buddhist discourse, the *bhūmis* are not only stages to liberation[39] but also stages that contain *kleśas*. The attainment at each *bhūmi* is the removal of a *kleśa*, which is an obstacle or impediment that obstructs progess on the path.[40] The *Daśabhūmikasūtra*, the *Bodhisattvabhūmi* and the *Saṃdhiniromocanasūtra* all mark the ten *bhūmis* by the removal of an obstacle. Indeed, the ten obstacles also feature widely in contemporaneous literature such as Vasubandhu's *Vijñāptimatratāsiddhi*, which charts the ten stages of the bodhisattva path (*daśabhūmi*). The functional counterstates[41] at the ten *bhūmis* are typically the six perfections (*pāramitās*) plus other states (e.g. *dāna*, *śīla*, *kṣānti*, *vīrya*, *dhyāna*, *prajñā*, *upāya*, *praṇidhāna*, *bala* and *jñāna*). As I discussed in Chapters 1 and 2, spiritual progress is not always conceptualized as a path; it can also be a ladder, a doorway, an awakening, the quenching of a flame and so on. Therefore, when we observe that another soteriology, Pātañjala yoga, specifies spiritual progress as a *bhūmi* or set of *bhūmis* (a *mārga*), this would appear to be significant.

The *Pātañjalayogaśāstra* refers to the concept of path in three instances. The first is a negation of the path: *unmārga*. *Unmārga* is the wrong path, which denotes having gone astray. It is the consequence of the blazing fires of *saṃsāra* that carry one out of one's path (PYŚ 2.33). At 2.26 the path to liberation (*mokṣamārga*) is described as the means of cessation, the burnt seed.[42] The other instance of *mārga* is the state one attains on hearing (*śravaṇa*) about *mokṣa*, when the seed of the knowledge of the difference (*viśeṣadarśanabīja*) begins to grow (*viśeṣadarśana* being a synonym for *vivekakhyāti*) (PYŚ 4.25).[43] Aside from these three explicit references to *mārga* in the *Pātañjalayogaśāstra*, there are also several conceptual references that reflect technical overlaps with yogācāra discourse. To start with, the most basic point to note is Patañjali's concept of the pinnacle of yoga practice as the cloud of dharma (*dharmamegha*). In Buddhist soteriology, the stage of the cloud of dharma (*dharmameghabhūmi*) is, most often, the culmination of the path of cultivation (*bhāvanāmārga*); that is, the tenth stage, the *bodhisattvabhūmi*, is the *dharmamegha* (O'Brien-Kop 2020). And so, if Patañjali points to the well-known cloud of dharma metaphor as the superlative outcome of yoga, it means that his text is, on the generic level, a *mārga* text that focuses on cultivation (*bhāvanā*) as the means. Patañjali's delineation of the path of yoga also intersects with that of the *Bhāvanāmayī Bhūmiḥ*. In the *Bhāvanāmayī Bhūmiḥ*, the seventh aspect of cultivation stresses the 'complete purification of all supramundane aspects', which is also the fourth stage of yoga, the *bhāvanāphala*.[44] The final component of *bhāvanāphala* contains three stages of samādhi:

> the acquisition of concentration (*samādhilābha*),
> the fulfilment of concentration (*samādhiparipūri*),
> the mastery of concentration (*samādhivaśitā*).

Entering *samādhi* means attaining the stage immediately preceding the first *dhyāna*: one must attain one of the main (*maula*) *dhyāna*s and finally master *samādhi* (*samādhivaśitā*), which then allows one to enter and exit the *dhyāna*s at will. There are twenty obstacles (*antarāya*s) that hinder the initial *samādhilābha*, entry into *samādhi* – and the appropriate counterstates are prescribed. Next, the fulfilment process (*samādhiparipūri*) is one of entering deep meditation in isolation by focusing on tranquillity practices. Finally, the mastery of concentration is attained by practising ascetic austerity to devote oneself to the practice. In this sense, isolated ascetic practice is clearly privileged as the highest practice, representing the culmination of the four stages of yoga.

We find echoes of these threefold stages of *samādhi* in the *Pātañjalayogaśāstra*, when it refers twice to *samādhilābha* and *samādhiphalam* as a pair of attainments or stages. In a discussion of *asaṃprajñāta samādhi* (non-cognitive concentration), *samādhilābha* is clearly set out as a goal: *samādhilābhaḥ samādhiphalaṃ ca bhavatīti* (PYŚ 1.21; Āgāśe 1904: 24). '*Samādhi* is obtained, and there are the fruits of *samādhi*.' And the commentary to the next *sūtra* explains how effort can be mild, medium or intense: *tasmād adhimātratīvrasaṃvegasyādhimātropāyasy āpy āsannatamaḥ samādhilābhaḥ samādhiphalaṃ ceti* (PYŚ 1.22; Āgāśe 1904: 25) 'Due to this distinction even among the closer [means], he who is zealously intense is the most near, and *samādhi* and the fruits of *samādhi* are obtained.' A third instance in Patañjali's text discusses *samādhilābha* in terms of failure: *alabdhabhūmikatvaṃ samādhibhūmer alābhaḥ* (PYŚ 1.30; Āgāśe 1904: 34) 'The state of non-attainment of the stages (*bhūmi*) is not attaining the stage of *samādhi*'. If there is non-attainment in the stage (*bhūmi*) of yoga which is *samādhi*, there is overall failure. Here, *samādhibhūmi*, which indicates attainment, is suggestive of the *samādhivaśitā* of the *Bhāvanāmayī Bhūmiḥ*.[45]

The ninefold path

In the formulation of the nine obstacles (*antarāyas*), there is a further account of Pātañjala yoga as a counterstate to impediments on the path. The nine obstacles are disease, stupor, doubt, negligence, idleness, non-abstention, confused knowledge, non-attainment of the stages (*bhūmis*; discussed above) and incapacity to remain/ endure (YS 1.30). These nine obstacles are first introduced at YS 1.29 in relation to devotion to *īśvara* (*īśvarapraṇidhāna*).[46] The commentary explains that when the nine obstacles are removed, one can perceive one's own form as *puruṣa*. Here, the obstacles are directly linked to the state of mental fluctuation (*cittavṛtti*); when the obstacles exist, the mind (*citta*) still undergoes modification. Conversely, concentration (*samādhi*) is attained when the mind is steady. This description is reminiscent of the *Bhāvanāmayī Bhūmiḥ*'s account of how a steady mind (*cittasthiti*) is attained when the obstacles (*antarāya*) to realization of the truth (*satyābhisamaya*) are removed (BhāvBh 7; Sugawara 2013: 804–5). Patañjali's nine impediments to yoga, *yogāntarāyas* (YS 1.31),[47] are followed by nine practices that constitute counterstates to dissolve these obstacles. Clearly, the *antarāyas* at YS 1.31 are directly linked to the set of practices that surround them (PYŚ 1.29–39): these impediments on the path can only be removed by the application of a set of yogic techniques that act as counterforces to move the obstacles from the path. These are counterstates (*pratipakṣas*):

1. devotion to Īśvara (*īśvarapraṇidhāna*) (YS. 1.29),
2. one-pointed concentration (*ekatattvābhyāsaḥ*) (YS 1.32),
3. the four (*brahma*)*vihāras*[48] (YS 1.33),
4. breath control (YS 1.34),
5. object-centred sense redirection (YS 1.35),
6. sorrowless luminosity (*viśoka jyotiṣmatī*) (YS 1.36),
7. contemplation on dispassion (*vītarāgaviṣayam cittam*) (YS 1.37),
8. knowledge of dream and sleep (YS 1.38),
9. absorption (*dhyāna*) (YS 1.39) (subdivided into four *samāpattis*).

This list, linked by the particle *vā* (or), is clearly presented as a list of optional practices in Pātañjala yoga, and they are the *pratipakṣas* to the nine obstacles,[49] constituting a path structure of nine stages. The paradigmatic context of these optional practices in the chapter on concentration (*samādhipāda*) can only be properly clarified by relating them to similar paradigms in Buddhist texts. Both the *Bodhisattvabhūmi* and the *Pātañjalayogaśāstra* agree that the desired state is to be without obstruction (*anāvaraṇa*).[50]

Another way to frame this argument is to look at the role of *bhāvanā* in this run of *sūtras* (YS 1.29–39) and beyond. In the above list of nine counterstates, the term *bhāvanā* appears as follows: *bhāvanā* describes quiet recitation (*japa*) of the syllable *oṃ* (YS 1.28, YSBh 1.28), the obstacle (*antarāya*) of carelessness (*pramāda*) is the lack of cultivation (*abhāvanā*) of the practice directed towards concentration (*samādhisādhana*) (PYŚ 1.30) and the cultivation (*bhāvanā*) of the four *brahmavihāras* clarifies the mind (YS 1.33). These three instances alone are enough to illustrate that the context of Patañjali's 'nine' alternative practices conveys the structure of *pratipakṣabhāvanā*, cultivation of the opposite states to the obstacles. If we require further evidence, the remainder of the instances of *bhāvanā* in the *Pātañjalayogaśāstra* underline this point. *Bhāvanā* appears in the following chapters in these contexts: the cultivation of *samādhi* (YS 2.2); cultivation of the opposites (*pratipakṣabhāvanā*) (YSBh 2.4; YS 2.33; YS 2.34 and YSBh 2.34); cultivation of the *brahmavihāras* (YSBh 3.33); the fourth stage of yoga practitioner, the one who has gone beyond cultivation (*atikrāntabhavanīya*) (YSBh 3.51); firm cultivation of a narrated counterstate (YSBh 3.51); and ceasing meditation on one's own self (***ātmabhāvabhāvanānivṛttiḥ***) (YS 4.25 and YSBh 4.25). Across these contexts in the *Pātañjalayogaśāstra*, *bhāvanā* consistently refers to the cultivation of particular mental states in meditation that lead to *samādhi*. In many ways, *bhāvanā* is the central technique of Patañjala yoga; there seems to be little to this yoga that is not *bhāvanā*.

The sevenfold path

In yoga and yogācāra, it is not only the paradigm of the obstacles that overlaps but also the positive description of the path structure itself. Another of the lesser studied path structures in the *Pātañjalayogaśāstra* is that of the sevenfold path of the yogin (PYŚ 2.27, 3.51). This sevenfold path of wisdom, offset against four levels of practitioner, bears structural resemblance to the *Śrāvakabhūmi*'s sevenfold stages of wisdom, offset against three levels of practitioner.

Pātañjalayogaśāstra 3.51 relates how the yogin is tempted by the gods to partake in heavenly delights. In this case, the counterstate is a narrated contemplation that directly addresses the details of the heavenly mirage one by one in order to 'neutralise' them.[51] The contemplative counterstate to the false allures of heaven appears within an exposition of the four stages of yoga:

1. the beginner (*prathamakalpika*),
2. the honeyed stage (*madhubhūmika*),

3. the light of knowledge (*prajñājyotis*),
4. one who has surpassed what is to be cultivated (*atikrāntabhavanīya*) (PYŚ 3.51).[52]

Within these four stages, the inclusion of a '*yogabhūmi*' (the *madhu-bhūmi* of yoga) perhaps hints at the *yogācārabhūmi* literature. Furthermore, in Patañjali's scheme, the fourfold level of practitioner is correlated to the sevenfold path stages, the *saptavidhā*. Only by advanced cultivation (*atikrāntabhavanīya*) can one reach the final stage of wisdom (*prāntabhūmiprajñā*) (see Table 4.2).

Not only do the first four stages here appear to reference the paradigm of the four noble truths,[53] but Patañjali's fourth and highest level of practitioner, the *atikrāntabhavanīya*, is resonant of the highest stage of practitioner in the *Śrāvakabhūmi*, *atikrāntamanaskāra* (see Table 4.3).

On the supramundane path of the *Srāvakabhūmi*, there are three stages[54] of practitioner:

1. the novice (*ādhikarmikaḥ*),
2. the adept (*kṛtaparicayaḥ*),
3. the one who has gone beyond contemplation (*atikrāntamanaskāra*).

Table 4.2 Patañjali's seven stages of wisdom paraphrased (*Pātañjalayogaśāstra* 2.27)

1	What is to be escaped has been fully examined	*parijñātaṃ heyaṃ*	Fourfold freedom from knowledge of anything left to be done
2	The causes of what is to be escaped have dwindled and do not need to be destroyed	*kṣīṇā heyahetavo na punar eteṣāṃ kṣetavyam asti*	
3	Abandonment by means of *nirodhasamādhi*	*nirodhasamādhinā hānam*	
4	Perfection of discriminating perception	*bhāvito vivekakhyātirūpo hānopāya iti*	
5	*Buddhi* has completed its function.	*caritādhikārā buddhiḥ*	Threefold freedom of the mind
6	The *guṇas* turn towards dissolution (like rocks falling from a mountain) and along with them comes everything else. The *guṇas*, dissolved, do not reappear	*guṇā giriśikharataṭacyutā iva grāvāṇo niravasthānāḥ svakāraṇe pralayābhimukhāḥ saha tenāstaṃ gacchanti.na caiṣāṃ pravilīnānāṃ punar asty utpādaḥ prayojanābhāvād iti*	
7	In the state beyond the *guṇas*, *puruṣa* is solitary and self-illuminating	*etasyām avasthāyāṃ guṇasaṃbandhātītaḥ svarūpamātrajyotir amalaḥ kevalī puruṣa iti*	

Note: PYŚ 2.27; Angot (2012: 468).

Table 4.3 Asaṅga's seven stages of contemplation (*Śrāvakabhūmi* 3.28.2.1.1–8)

1	Contemplation perceiving characteristics	*lakṣaṇapratisaṁvedī manaskāraḥ*
2	Contemplation leading to/characterized by conviction	*ādhimokṣiko manaskāraḥ*
3	Contemplation engendering separation	*prāvivekyo manaskāraḥ*
4	Contemplation comprising delight	*ratisaṁgrāhako manaskāraḥ*
5	Contemplation of enquiry	*mīmāṃsā manaskāraḥ*
6	Contemplation attaining fulfilment of the practice	*prayoganiṣṭho manaskāraḥ*
7	Contemplation representing the fruit of the fulfilment of the practice	*prayoganiṣṭhāphala manaskāraḥ*

Note: The English translations of the stages draw on Deleanu (2006, 1: 29–30).

In the *Śrāvakabhūmi*, only the highest stage of practitioner, the *atikrāntamanaskāra*, can attain the seventh stage of contemplation (*manaskāra*), which is the end goal, the fruit of the culmination of the practice (*prayoganiṣṭhāphalo manaskāraḥ*) (ŚBh 3.15).

The structural correspondences in these two schemes between the levels of practitioner and the seven levels of contemplation are striking. In yogācāra, the stage of *atikrānta* is particularly associated with the *bodhisattva* and is a frequent qualifier of *bodhisattva* status in the *Bodhisattvabhūmi*.[55] The classification of seven levels of wisdom is typical of the early Buddhist and Abhidharma-style classification in this period.[56] A sevenfold path to wisdom (*prajñā*) is present in the *Pātañjalayogaśāstra* but is not evident in other key Brahmanic texts on yoga. The *Pātañjalayogaśāstra* and the *Yogācārabhūmiśāstra* thus share a path structure of seven-stage yoga training that has as its most advanced level the *atikrāntamanaskāra* (ŚBh) or the *atikrāntabhāvanīya* (PYŚ), both of which paths have as their goal the attainment of *prajñā*.

In sum, in an image-schema that relies on the conceptual metaphor SPIRITUAL PROGESS IS A PATH, Pātañjala yoga and yogācāra both propose a seven-stage path of the adept and a correlative technique to remove impediments on the path, *praktipakṣabhāvanā*.

3. Yoga is clear vision: Errors of perception and the visual field

The metaphor YOGA IS CLEAR VISION rests on the root metaphor SEEING IS KNOWING. In this model, the undesired factor is that which obscures vision, either in the form of a 'block' in the field of vision or as the limiting condition of darkness (producing *avidyā*, *moha*, *mithyājñāna*, etc.). This is an epistemological model, which was generated to theorize how knowledge operates. This model deals with cognition, ignorance and knowledge and is often expressed as veiling/unveiling the truth or covering/uncovering the light of knowledge, for example, 'the lamp of yoga' (PYŚ 3.51).

Yoga as the correct type of vision is, of course, central to Sāṃkhya soteriology, in which one is liberated by perceiving the true self as *puruṣa* (and not falsely perceiving the self as *prakṛti*). However, there is at least one other instance of the conceptual metaphor YOGA IS CLEAR VISION, which intersects specifically with a Buddhist paradigm. Patañjali's account of *kriyā yoga* contains a discussion of the counterstate in relation to the four errors of perception. These four misperceptions constitute the foundation of ignorance (*avidyā*), the master affliction from which the other *kleśa*s spring:

> ***Avidyā* is [seeing] permanence, purity, happiness, and perception of self as impermanence, impurity, suffering, and non-self.** (YS 2.5)[57]

This paradigm appears to refer to 'the four errors' or misperceptions (*viparyāsa*) of Buddhist thought, also called the four *ākāras*.[58] These four misperceptions are also evident in the *Bhāvanāmayī Bhūmiḥ*, where they are accompanied by contemplations that are designed to counter the four errors of perception regarding the nature of reality. Three of the four errors are included in the *Bhāvanāmayī Bhūmiḥ*'s list of the ten counterstates (I discussed these in Chapter 3).[59] According to these errors, the conditioned nature of *saṃsāra* is misunderstood as permanent, pure, blissful and self – the same formula that we find in the *Pātañjalayogaśāstra*. So, what is the rationale behind these four errors in Buddhism? The four misperceptions began as the three marks of existence (*trilakṣaṇa*) in the early teachings of the Buddha: *anitya*, *duḥkha* and *anātman* – all conditioned things are impermanent, all conditioned things are therefore unsatisfactory and all knowable things are not-self (e.g. *Dhammapada* 277–9). The three marks, however, are perverted by the delusion or nescience (*moha*; *avidyā*) of the human mind, which can only be corrected by apprehension of the noble truths and practice of the noble eightfold path.[60] When the three *lakṣaṇa*s (*anitya*, *duḥkha*, *anātman*) were extended, the fourth component was 'impurity', understood as *aśuci* (unclean) or *aśubha* (disagreeable). In fact, it is the addition of *aśubha* that causes the perversion of the three *lakṣaṇa*s into the four misperceptions. However, *aśubha* meditation can also restore the true perception of the three *lakṣaṇa*s – the truth of the body as impermanent, filled with suffering and characterized by non-self. Yogācāra philosophy adds emptiness (*śūnyatā*) as a fourth element (instead of *aśuci* or *aśubha*), to indicate that it is the essential teaching underlying the three marks. The *Śrāvakabhūmi*[61] includes emptiness in its description of the paradigm of the four forms in the supramundane path (*lokottara mārga*): the truth of suffering (*duḥkhasatya*) (the first of the four noble truths) is inspected through the four *ākāra*s of impermanence (*anityatā*), suffering (*duḥkhatā*), emptiness (*śūnyatā*) and non-self or non-substantiality (*anātmatā*).[62] However, at another instance the formula is cited with *śuci* rather than *śūnyatā* (ŚBh 10A.3-2a; Wayman 1960: 98).[63] In all of these cases, whether Brahmin or Buddhist, the error in perception is mistaking the doctrinally rejected state for the ideal state.

In comparison to the Buddhist paradigm of the four *ākāras*, how does Patañjali propose that clear vision be attained? It is not by removing the obscurant in the field of vision, nor by increasing the light. Rather we return to the technique of the counterstate as a cultivated visual image that negates its opposite. For example, Patañjali's description of the state of impurity contains the false perception of beauty in a woman's form:

> Because in the impure, purity is perceived. It is as when a young girl, like the curved moon, might lead [one] to love with her limbs as if made from honey and nectar, known as if her appearance has burst forth (*bhittvā*) from the moon; with eyes like the petals of the blue lotus, she consoles the living world with alluring gestures and glances. Of whom and to what is the relationship? Thus there exists in impurity the erroneous idea of purity. (PYŚ 2.5)

This erroneous perception is countered with a quoted verse that illustrates the *aśubha* state of the body, which is in fact impure (*aśuca*) and disgusting to the utmost degree (*paramabībhatsa*). The *Pātañjalayogaśāstra* quotes,

> 'Because of its state, its origin (seed), its excitation/strength, its emissions, its death, and its assignation to [becoming] pure, paṇḍits know the body to be impure.' (PYŚ 2.5)[64]

It is difficult to arrive at any other conclusion than Patañjali's formula is a response to the Buddhist doctrine of the four errors, in which *aśubhabhāvanā*,[65] a distinctly visual form of meditation, is a counterstate to the problem of misperception. Of course, the doctrinal underpinnings in the *Pātañjalayogaśāstra* and the *Yogācārabhūmiśāstra* are different, in that Sāṃkhya proposes a world that *is* permanent and has a fixed self. Yet both texts share a paradigmatic presentation of the four errors of perception using the structural metaphor YOGA IS CLEAR VISION.

The above comparison of intertextual metaphors and paradigms shows that Pātañjala yoga and yogācāra shared a view of *yogabhāvanā*, or yogic cultivation, as the meditative application of a counterstate to an unwanted state. Both the *Pātañjalayogaśāstra* and the *Yogācārabhūmiśāstra* promote practices that are designed according to common understandings of goal and process. What is one doing in yoga discipline? One is remedying the self of psychological poisons (YOGA IS AN ANTIDOTE), applying oneself in forward motion towards an end destination (YOGA IS A PATH) and increasing the clearness of one's mental perceptual field (YOGA IS CLEAR VISION). In the seed metaphors examined in Chapter 2, we also saw the mechanism of the counterstate at work: for example, in the injunction to uproot bad growth in the self and to replace it with good growth or to replace the propagative seeds of *kleśa* with ones that are sterile. In combination, these conceptual metaphors centred on '*yoga*' and '*kleśa*' created a conceptually integrated scheme, the cultivation of the counterstate (*pratipakṣabhāvanā*).

Conclusions

The conceptual models of SEED/ANTIDOTE/PATH/VISION are not exclusive and demonstrate some conceptual inconsistencies – but they do share a common entailment: an unwanted factor can only be removed by applying the *appropriate* counterstate. In this sense, we may think of *pratipakṣabhāvanā* as a practice of applying an appropriate counterstate continuously or repeatedly. Overall, the presentation of yoga as the overcoming of the obstacles appears to draw on two different strands of ascetic-philosophical thought. We are returned again to the notion of at least two traditions compounded in the *Pātañjalayogaśāstra* – and reminded of Sarbacker's categories of the numinous and the cessative (Sarbacker 2005). One paradigm of 'obstacles' is epistemological and appears to be more archaic: it is the discourse that frames the obstacle in terms of knowledge and ignorance and terms it *āvaraṇa*, the obstruction of vision. The other discourse is ontological and appears to be a subsequent innovation: it is the discourse that frames the obstacles as impediments to progress on the path, and both yoga and yogācāra conceive of the problem as obstacle (*antarāya*), specifically a physical impediment. In the *Pātañjalayogaśāstra*, the context of the *antarāya*s is closely connected to that of *pratipakṣabhāvanā* and the *mārga* soteriology of Buddhism, while the context of the *āvaraṇa*s (obscurants) is more closely associated with Sāṃkhya philosophy, which rests on liberation as correct or clear perception.

This chapter has highlighted how the soteriological discourse of the *Pātañjalayogaśāstra* and the *Yogācārabhūmiśāstra* are intricately intertwined through shared conceptual metaphors and image-schema. This is particularly reflected in a mutual understanding of yogic meditation as the (mental and ethical) cultivation of the opposites, *pratipakṣabhāvanā*. The structural and textual parallels that I have outlined in this chapter, in relation to a theory of yoga as *pratipakṣabhāvanā*, suggest that Patañjali may have had access to or knowledge of earlier independent yogācāra texts in circulation, such as the *Śrāvakabhūmi*, the *Bhāvanāmayī Bhūmiḥ* or the early **Yogācārabhūmi* of Saṅgharakṣa.

5

Who put the classical in 'classical yoga'? The inadequacy of an analytical category

Introduction

Having established that the *Pātañjalayogaśāstra* co-evolved conceptually in relation to a range of Buddhist texts – from Abhidharma *śāstra* literature to yogācāra meditation manuals to Mahāyāna *sūtra*s – I will now take a wider purview on the term 'classical yoga'. 'Classical yoga' is a ubiquitous category not only in the study of South Asian religion and philosophy or the coalescing academic field of 'yoga studies' but also in global yoga culture. 'Classical yoga'[1] is broadly used to refer to the *Yogasūtra* of Patañjali and hence to a 'singular' concept and practice of yoga in South Asia in the early first millennium CE. Here, I interrogate the category of 'classical yoga' by identifying its historical provenance as an anglophone term and questioning its historical appropriateness for the South Asian context. A thorough deconstruction of the term 'classical yoga' in contemporary culture is a subject for future research, but this chapter examines historical evidence to show that the primary criteria implicit in 'classical yoga' are a poor match for the distinctiveness of South Asian culture and history. In the closing chapter of this book, I explore alternative epistemic criteria for discussing what is and is not 'classical yoga'.

'Classical yoga' is a Eurocentric category of Indian religion and philosophy that has maintained intellectual currency from oriental scholarship to present-day contexts. Although Singleton (2008) has directly addressed historical factors in the affirmation of the *Pātañjalayogaśāstra* as a classical text in order to make it 'a fit participant in an explicitly European hermeneutic and philosophical colloquy' (Singleton 2008: 82), to date scholarly critiques of the category of 'classical yoga' have been limited. This chapter explores how the category of 'classical yoga' came to be as an anglophone scholarly label during the colonial era. The development of this label was shaped by the interplay of divergent cultural forces, motivations and ideologies, and there were separate strands of 'classical yoga' as a historical, religious, philosophical, aesthetic and cultural signifier, not only 'externally' applied as a retrospective orientalist label but also 'internally' generated and utilized within modern anglophone Indian literary, religious and philosophical discourse.

In unravelling the formation of the category of 'classical yoga' in the European scholarly imagination, this chapter traces the impact of nineteenth-century discussions by European figures such as Colebrooke and Hegel upon the early-twentieth-century scholarship of modern Indian philosophers such as Radhakrishnan and Mukerji. This entails examining how the orientalist category of 'the classical' intersected with Indian value systems of 'high culture', including the cultural status of Sanskrit, the intellectual privileging of *śāstra* literature, medieval doxographies of the philosophical systems, the representation of the Gupta period in Indian history as a 'golden age' and late-nineteenth-century Indian nationalist motivations. The category of 'classical yoga' as a Eurocentric label appears to have gained currency *implicitly* in the late-eighteenth-century European comparisons of Indian philosophical texts to Greek counterparts. This epistemic imposition was, in part, a reflection of the neoclassical trend in European culture and was an attempt to positively appraise the merit of Indian philosophy and literature and to tame its 'otherness' by assigning it a familiar Eurocentric qualitative value. Indeed, the category of 'classical yoga' remained implicit for much of the early nineteenth century, since European enquiries into the philosophy of yoga were either focused on Sāṃkhya as a 'pure' and superior form of philosophy (e.g. Colebrooke's analysis)[2] or were focused on yoga in the *Bhagavad Gītā*. The *Yogasūtra* itself did not garner significant critical attention until its translation into European languages began in the mid-nineteenth century by Ballantyne and Shastri. It was not until the early twentieth century that the label 'classical yoga' began appearing explicitly, concurrently in the works of anglophone Indian philosophers and European indologists. Contrary to my initial working hypothesis, the academic category of 'classical yoga' did not arise in the discourse of study of religions but rather in disciplinary approaches of literature and philosophy.

The first part of this chapter traces the historical development of the term 'classical yoga' in European colonialist discourse, and the second part considers developments in Modern Indian Philosophy that employed the conservative descriptor 'classical' as a tool for reconfiguration of the international philosophical canon – albeit one that would not bear fruit for years to come.

The yoga 'canon'

Within academic scholarship on and popular conceptions of yoga, there is a transnational canon of key texts. Alter broadly defined this canon as the *Yogasūtra*, the *Yoga Upaniṣads*, the *Bhagavad Gītā*, the *Haṭhayogapradīpikā*, the *Śivasaṃhitā* and the *Gherandasaṃhitā* (Alter 2004: x), pointing to the constructed, that is, artificial, nature of such a canon:

> Yoga philosophy has never existed as a fixed, primordial entity, even though the canonical status of a few primary texts gives this impression. (Alter 2004: 4)

Embedded within such canonization is the myth of continuity. One of Alter's questions from 2004 still holds true: how do we tackle 'the assumption in all Orientalist scholarship' that 'the classical texts dealing with Yoga provide a "gold standard" that can be used to measure the relative authenticity of various kinds of practice'? (Alter 2004: 18). Such canonical hegemony has recently been addressed in several research projects. The Haṭha Yoga Project[3] sought to expand the narrow definition of a premodern ('classical *haṭhayoga*') canon by creating accessible critical editions of hitherto unexamined texts that may have had significant cultural impetus (Mallinson 2020a and 2020b; Birch 2019a and 2019b). This project also sought to blur the religious demarcation of the yoga canon by positing that the earliest textual record of codified *haṭhayoga* practices occurs not in the Hindu tradition but in the *Amṛtasiddhi*, a Buddhist Vajrayāna source from *c.* the eleventh century (Mallinson 2020b).[4] Other ongoing research seeks to disrupt the hegemonic role for Sanskrit in both Eurocentric and Indocentric canons of yoga texts (e.g. Cantú 2021, which examines Bengali and Tamil works on yoga).

What does the 'classical' in 'classical yoga' *mean*?

There are several ways in which the Eurocentric term 'classical' operates in the category of 'classical yoga': as a descriptive bracket of historical periodization, as a means of alignment to 'classical' Greco-Roman philosophy and as a value-laden aesthetic cultural category in European neoclassicism. All of these attributions are problematic. Firstly, periodization is itself a controversial process. Secondly, the identification of 'classical' yoga was part of a larger enterprise of categorizing religion and philosophy, fuelled by the Enlightenment emphasis on creating individuated disciplines of knowledge. Thirdly, neoclassical fashions in Europe were bound up with the values of colonialism's 'civilizing' force. Therefore, we should question the appropriateness of the European parameters of the 'classical' for Indic history.

What does the 'yoga' in 'classical yoga' *mean*?

I have identified three major premises that underpin the general use of the term 'classical yoga' in transnational scholarly thought:

1. 'Classical yoga' has been associated with one text, the *Yogasūtra* of Patañjali or the *Pātañjalayogaśāstra*.[5] Despite the narrowness of Alter's overall yoga canon, the canon for 'classical yoga' is even more delimited and is populated by just one text: the *Yogasūtra* of Patañjali.[6] This chapter highlights key historical processes by which the *Yogasūtra* came to be designated as *the* text of 'classical yoga' and questions the exclusiveness of this association.[7] (It's important to note that my discussion of 'classical yoga' as a modern anglophone category is a distinct issue from the *Yogasūtra*'s status as a root text in the orthodox philosophy (*āstika darśana*), a later doxographical designation in Indian scholasticism – and which is not being addressed here. For more on this topic, see Nicholson 2010.)
2. The *Pātañjalayogaśāstra* is identified as the first systematized account of yoga, which distinguishes it from pre-systematized accounts. In this book, Chapters 3, 4 and 5 argue that systematized accounts also exist in Buddhist literature and may predate the Brahmanical formulations in Patañjali's *sūtra* text.
3. The *Pātañjalayogaśāstra*, and thus 'classical yoga', has been associated primarily with the Brahmanic-Hindu religious continuum.

In order to broaden, interrogate and challenge the application of the category 'classical yoga', this study proposes a revision of these premises to produce the following assertions:

1A. 'Classical yoga', as a modern anglophone category, can refer not only to the *Pātañjalayogaśāstra* but also to the *Yogācārabhūmiśāstra* and to other soteriological texts in the early Common Era concerned with aspects of yoga and meditation.

2A. The first systems of yoga discipline are found in a range of texts in the early Common Era, including yogācāra texts (and are somewhat overlapping).

3A. The *Pātañjalayogaśāstra* and other texts of 'classical yoga' reflect input and influence from Brahmanism, Buddhism and Jainism in combination.

Classical periodization and the 'theft of history'

One of the primary functions of the label 'classical' in relation to yoga is historical periodization. By 'classical yoga', we refer to a historical phenomenon (yoga) that thrived in a period designated as the classical era of Indian history. However, within the apparently straightforward identification of such epochal divisions, the label 'classical' is not self-evident but, rather, contested. Historical periods are not 'actual' but are concepts for ordering the past, and so periodization is itself a controversial process: who is authorized to say where the 'classical' period should begin or end in South Asia, and how does this anglophone label relate to Indocentric analyses of history?

The longstanding apparent infallibility of European classicism has been thoroughly deconstructed. For example, in 1970 Foucault's *The Order of Things* critiqued the classical as a historical designation that does not acknowledge ageing and development. Furthermore, since the classical episteme allows no role for time in its view of nature, it was hence suitable for the de-agented 'timelessness' of the colonial conception of the Indian subcontinent (Said 1978). The historian Thapar has also highlighted the implicit biases in this Eurocentric periodic category. She refers to the myths of 'high cultures' and 'golden ages' in European classicism and insists on the likelihood of a plurality of 'classical' periods in any regional history (Thapar 2003: 280–2). Contemporary historiography and critical theory continue to challenge assumptions of classical periodization. Conrad notes that even in the contemporary global history approach, generalization occurs at the expense of local specificities:

> A global history approach cannot be projected indiscriminately; it makes more sense for some periods, places, and processes than for others. Any attempt to contextualise globally needs to consider the degree and quality of the entanglements in its purview. (Conrad 2016: 13)

Moreover, Goody critiques the 'theft of history' by Eurocentric chronologies and 'the way that Europe has stolen the history of the East by imposing its own versions of time (largely Christian) and of space on the rest of the Eurasian world' (Goody 2006: 286).

> [In] the attempts at periodization that historians have made, dividing historical time into Antiquity, Feudalism, the Renaissance, followed by Capitalism ... the west assumes a superiority (which it has obviously displayed in some spheres since the nineteenth century) and projects that superiority back in time, creating a teleological history. (Goody 2006: 286)[8]

South Asian scholars in the colonial period were well aware of these epistemic distortions and foregrounded the arbitrary divisions of historical periods. In his 1923 *History of Indian Philosophy* Volume 1, Radhakrishnan wrote,

> In the absence of accurate chronology, it is a misnomer to call anything a history. Nowhere is the difficulty of getting reliable historical evidence so extreme as in the case of Indian thought. The problem of determining the exact dates of early Indian systems is as fascinating as it is insoluble, and it has furnished a field for the wildest hypotheses, wonderful reconstruction and bold romance. (Radhakrishnan 1923: 9)

The lack of material evidence for texts in early South Asia makes dating and chronology challenging, but this is compounded by Eurocentric labels. Even in a volume dedicated to this issue, *Periodization and Historiography of Indian Philosophy*, Franco notes that consensus is absent – although he surely overstates the case:

> When we come to Indian philosophy we do not even have an established terminology upon which to disagree. No one would know, for instance, what I have in mind if I speak of 'Indian Philosophy in the classical period', or 'in the medieval period', or 'in the scholastic period'. (Franco 2013: vii–1)

'Early', 'middle' and 'late' are often used to sidestep Eurocentric periodization. When categories of religion are added in, however, there are further nuances and benchmarks to consider: 'classical Hinduism' often refers to the *Purāṇas* onwards, while the same period in Buddhism is often called the 'middle period'. Language can represent a watershed, with Jainism divided into a canonical Prakrit and a para- or post-canonical Sanskrit period. For European scholars, the way in which 'classical' was employed to denote a period was intertwined with how the term 'classical' was applied to Sanskrit language and literature – often determined by regularity and rigour in grammar and metrical patterns (e.g. Deussen 1914: 3). Such speculative periodization is typified in indology by Deussen's distinction between the Vedic period and the later classical Sanskrit period, with the intervening period as epic (Deussen 1914: 2–3). Samuel highlights the link between periodization and philology to create 'orthogenetic' narratives of the history of religion, which emphasize chronological continuity and the arrangement of 'texts in a presumed historical sequence of development' (Samuel 2008: 18). On the basis of historical periodization alone, then, we have reason to question the validity of the application of the European 'classical' to categorize a yoga philosophy tract produced in South Asia *c.* the fourth century CE.

Setting these theoretical problems aside for now, what does the 'classical' bracket point to for our context? Despite Franco's misgivings about scholarly consensus, there are broad agreements about the classical period of South Asian history. 'Classical' is typically used to designate a time period of roughly a millennium, from around the second century BCE to the tenth century CE. In this volume, the 'classical' broadly points to the period of the predominant production of the *sūtra*s and *śāstra*s from approximately third century BCE to seventh century CE but before the flourishing of the commentarial tradition. This is, more than anything, a practical working definition and not intended to be delimiting. Yet even within these broad brushstrokes of periodization, there is a great deal of variation, both among and between Western scholars and South Asian scholars. For Ram-Prasad (2001), the classical age is bounded by the dates for the root *darśana* texts, including Buddhist systems. For Dundas, it is the period from the Mauryan to Gupta empires in which 'classical Jainism' emerges (Dundas 2006: 406). For Mohanty (2000), the classical proceeds up to 900 CE. Larson classifies Vācaspatimiśra as a classical rather than a medieval scholar and describes the period of the classical as extending from 100 CE to the early eleventh century CE (Larson 2018: 6–7).[9]

The classical period of India is often taken to be synonymous with the reign of the Guptas, a period frequently framed as an apex of cultural achievement by Indian and European historians. At its height, the Gupta Empire (319–543 CE) stretched across the northern subcontinent from modern day Assam and Bengal to Gujarat. The Guptas both valorized the past and also embraced sweeping innovations in religious culture, venerating the 'new' gods Viṣṇu and Śiva over the Vedic gods and consciously promoted the 'building of temples and the plastic art, both of which could be used for royal representation' (Witzel 2006: 493). Their reign is presented as a time of flowering of Sanskrit culture, the performing arts, poetry, architecture, canonization of texts such as the *Mahābhārata* and developments in knowledge and learning – including mathematics and the founding of the university of Nālanda. For some Indian historians, the Gupta period was a 'golden age' of India and Hinduism (e.g.

Basham 1975: i; Khandalavala 1991: 8) – or, in more critical Marxist analyses, a period of Gupta imperialism. Depictions of the Gupta era as a classical golden age have also been prevalent in European scholarship:

> For two centuries the Gupta empire dominated India, and this domination marks the high point of classical Indian civilization ... With the coming of the Guptas we find, therefore, socio-economic stability, prosperity, Buddhism a major academic (and land-holding) institution, a dynamic resurgent Hinduism in its classical form, and an environment of intellectual brilliance and sophistication. (Williams 2001: 77–8)

To sum up, given that the classical epoch is conceptually Eurocentric, it is a form of teleological reckoning of time as progressive, in which the start and end points of historical chronology are European superiority (Ancient Greco-Roman culture and capitalism) (Goody 2006: 286). It would therefore be more useful to link India's cultural output in this period to its own historical and self-referential discourses and categories and not to those of Greco-Roman culture.

Classical yoga in empire

Within contemporary scholarship on Indian religions, there has been a compelling postcolonial critique of the notion of classical religion as a construct of the Enlightenment epistemology of orientalism.[10] Said's landmark study in 1978 posited 'Orientalism' as equal to imperialism. Since then, there has been considerable effort to tease apart these two categories (e.g. see Halbfass 1988). However, as Clarke notes, Europe's initial fascination[11] with Indian religions in the late eighteenth century coincided with the expansion of empire, and the European acquisition of cultural knowledge was part and parcel of the acquisition of material resources and land in colonized territories (Clarke 1997: 26).[12] Let us now look at the early European encounters with the *Yogasūtra* to assess how it was initially understood by scholars to fit within the contemporaneous frame of classical European religion and philosophy.

The conception of 'classical yoga'

White (2014) has described the translation and reception of the *Yogasūtra* in European languages and the effect this had on European 'high society'. However, although White looked at the reception history of the *Yogasūtra* and its canonization in the Western academy, he did not trace the specific discursive construction of this text in relation to the 'classical'. I will attempt to do that here.

The earliest translation into English of the *Yogasūtra* was Ballantyne's partial translation of the first two chapters in 1852–3 with 'illustrative extracts' from the commentary of the tenth-century commentator Bhojarāja. In his preface, Ballantyne refers to the 'great body of Hindu Philosophy' comprised of 'six sets of very concise Aphorisms' (Ballantyne 1852: i), but he makes no mention of a 'classical yoga'. Banerjee and Mullins compiled summaries of yoga from Ballantyne's version, but the translation itself was finished by Govinda Shastri Deva in 1871 and published in a Benares magazine called *The Pandit*.[13] In 1883, Rajendralal Mitra's learned introduction to his translation of the *Yogasūtra* for the Royal Asiatic Society makes no mention of Pātañjala yoga as 'classical'. He does, however, contribute to the nineteenth-century trend of situating Patañjali's text in relation to classical Greek authors – for instance, by comparing 'purusha, chitta and ahankāra' (consciousness, mind and ego) to concepts of Plato and Aristotle (Mitra 1883: lviii-lix). To understand the European construction of 'classical yoga', then, we need to first consider another text.

Bhagavad Gītā, the classical and yoga

The earliest European discussions of the topic of yoga in Indian religion and philosophy were focused not on the *Yogasūtra*, but on the *Bhagavad Gītā*, and we must consider the European reception of these two texts as intertwined in relation to 'classical yoga'. The first direct translation of a Sanskrit work into a European language was British scholar Wilkins's *Bhagavad Gītā* into English in 1785. Wilkins's choice of translating the *Bhagavad Gītā* section of the *Mahābhārata* reflects the high value placed upon this text by the Brahmins with whom he worked in Benares. In the introduction, Wilkins wrote, 'The Brahmans esteem this work to contain all the grand mysteries of their religion' (Wilkins 1785: 23). The preface to Wilkins's translation was written by the first governor general of British East India (Bengal), Hastings, who was, in general, laudatory about the literary merits of the *Bhagavad Gītā*, contextualizing it with the epic and classical works of Europe:

> I should not fear to place, in opposition to the best French versions of the most admired passages of the Iliad or Odyssey, or of the 1st and 6th books of our own Milton, highly as I venerate the latter, the English translation of the Mahābhārat. (Wilkins 1785: 10)

Wilkins's *Bhagavad Gītā* was quickly translated into other European languages including German, where the text was championed in the early Sturm und Drang of German Romanticism.[14] Meanwhile Lanjuinais translated the text into French, commenting:

> It was a great surprise to find among these fragments of an extremely ancient epic poem from India, along with the system of metempsychosis, a brilliant theory on the existence of God and the immortality of the soul, all the sublime doctrines of the Stoics, the pure love which bewildered Fénelon, a completely spiritual pantheism, and finally the vision of all-in-God upheld by Malebranche. (cited in Schwab 1984: 71)[15]

Following Schlegel's positive appraisal of Indian religious literature,[16] Humboldt lectured on the *Gītā* in 1825–6 at the Royal Prussian Academy of Sciences, Berlin.[17] In these lectures, Humboldt praised the *Gītā* as a work 'so rich of philosophical ideas' and 'the most beautiful, presumably the only real philosophical poem of all known literatures'.[18] At the beginning of the nineteenth century in Europe, then, the text of the *Bhagavad Gītā* and its inherent doctrines on yoga was held in high esteem by European scholars, who both associated this yoga text with the classical eminence of Greco-Roman literary and philosophical works and also identified the *Gītā* as part of a primordial and pure *ur*-culture that had given birth to all other cultures. It is worth emphasizing that, by far, the predominant notions of 'classical' and 'yoga' in association were centred on the *Gītā* and not on the *Pātañjalayogaśāstra*.

'Fanatical' not 'classical'

The first record of situating Patañjali's text in relation to the European classical is found in the writings of Jones,[19] who in an absurdly forced comparative frame, likens yoga to stoicism and Patañjali to Zeno:[20]

> Of the philosophical schools it will be sufficient here to remark that this first Nyāya seems analogous to the Peripatetic; the second, sometimes called the Vaiçeshika, to the Ionic; the two Mímámsás, of which the second is often distinguished by the name of Vedânta, to the Platonic; the first Sánkhya, to the Italic; and the second or Pátanjala, to the Stoic philosophy: so that Gautama corresponds with Aristotle; Kanâda with Thales; Jaimini, with Socrates; Vyása, with Plato; Kapila, with Pythagoras; and Patanjali, with Zeno. But an accurate comparison between the Grecian and Indian schools would require a considerable volume. (Jones 1799, 1: 360–1)

However, the introduction of Patañjali's *Yogasūtra* to European audiences in any detail began in 1823 when Colebrooke[21] initiated a series of lectures titled 'On the Philosophy of the Hindus' to the Royal Asiatic Society in London, in which he outlined the systems of philosophy, or *darśanas*.[22] Colebrooke's first description of the *Yogasūtra* in his lectures was far from positive. In contrast to the proper philosophy of Sāṃkhya, he denounced the *Yogasūtra* as 'fanatical' and he labelled the yogin 'a vulgar apprehension, a sorcerer' (Colebrooke 1858: 158).[23] This characterization of the *Yogasūtra* as debased, fanatical magic was quite remote from the classical compliments showered on the *Bhagavad Gītā*. Yet, despite his denigrating tone, the seed for the association of the *Yogasūtra* with the high culture of the classical was also present.[24] In Colebrooke's mind there was no doubt of a cultural transmission between Greek and Indian thought, with the Greeks 'indebted to Indian instructors' (Colebrooke 1873: 436–7). The cosmologies of Greece and India aligned so that Pythagoras and Ocellus 'agree precisely with the Hindus' (Colebrooke 1873: 441), and 'Pythagoras and his successors held the doctrine of metempsychosis, as the Hindus universally do the same tenet of transmigration of souls' (Colebrook 1873: 442). However, in particular, Colebrooke was interested in parallels between Greek and Sāṃkhya systems:

> Like the Hindus, Pythagoras, with other Greek philosophers, assigned a subtle ethereal clothing to the soul apart from the corporeal part, and a grosser clothing to it when united with the body; the *súkshma* (or *linga*) *çarira* and *sthúla çarira* of the Sánkhyas and the rest. … I should be disposed to conclude that the Indians were in this instance teachers rather than learners. (Colebrooke 1873: 442)

This idea of Indian origins for specific Greek tenets gained traction in Europe over the nineteenth century. Wilson also speculated, in his 1837 preface to Colebrooke's translation of *Sāṃkhyakārikā* and in Wilson's own translation of the commentary by Gauḍapāda, that Indian systemic thought lent ideas to the Greeks. Wilson was curious to which 'degree the speculations of Plato and Aristotle correspond with those of Kapila and Gautama' (Wilson 1837: ix):

> As far as we are acquainted with the tenets of the Ionic and Italic schools, it is with them that Hindu philosophy, unalloyed with Hindu pantheism, seems to claim kindred, rather than with the mysticism of Plato, or the subtleties of Aristotle. (Wilson 1837: x)

Such comparisons gained impetus in ensuing decades; for instance, Barthelmy's *Premier Mémoire sur le Sânkhya* in 1852 continued to argue that Greek philosophy was influenced by Indian (Barthelmy 1852: 512–13; 521–2).

The ambivalence in the European classification of yoga as both 'fanatical' and 'classical' is most visibly reflected in the work of Hegel. In 1827, Hegel published two essays on the *Gītā* in which he not only critiqued Humboldt's positive assessments but also drew on Colebrooke's 'On the Philosophy of the Hindus' to incorporate reflections on the *Yogasūtra*. There is a significant difference between Hegel's attitude to yoga in the essays published as 'First Article' and 'Second Article', and the development of his analysis on the subject is made evident by highlighting some key passages. In the first essay, Hegel dismissed Indian soteriology[25] and strongly denied the fitness of any comparison with the Greeks. He characterized Indian thought as immature and superstitious and not as philosophy proper – yoga was religion and Sāṃkhya was philosophy:

> The path which philosophy is directed to, shows itself entirely peculiar and valuable when comparing it with the path which Indian religion partly prescribes, partly compromisingly tolerates when itself taking the turn to the elevation of the Yoga conception. Hence one would do utterly wrong to Indian philosophy, which is Sāṅkhya doctrine, if one would judge it and its procedure by that what has been said above, what is called Sāṅkhya doctrine in the Bhagavad-Gītā and what does not go beyond the common, popular-religious views. ('First Article', trans. Herring 1995: 29)

In the second essay Hegel identified yoga as the central doctrine of the *Bhagavad Gītā*.

> The informations [*sic*] which the lecture at hand contain are all the more interesting as they do not deal with some particular aspect of the immense manifold of Indian mythology, but predominantly with the *Yoga doctrine*, the nucleus of the religion of this people, which comprises the essence of their religion as well as its most sublime concept of God. This doctrine is the fundamental idea prevailing throughout the entire poem. ('Second Article', trans. Herring 1995: 33)

However, Hegel dismissed any 'misunderstanding' that this yoga doctrine is systematically developed; rather it is 'a mystical doctrine' that 'embraces only a few statements and assertions' ('Second Article', trans. Herring 1995: 33).[26] Yet Hegel's final assessment of yoga in his writings was to place it at the centre of Indian religion *and* philosophy ('Second Article', trans. Herring 1995: 39), even offering a somewhat modern caution on the inappropriate use of terms such as 'penance' to translate ascetic acts, *tapas*.[27] The extent of Hegel's volte-face on Indian thought was such that he even compared the *Gītā* to classical Greek literature (Homer),[28] and by his works of 1829–30 he conceded that the fourth chapter of the *Yogasūtra* could be regarded as philosophical.

Such comparison of the *Bhagavad Gītā* with Greco-Roman culture - as expressed by Colebrooke, Hegel and other European scholars - was the first primary driver behind the generation of the concept of 'classical' yoga; more so than a form of periodization, it was used as a standard to measure cultural value. Through its shared topic of yoga with the *Bhagavad Gītā*, the *Yogasūtra* was drawn into this frame of classical cultural comparison, which initially focused on literature, language and philosophy. In addition, the *Yogasūtra* also incurred the value of the classical by its association with the classically designated philosophy of Sāṃkhya. However, as we have seen, the *Yogasūtra* itself was more popularly understood as expressing religion and a fanatical form of religion at that. Even by 1859, Fitzedward Hall's *A Contribution towards an Index to the Bibliography of the Indian Philosophical Systems* reflected a deep resistance to the integration of yoga works into religious decency:

> As few of the twenty-eight Yoga works which have fallen under my inspection are at present read, so, one may hope, few will ever again be read, either in this country or by curious enquirers in Europe. If we exclude the immundities of the *Tantras* and of the *Kāma-śāstra*, Hindu thought was never more unworthily engaged than in digesting into an economy the fanatical vagaries of theocracy. (Hall, *Contributions*, XI; cited in Mitra 1883: lv–lvi)

Yet as the nineteenth century progressed, there was a growing European interest in the *yoga darśana* as philosophy, and so the trend of Greco-Roman comparison continued apace.

Classical literature and the Indo-Greek debates

In his influential 'Six Systems of Indian Philosophy' in 1899, Müller wrote that 'the real object of what was originally meant by philosophy' was 'an explanation of the world'. He added:

> This determining idea has secured even to the guesses of Thales and Heraclitus their permanent place among the historical representatives of the development of philosophical thought by the side of Plato and Aristotle, of Des Cartes and

> Spinoza. It is in that Walhalla of real philosophers that I claim a place of honour for the representatives of the Vedânta and Sâmkhya. (Müller 1919: xvi)

Here, again, we see the emphatic identification of Indian schools of thought with the classical Greek tradition. Müller's assessment of the status of yoga as a philosophical activity – gleaned from his 'native' informant – was that yoga was 'neglected ... except in its purely practical and most degenerate form' (Müller 1919: xviii). Yet in his rebuttal of Weber's argument that the Greek concept of *logos* was derived from the Indian *vāc*, Müller separated Greek and Indian thinkers, referring to 'classical *and* Sanskrit scholars' (Müller 1919: 56, my emphasis). Müller therefore reserved the term 'classical' primarily for Indian literature, particularly the Vedic Upaniṣads (in order to distinguish them from the later Upaniṣads). In a section titled 'Literary References in the Upanishads', he stated,

> Of the technical names of the six systems of philosophy, two only occur in the classical Upanishads, namely Sâmkhya and Yoga, or Sâmkhya-yoga. (Müller 1919: 84)[29]

Yet even though he applied the term 'classical' only to literary texts, the above passage reflects the implicit designation of Sāṃkhya and Yoga as part of the classical domain.[30] Müller did refer to the 'six classical or orthodox systems' (Müller 1919: 91) and 'the six classical philosophies of India' (Müller 1919: 114),[31] but in all instances he used the label 'classical' at the generic level of a corpus (Upaniṣads; the six *āstika* systems) and not in relation to an individual school of thought, including yoga.

Similarly, in his 1896 essay 'Sāṃkhya and Yoga', Garbe referred to 'klassischen Sanskritlitteratur' on several occasions but not to classical yoga – even if he was convinced that Sāṃkhya-Yoga exerted an influence on Neo-Platonism. What is interesting about Garbe's contribution, however, is that it was part of a wider conversation in the 1890s, which we might refer to as the Indo-Greek debates. These were arguments that went much further than the earlier fledgling claims by Colebrooke, Wilson and Barthelmy that Indian thought had influenced Greek; rather there were intensified and more granular claims about similarities in the concepts of Indian and Greek sources and vexed discussions about which came first. Garbe was firmly of the view that Greek ideas were derived from Indian. In *Philosophy of Ancient India*, he devoted a whole chapter to 'The Connexion between Indian and Greek Philosophy':

> It is a question requiring the most careful treatment to determine whether the doctrines of the Greek philosophers ... were really first derived from the Indian

> world of thought, or whether they were constructed independently of each other in both India and Greece, their resemblance being caused by the natural sameness of human thought. For my part, I confess I am inclined towards the first opinion. (Garbe 1897: 37)

Focusing on the Eleatics and Epicurus as probably influenced by Indian concepts, Garbe had 'no doubt' about Pythagoras's dependence on Indian thought, 'and all the more so, as the Greeks themselves considered his doctrines as foreign' (Garbe 1897: 39). Drawing on Lassen's work, Garbe was assured of connections between Indian philosophy and both Christian Gnosticism and Neo-Platonism, due to 'lively relations between Alexandria and India' (Garbe 1897: 46). However, where Lassen argued for the influence of Buddhism on the cosmogony of Christian Gnosticism and on the doctrines of soul and matter, Garbe disagreed and suggested instead that such influence should, in fact, be credited to Sāṃkhya (Garbe 1897: 47). Garbe, then, went further to claim that beyond obvious reliance of Plotinus on the '*pure* Sâṃkhya' doctrine (his italics),[32] there existed 'an even closer connexion' with '*that* branch of the Sâṃkhya philosophy which has assumed a theistical and ascetical character, and has, under the name of the Yoga philosophy, acquired an independent place among the Brahman systems' (Garbe 1897: 50). Hence, for Garbe, Yoga was a branch of Sāṃkhya and most likely the direct source of influence on Neo-Platonism:

> Plotinus pronounces all *worldly* things to be vain and void of value, and he therefore calls upon us to throw off the influence of the phenomenal world. If we keep off all external impressions and by way of concentration of thinking overcome the multiplicity of ideas, resulting from these impressions, the highest knowledge will fill our mind, in the form of a sudden, ecstatic perception of God. (Garbe 1897: 51)

The 'union with the deity' as described by Plotinus relates directly to the flash (*prātibha*) of knowledge in the *Yogasūtra* (YS 3.33), and it is from the 'Yoga-praxis' that the later Neo-Platonist Abammon derived his idea 'that people who are filled with a holy enthusiasm attain miraculous powers' (Garbe 1897: 52–3). Crucially, Garbe stressed that even though there was a Sāṃkhya influence on Neo-Platonism, Indian philosophy had as a whole been 'entirely omitted' from the Western histories of philosophy. He accounted for this omission thus:

> An explanation of this indifference may be found in the fact that the Indian systems became known in Europe and America only in their roughest outlines

> in this century, and that even now only Buddhism and two Brahman systems, Vedânta and Sâṃkhya, have been laid open to study by detailed works. (Garbe 1897: 55)

Despite, then, the wave of scholarship that drew parallels between Greek and Indian philosophy – with a large contingent of indologists arguing for the derivation of Greek concepts from Indian – Garbe indicates that the academic study of Patañjali's text in European languages had *not* been strongly established by the end of the nineteenth century. Therefore, we shall have to wait until the early twentieth century to see the forging of the anglophone label 'classical yoga'.

Neoclassical literary aesthetics and religious texts

Let's now turn to how the label 'classical' embeds the neoclassical as an aesthetic. The development of late-eighteenth-century orientalist scholarship was also underpinned by the fashion for and cultural aesthetic of the 'neoclassical'. Neoclassicism, a hearkening back to an ideal culture of ancient Greece or Rome, was prominent in European literature, art and archaeology from the seventeenth to the early nineteenth century. Neoclassical literature was strictly codified to follow the rules of Greek poetics, and the literary aesthetic of the period valued simplicity, form, order, harmony, balance, clarity, decorum, restraint, serenity, unity and proportion – together with an emphasis on reason. Classicism in literature held that a writer must be bound by rules, convention and models rather than inferior inspiration. A classical work was seen as a work of 'the highest class' or an unsurpassed model of excellence (Baldick 2001. It is essential to consider these aspects of the category 'classical' in nineteenth-century Europe, because orientalist scholars were investigating Asian religions almost exclusively on the basis of texts, and their attitudes to a text's form, style, content and generic identity were thus filtered through a European lens – as Said stated, orientalism was a 'textual attitude' (Said 1978: 93–4). To understand the background of the category of the 'classical' in religion and philosophy, then, we should review something of the application of this category in literature. What we find is that the aesthetic basis of the category 'classical' was infused with a range of assumptions and values, some of which directly contradicted key features of Indian śāstric literary culture.

In the eighteenth century, Europe's literary culture was awash with homage to ancient classical culture,[33] and this predominant intellectual aesthetic was also reflected in the scholarly output. German literary criticism looked back to the ancient models of texts and to rationality, optimism and 'natural law' as well as 'notions of common sense, normality, probability, nature, imitation and rule. Here again beauty, goodness and truth became equated, thus fostering the didactic purpose of literature' (Secretan 1973: 70). In the minds of European intellectuals, such as Gottsched (1700–1766), a promoter of German as a literary language, there was a continuity from ancient Greco-Roman culture to the present day: 'The nature of man and the strength of his mind is the same as it was two thousand years ago: consequently, the way to poetic pleasure must be the same as that which the ancients chose so appropriately' (cited in Secretan 1973: 70).

Against this backdrop, the translation of Sanskrit works took place not only into other classical languages – the Upaniṣads were first translated into Latin after all[34] – but also into classical form. For his own collection of verse, Jones adapted the European poetic mode of the ode to render Sanskrit hymns to Viṣṇu. Since the ode is a classical form in Greek literature, we can analyse this as part of the colonial project of 'anglicizing' Hinduism in part through 'literary annexation' (Teltscher 1995: 210–11), making Hinduism 'familiar' as part of an epistemic takeover (Johnson 2011: 51–2). In the preface to his 'translation' of a Vedic hymn to the sun god Sūrya, Jones wrote that the 'personification of the Sun will account for nearly the whole system of the *Egyptian*, *Indian* and *Grecian* polytheism' (Jones 1807, XIII: 365). Nonetheless, Jones became tired of the 'recycled classicism' of European poetry (Johnson 2011: 49) and explicitly aimed to expand European classicism to include 'the East'. He suggested repeatedly 'that a Europe deadened by its obsession with classical Greece and Rome look further east, to Persia and India, for new inspiration' (Mulholland 2013: 23).[35] The designation of an Indian text as 'classical' conveyed an aesthetic judgment of a work as harmonious, well-proportioned, balanced, unified and simple. Such neoclassical markers affected style, form and language in translation from Sanskrit. This was true beyond the work of Jones; in Schlegel's rendering of 'about one-fifth of the *Gita* in metrical German', the 'pattern of his selections and omissions is significant' (Davis 2015: 90). Amongst other themes, Schlegel omitted the teaching on *bhakti yoga* and emphasized *jñana yoga* – thus highlighting the rational aspect of yoga (in line with neoclassical values) 'uncluttered by conflicting perspectives' (Davis 2015: 90).

On the surface, the applicability of neoclassical aesthetic markers to a Brahmanical *sūtra* would appear commensurable; a *sūtra* text is, after all, set out as a logical and well-formed discourse that crystallizes and encapsulates a field of thought. Nonetheless, there are core features of śāstric literary and intellectual culture that cannot be expressed within the narrow limits of Eurocentric aesthetics. The *Yogasūtra* is not an epitome of classical coherence as dictated by European ideals; rather its formal efficacy is defined by other factors – such as synthetic stratification, conceptual condensation and formal reasoning in the Indian tradition. Indic texts in this period often collated different strata of material, and the *śāstra* genre bolstered authority by aligning itself to precedent. Thus, the *Pātañjalayogaśāstra* has a composite editorial character and, accordingly, does not present a monolithic or singular definition of yoga. Indeed, the text's description of yoga is more plural and polyvalent than is often asserted. We encounter *nirodha*, *kaivalya*, *kriyā yoga*, *aṣṭāṇga yoga*, *asaṃprajṇāta samādhi*, *nirbīja samādhi*, *saṃyama*, *cittam ekāgram*, *dharmameghasamādhi*[36] – all presented as paramount techniques of yoga. Yet these techniques often jostle for primacy and do not necessarily sit together in a neat synthetic unity, and because the purpose of *śāstra* was often to function as a compendium, there is no reason why the contents of the *Pātañjalayogaśāstra* should be internally 'absolutely' unified. Furthermore, the 'simplicity' that we encounter in a *sūtra* text is disarming – since the brevity is not a marker of accessibility, but rather a paradoxical concealment of greater depth and complexity. The brevity of the *sūtra* format is a pragmatic tool for memorization of an extended body of teachings, hence behind the concise *sūtra* floats a mass of conceptual content which only the privileged can gain access to historically (e.g. those with knowledge of Sanskrit, those who were literate, those with access to particular teachers, those who lived in particular time periods, those who belonged to the right social class). Thus European 'classical' aesthetic markers such as coherence and simplicity may indeed apply to a śāstric text, but only in a somewhat superficial way. The cultural significance of such values was vastly different between, say, the medieval Indian doxographers and the early oriental scholars. Both communities of scholars venerated the 'high culture' to which the *Yogasūtra* belonged but qualified that high culture along entirely different lines.

The omission of Buddhist texts from 'classical yoga'

There are two sides to this line of investigation: the promotion of Pātañjala yoga as 'classical' rested on the neglect, omission or denial of the contemporary Buddhist *Yogācārabhūmiśāstra* as equivalently classical.

There are several key factors in Indian cultural history that informed the categorical separation of Buddhist yogācāra from Pātañjala yoga. This included both the way in which yogācāra developed more formally as a philosophical school from the middle of the first millennium CE, as well as the cultural import of the Indian doxographies. The premodern Indian doxographies were texts that systematically ordered Indian religious and philosophical bodies of thought into clearly demarcated schools. In these doxographies, six orthodox (*āstika*) *darśanas* were identified and each had its own root text, which was a *sūtra* (Nicholson 2010; Maas 2013). These doxographies placed Buddhism as an unorthodox (*nāstika*) philosophy in a different category – although scholars have recently challenged this neat distinction of *āstika* and *nāstika* in doxographical Hinduism (Nicholson 2010).

One basis for the European understanding of 'yoga' in South Asian traditions was through the prism of Indian doxographies which 'segregated' Buddhist thought from *āstika* schools. Another basis was the interaction of the orientalists with Brahmin scholars who may have had mixed attitudes in representing Buddhist texts to Europeans – Buddhism having long since declined as a major cultural force on the subcontinent. The weak identification of 'classical' Buddhist texts in the Eurocentric frame may also have been due to literary style; while a Brahmanical *sūtra* text was perceived to conform to neoclassical parameters, the more florid and expansive Mahāyāna *sūtra* style did not quite fit with the European classical aesthetic. Indeed, the sprawling and extensive format of the *Yogācārabhūmiśāstra* would not have easily lent itself to the aesthetic criteria of the neoclassical as a streamlined and uncluttered cultural artefact. Additionally, in orientalist scholarship, Buddhism was excluded from discussions of yoga, in part, due to the post-Enlightenment taxonomy of religions in which the emphasis was on distinct dividing lines rather than imbricated worldviews and practices.[37] Indeed, orientalist scholars represented Indian Buddhism in a different way than Hinduism; Buddhism was seen to be more relatable to the orientalist scholars' own cultural framework, which identified Protestantism as a rational, reformed Christianity that morally superceded the older, corrupt and non-rational Catholicism (Schopen 1991). Accordingly, oriental scholars who discussed 'classical Buddhist religion' prioritized Theravāda texts, perceived to be earlier and more original than the 'later' Mahāyāna stream of Buddhism, to which the *Yogācārabhūmiśāstra* belongs.[38] Nevertheless, such cultural factors in colonial times do not fully account for the oversight of the *Yogācārabhūmiśāstra* in formulations of 'classical yoga', which is a more complex story rooted in the development of academic yogācāra studies.

Wrestling with the *Yogācārabhūmiśāstra*

In comparison to the *Yogasūtra*, the *Yogācārabhūmiśāstra* was encountered by European scholars at a later date and was characterized by a range of distinct features that limited its accessibility – even until the present day. As discussed in Chapter 3, the *Yogācārabhūmiśāstra* is a voluminous treatise and in any language is, as Delhey describes it, 'bulky' (Delhey 2013: 498), making it a challenging text to analyse in comparison to the compact *Yogasūtra* or even the *Pātañjalayogaśāstra*. Furthermore, the *Yogācārabhūmiśāstra* is not fully extant in Sanskrit; Delhey recently estimated that only around 50 per cent of the text had survived in Sanskrit manuscripts (Delhey 2013: 508).[39] Rather, this *śāstra* has been preserved in full in Chinese and Tibetan. Hence, the study of this text has been somewhat limited to scholars of Buddhism who had access to the requisite languages.[40]

The first attempts at critical editions of the extant portions of the *Yogācārabhūmiśāstra* date to Wogihara's edition of the *Bodhisattvabhūmi* in the 1930s, some years after he had first begun transcribing the manuscript at Cambridge. (See Appendix 3 for a list of all sections of the *śāstra*.) Subsequent key critical editions in Sanskrit were Bhattacharya's partial edition of the *Yogācārabhūmi* in 1957 (containing the first five books/foundations, or *bhūmi*s, out of seventeen) and Wayman's 1961 partial edition and analysis of the *Śrāvakabhūmi*. These editions became outdated as more manuscripts and manuscript fragments were discovered in the latter half of the twentieth century. However, even today, one cannot simply pick up a Sanskrit critical edition – or even an English translation – of the *Yogācārabhūmiśāstra* but rather has to piece it together from a range of works, articles and chapters that contain published critical editions of sections of the work.[41] Equally, scholarship on the *Yogācārabhūmiśāstra* has remained piecemeal and fragmented, often concentrated in Japanese or Korean language scholarship.

Twentieth-century academic study of the *Yogācārabhūmiśāstra* was therefore dogged by the lack of extant manuscripts, legibility of manuscripts, restricted access even to poor quality photos of manuscripts and incomplete critical editions that were published slowly, often over decades. A further complicating factor was that the Indian commentaries on the *Yogācārabhūmiśāstra* did not survive and, as Delhey states, 'a significant amount of the vocabulary of the YoBh is not covered by the general dictionaries of the Sanskrit language' (Delhey 2013: 514), necessitating scholars to rely on other resources such as Edgerton's *Buddhist Hybrid Sanskrit Dictionary* or Bechert et al.'s *Sanskrit-Wörterbuch der buddhistischen Texte aus den Turfan-Funden und der kanonischen Literatur der Sarvāstivāda-Schule.* All of these factors of effort meant that, in the twentieth-century, study of the *Yogācārabhūmi* was the preserve of those who were willing to go to great lengths to create critical editions or to be proficient in a range of Asian languages to access not only the two intact premodern editions in Tibetan and Chinese[42] but also the secondary scholarship in Japanese and Korean. Today the situation has improved, and there are numerous translations and editions in Asian languages as well as digital editions. The most recent extensive contribution to the field in English has been Kragh's weighty edited volume in 2013, which rivals the *Yogācārabhūmisāśtra* in its comprehensiveness.

Orientalism, 'Jôgâtschâra' and the 'Jôgâtschâryabhûmi çâstra'

There was, then, a significant time lapse in the reception histories of Brahmanical yoga and Buddhist yogācāra in Europe; as discussed above, knowledge of the *Bhagavad Gītā* was assimilated into European academic discourse from the early nineteenth century and part-translations of the *Yogasūtra* were published from the mid-nineteenth century. In contrast, although Burnouf had been translating Pāli texts since the 1820s and wrote the influential 'Introduction a l'histoire du Bouddhisme Indien' in 1844, there was by the mid-nineteenth century only a 'dim knowledge' of the contents and significance of Asaṅga's *Yogācārabhūmiśāstra* among European scholars (Delhey 2013: 504). One example of such limited understanding was the analysis by indologist Koeppen, who included a discussion of Asaṅga's work in his 1859 *Die Religion des Buddha, Volume 2.* Koeppen's skewed assessment was that Asaṅga's *śāstra* was the first source to harmonize the yoga teachings of the Brahmanical Shaivas, characterized by 'magic and mythology', alongside both Mahāyāna philosophy and its theory of meditation (Koeppen 1859: 32). As Delhey points out, Koeppen misunderstood many facets of Buddhism, including mixing up yogācāra with both Buddhist and Shaiva tantra (Koeppen 1859: 25; Delhey 2013: 504 fn 18) and yet Koeppen's views are also interesting. Firstly, they affirm the mid-nineteenth-century European understanding of yoga texts as characterized by 'magic and mythology' and tantra (in this case Shaiva tantra) and the contrastive status of Buddhism as a discipline of reason or philosophy. Koeppen refers to Jôgâtschâra both as a 'school' (Koeppen 1859: 32) and a 'system of mysticism' (Koeppen 1859: table of contents), the latter presumably by association with 'yoga'. He misrepresents yogācāra as a blend of Shaivism and the theory of 'Dhyâni-Buddhas' (Koeppen 1859: 25), that is, the five Buddhas of Vajrayāna Buddhism. Crucially, Koeppen did not have direct access to the *Yogācārabhūmisāśtra* but was piecing together a derivative understanding from other tangential studies.

During the second half of the nineteenth century, European scholarship on yogācāra did not advance significantly. As Wangchuk describes, British indologists such as Hodgson and the Wright brothers collected Sanskrit manuscripts from Nepal throughout the nineteenth century, but it was not until 1883 that they were catalogued by Bendall in the Cambridge University collections (Wangchuk 2007: 357–9). Among these manuscripts was a palm-leaf copy of the *Bodhisattvabhūmi* (one of the earliest and the largest books or portions of the *Yogācārabhūmiśāstra*). It was a Japanese scholar, Wogihara, who first took interest in this manuscript, incorporating it into his dissertation for Strassburg University and eventually publishing the first critical edition of the *Bodhisattvabhūmi* in 1930–6. Meanwhile another *Bodhisattvabhūmi* manuscript, this time on paper, was discovered by Japanese scholar Sakaki in 1914 and was taken to the Kyoto University Library. A further palm-leaf manuscript of the *Bodhisattvabhūmi* – this time along with the *Śrāvakabhūmi* (the likely earliest layer of the *Yogācārabhūmiśāstra*) – was found and photographed in a Tibetan monastery in 1938 by an Indian scholar, Sāṅkṛtāyana, and this *Bodhisattvabhūmi* was again photographed by Italian scholar Tucci in 1939. What is significant about this trajectory of the *Yogācārabhūmi*, or portions thereof, into worldwide scholarship is that

1. Any awareness of Sanskrit manuscripts occurs almost a century after Colebrooke's first paraphrasis translations and expositions of the *Yogasūtra* in English. This also means that the secondary scholarship on Asaṅga's text in European languages only took off from the mid-twentieth century, for example, in the works of de La Vallée Poussin or Demiéville.
2. The earliest work was carried out by Japanese scholars and hence established Japan as a main centre for scholarship on yogācāra outside of India.
3. Since Buddhism was a minority religion in India in the nineteenth century the interest of Indian scholars was somewhat limited, so that although Sāṅkṛtāyana deposited his negatives in the Bihar Research Society in Patna,[43] it was not until 1966 that Nalinaksha Dutt published the first critical edition of the *Bodhisattvabhūmi* to be produced in India.

This different, fragmented and protracted way in which scholarship on the *Yogācārabhūmiśāstra* developed is one key reason why early yogācāra was not discussed within the Eurocentric category of 'classical yoga' as it developed over the nineteenth century.

To sum up, various factors determined the omission of sustained scholarly discussion on Buddhism and yoga in early South Asia, including the precedents of Indian doxography, the attitude of Hindu informants towards Buddhist texts during colonialism, the separatist Enlightenment taxonomy of religions, the slow pace of critical editions and translations into European languages throughout the nineteenth and twentieth centuries, the privileging of Theravāda over Mahāyāna forms of Buddhism in orientalist scholarship, the late-nineteenth-century dismissal of yoga as fanatical religion and its marginalization as a topic for philosophical study, and the literary specificity of Buddhist yogācāra treatises that did not conform to the European neoclassical aesthetic markers.

Modern Indian philosophy and the category of 'classical yoga'

Let's now turn our attention to anglophone Indian scholarship. Within the nineteenth-century Hindu intelligentsia, nationalist concerns fused with the colonial representations of yoga to consolidate the anglophone canonical status of the *Yogasūtra*. Singleton has noted the interplay between orientalist and nationalist motivations:

> The installation of the YS as the Classical Yoga text in the modern age is bound up with several dialectically interlinked, ideological currents. These include colonial translation projects intended to inculcate the critical habits and values of European philosophy in Indian minds via Hindu scripture and subsequent reclamations of these texts by Indian cultural nationalists seeking to identify and interpret the definitive canon of modern Hinduism. (Singleton 2008: 77)

Here, Singleton is pointing to the projects of Indian cultural nationalism that both drew on traditional doxographic models and converged with the European attention to Sanskrit texts in orientalist taxonomy to locate classical yoga as part of Hinduism and not Buddhism. In the early twentieth century, there were fewer and less compelling cultural motives for Indian scholars to point to yogācāra as part of a 'classical' yoga. The religious focus in public discourse was rather on Hinduism, Islam and Christianity and their complex relationships in the crumbling empire and burgeoning Indian nation state. However, it is within this cultural frame that we encounter the first explicit uses of the descriptor 'classical yoga' for Pātañjala yoga.

The 1920s and early 1930s were a prolific time for Modern Indian Philosophy and saw the publication of encyclopaedic multivolume compendia that would inform the anglophone study of Indian philosophy for much of the twentieth century – for example, works by Radhakrishna, Dasgupta, Hiriyanna, Ranade and Bhattacharya. The emergence of Modern Indian Philosophy was linked to the building of an independent cultural identity for a proposed Indian nation state:

> Anglophone Indian philosophy coincides with and contributes to the Indian Renaissance (or Resurgence, as Vivekananda chose to characterize it). Traditional philosophical concerns were linked to the social and political movements that swept India during this period. (Bhushan 2011: 178)

As early as 1909, the philosopher Coomaraswamy stated, 'Our struggle is part of a wider one, the conflict between the ideals of Imperialism and the ideals of Nationalism' (Coomaraswamy 1909: 2). Indeed, Bhushan describes the colonial occupation by the British as one of the key 'axes that produced Anglophone Indian philosophy' generated from a 'politico-cosmopolitan awareness and a distinctive approach to imagining the modern Indian nation in academic and nonacademic philosophical circles' (Bhushan 2011: 170). The early-twentieth-century compendia by Indian scholars often had a comparative agenda to bring Indian and European philosophy into constructive dialogue by (a) showing how European philosophy can be understood through concepts from Indian philosophy[44] and (b) 'prestige showcasing' Indian philosophy in its antiquity. Eventually, this historical trend would be critiqued by Mukerji who wanted simply to 'do philosophy' with Indian traditions and tools and to subject both Indian and European claims to critical scrutiny (Mukerji 1938). Bhushan refers to the early decades of the twentieth century as 'the hey dey of philosophical comparisons' (Bhushan 2011: 174), and I want to suggest that the term 'classical yoga' is a product of this period of cross-cultural comparison – having been implicitly developed by Indian and European scholars and translators in the nineteenth century, the term 'classical yoga' was only explicitly applied and foregrounded by Indian philosophers in the early twentieth century. We will now survey some of these key philosophical works in the modern Indian anglophone tradition.

Let us start with the omissions and variations, which are informative in themselves. Some key works from this period make no mention of classical yoga. Despite dedicating a whole book to Pātañjala yoga – *The Study of Patañjali* in 1920, replete with references to the classical – Dasgupta did not employ the term 'classical yoga'. In his subsequent *A History of Indian Philosophy, Volume 1* (1922), Dasgupta reserves the label 'classical' for Sāṃkhya, especially the *Sāṃkhyakārikā*. Occasionally, he also uses 'classical' in relation to Sanskrit or the Upaniṣads. However, yoga is often implied in Dasgupta's understanding of 'classical Sāṃkhya'. For example, one of his chapters is titled 'The Kapila and Pātañjala Sāṃkhya', which reflects his regard of Pātañjala yoga as a specific type or branch of Sāṃkhya, rather than an independent 'school'. Other omissions are also telling. In Belvalkar and Ranade's *An Encyclopedic History of Indian Philosophy, Volume 2* (1926) the term 'classical' is used often in relation to the Upaniṣads as a genre, but also to describe yoga in *Svetāśvatara Upaniṣad*: 'The second chapter contains a classical description of yoga' (Belvalkar and Ranade 1926: 12). Here, classical yoga was associated with late Vedic traditions, rather than Patañjali's (as it was for many of the nineteenth-century indologists).

However, when we turn to Radhakrishnan's *History of Indian Philosophy* (published in two volumes in 1923 and then revised in 1927 and 1929), we find something different. Radhakrishnan's text is vital to our discussion, since not only does he appear to be the first scholar (that I have so far traced) to use the term 'classical yoga' to refer to Patañjali's text, but he also asserts straightforwardly that yogācāra is a Buddhist expression of yoga. For Radhakrishnan there is no division between yoga and Buddhism. In discussing the Vedic developments of yoga, he states,

> Buddha practised Yoga in both its senses. He underwent ascetic austerities and practised the highest contemplation. According to *Lalitavistara*, numberless forms of ascetic austerities were in vogue in Buddha's time. Some of the teachers of Buddha, like Ālara were adepts in Yoga. The Buddhist Suttas are familiar with the Yoga methods of concentration. The four states of dhyāna of Buddhism correspond roughly to the four stages of conscious concentration in the *classical Yoga*. According to Buddhism, the possession of the five qualities of faith, energy, thought, concentration and wisdom, enables one to attain the end of Yoga; and the Yoga accepts this view. The Yogācāra school of Buddhism openly combines Buddhist doctrine with the Yoga details. The later Buddhistic works assume a developed Yoga technique. (Radhakrishnan 1929: 339–40, my italics)

What is interesting here is that not only does Radhakrishnan see yoga as an independent school of thought that is taken up by Buddhism as much as by Brahmanism, but he also refers to the *Yogasūtra* as 'classical yoga' – he footnotes this term specifically in relation to *Yogasūtra* 1.17, which discusses the five 'qualities' of cognitive concentration. Given that Radhakrishnan first wrote the text in 1923 – and the 1929 edition only contains minor corrections (according to Radhakrishnan's preface) – we must then consider that this is the first explicit designation (or at least among the first) of 'Pātañjala yoga' as 'classical yoga'.[45]

For Radhakrishnan, yoga is a standalone discipline that travels between religious traditions: 'The Upaniṣads, the *Mahābhārata*, including the *Bhagavadgītā*, Jainism and Buddhism accept Yogic practices' (Radhakrishnan 1929: 340). Moreover,

> the ideals of yogic practice are different in different metaphysical systems. In the Upaniṣads it is union with or realisation of Brahman. In Patañjali's Yoga it is insight into truth. In Buddhism it is attainment of the Bodhisattva condition or realization of the emptiness of the world. (Radhakrishnan 1929: 360)

He evaluates yoga as ancient and doctrinally polymorphous, but 'when insistence on activity is attached to the Sāṁkhya philosophy, we get the classical type of Yoga' (Radhakrishnan 1929: 340). The relationship between yoga and Buddhism is reciprocal; Patañjali's *dhyāna* in the first *pāda* (chapter) is derived from the Buddhist fourfold model of *dhyāna* (Radhakrishnan 1929: 339). While the analysis of yoga as common to Buddhism and Brahmanism is not unique to Radhakrishnan,[46] his assessment of yogācāra as an expression of yoga is unusual in any anglophone academic discourse of the nineteenth or early twentieth century. Yet, Radhakrishnan's explanation of the connection between yoga and yogācāra remains limited. Referring to one of the multiple names of the yogācāra philosophical school,[47] he comments, 'The title Yogācāra brings out the practical side of the philosophy, while Vijñānavāda brings out its speculative features' (Radhakrishnan 1929: 537). His entire section on yogācāra deals with philosophy of mind and ontology – only at the end of the section does he return to the topic of yoga to state somewhat baldly:

> The Yogācāras practice yoga. Yoga helps us to acquire intuitive insight. Discursive understanding gives us dependent or empirical knowledge. The metaphysical truth requires yogic discipline. When the mind is clear of all prejudice or illusion, it reflects the truth. (Radhakrishnan 1929: 552)

Given Radhakrishnan's prior definitions of 'Patañjali's yoga' or 'classical yoga' as being a method to yield insight into truth, it is clear that the connection that he posits here is not to the Upaniṣads but to the *Yogasūtra*.

In European anglophone scholarship, the first instance I have traced of the term 'classical yoga' is in the 1925 publication by Keith, *The Religion and Philosophy of the Vedas and Upanishads Volume 2*. Here, we find the same references to classical philosophical systems as were apparent in the nineteenth-century sources. In analysing a *Rg Vedic* hymn (the 'Nāsadīya' or 'Creation Hymn'), Keith notes, 'While much of its content is repeated in the later philosophy, its spirit of doubt is totally alien to the classical philosophical systems of India' (Keith 1925: 435). Keith refers to the story of Śunaśepa as a 'classical legend' (Keith 1925: 460) and to both 'Sāṃkhya in its classical form' and 'classical Sāṃkhya' (Keith 1925: 539). However, in a discussion on the Upaniṣads, he explicitly employs the label 'classical yoga': 'The Śvetaśvatara, however, contributes an element which in the classical Yoga distinguishes it from the Sāṁkhya' (Keith 1925: 549). And on the same page, discussing a passage from the Upaniṣads about two birds in one tree,[48] Keith adds, 'In the classical Yoga this picture presents itself in the form of a god who is a special spirit untouched by the impurity of the world, by action and its fruits, and who promotes the freedom of unemancipated spirits' (Keith 1925: 549). In both instances, Keith is using the term 'classical yoga' to refer to Patañjali's treatise, but he also links this term to the early Upaniṣadic accounts. Even when Keith refers to the classical eight limbs of Patañjali, it is to draw a distinction from the six limbs in *Maitranīyana Upaniṣad* (Keith 1925: 539). Unlike the late-nineteenth-century indologists, Keith goes to considerable efforts to refute the 'India origins' claims by devoting a whole chapter to this topic, titled 'Greece and the Philosophy of India'.[49] So if Keith is not employing 'classical' in relation to Greek philosophy, where does his understanding of this label derive from? My suggestion is that he reproduces prior associations of the Upaniṣads as 'classical literature' in the 'classical language' of Sanskrit – rather than referring to any specific notion of classical philosophy or religion.

Subsequent to Radhakrishnan's and Keith's foregrounding of 'classical yoga' to refer to Pātañjala yoga, the label was unevenly used by anglophone Indian scholars. For example, there are not explicit mentions of 'classical yoga' in Hiriyanna's 1932 *Outlines of Indian Philosophy* but rather of 'dualistic yoga of classical times' (Hiriyanna 1932: 268) and of the standard 'classical Sanskrit' and 'classical Sāṃkhya'. In the same year, 1932, in *Akṣara: The Forgotten History of Indian Philosophy*, Modi employs 'classical yoga' but in relation to the *Mahābhārata* and the Upaniṣads (Modi 1932: 63), again affirming the prevalent use of 'classical' to denote literary genre and language mode. In an extensive discussion, Modi addressed the 'grave blunders' of indologists Hopkins,

Deussen and Edgerton in their lack of technical interpretations of this textual material (Modi 1932: 67), and he attempts to redress such errors. Yoga can be labelled a classical school (Modi 1932: 56), and Modi stresses the identification of Sāṃkhya and yoga in the *Mahābhārata* but adds, 'the doctrinal teaching is not the same in the two schools'[50] (Modi 1932: 56). Even if the term 'classical yoga' refers to Pātañjala yoga, in Modi's analysis the roots of this system are traced back to book 12, the 'Śānti Parvan', of the *Mahābhārata*:

> Just as the origin of the classical Sāṃkhya is to be traced to the rejection of the Higher Nature, so we find, according to the above interpretation of the L MBh., that the Origin of the Classical Yoga lies in the rejection of the traditional identity of the Jîva and Īśvara inherited from the days of the Earliest Prose Upaniṣads. (Modi 1932: 81)[51]

Modi concludes, 'The origin of the idea of God in the Classical Yoga is to be traced not to a superficial ascription of God to an atheistic Sāṃkhya system, but to a rejection of the Upaniṣadic oneness of God and the soul' (Modi 1932: 82). For Modi, classical yoga is a specific non-dual ontology that reconceptualizes the *ātman-brahman* identity of the Upaniṣads.

Although by the mid-1920s Radhakrishnan and Keith were early pioneers of the term 'classical yoga', even in the decade afterwards, the term did not crystallize in academic discourse. It floated semantically to indicate period, language, literature or, more specifically, yoga in the Upaniṣads or the *Mahābhārata*. It would take further decades before 'classical yoga' became firmly established in anglophone scholarship as the categorical shorthand for the *Yogasūtra* of Patañjali.

Conclusions

This chapter has sought to highlight the colonial European provenance of the analytical anglophone category of 'classical yoga' as a reflection of the aesthetics of neoclassicism that informed historical periodization. 'Classical yoga' was first used by orientalists in relation to literature, language and philosophy more so than religion and surfaced both in evaluative comparison of Indian culture to European and in later nineteenth-century debates on 'Indian origins' for elements of Greek philosophy. The application of the value and term 'classical' to yoga was initially implicit in two ways: (a) yoga was 'classical' because its texts were *like* and equal in standard to classical Greek thought, language and literature and

(b) yoga was classical by its association with 'classical Sāṃkhya' philosophy, of which it was classified as a sub-branch. While anglophone 'classical yoga' was not a Sanskritic classification, it was underpinned by the Indian doxographical values that accorded Sanskrit *sūtra* texts 'high-culture' status. Still riding out the wave of neoclassicism, there was an accelerated interest in late-nineteenth-century indology in India as the source, in part, of Greek philosophy. In the early twentieth century, the label 'classical yoga', which seems to have first been used by Radhakrishnan, was gradually taken up by Indian philosophers, within the discursive, conceptual and institutional struggle of Modern Indian Philosophy to engage on an equal footing with European philosophical thought.[52]

What we find, then, is that far from 'classical yoga' being circulated in early oriental scholarship, it was a modern invention that surfaced as an *explicit* analytical category in anglophone Indian scholarship. At the outset of orientalism, all notions of the classical in relation to yoga were restricted to the scope of the *Bhagavad Gītā*, and it was 'classical Sāṃkhya' that was the vehicle of interest for philosophical enquiry. Since the neoclassical aesthetic was concerned with rationality, yoga as religion (and hence irrational in post-Enlightenment thought) was not readily discussed in the emergent category of 'classical yoga'. In its inception as an analytical category, 'classical yoga' had little to do with the bodies, practices or beliefs of religion but was a category reserved for rational systemic thought (philosophy) and its erudite exposition in literary artefacts. Furthermore, the nineteenth- and early-twentieth-century philosophical significations of 'classical yoga' appear to have been subsequently forgotten by a reshaping of 'classical yoga' as a category in religious studies throughout much of the mid-to-late twentieth century (e.g. Eliade 1958).

We have established that there is a questionable basis for asserting that the *Pātañjalayogaśāstra* should conform to the conventions of classicism or neoclassicism as dictated by European ideals, having been produced in a different literary and philosophical culture and era. However, it is also important to acknowledge that the imposition of the term 'classical' on Indian religion did not operate in a vacuum, but was also a product of dialogic interaction between European and South Asian thought. Postcolonial scholarship has now moved on from the analysis of orientalism as a one-way force of oppression and erasure of Indian culture to a more nuanced understanding of how Indian agents co-constructed imperialist narratives about religion, sometimes in relationships of complicity and sometimes in relationships of subversion (Strube 2020). Thus, however ill-suited it may have been, the orientalist use of the label 'classical' was an attempt to respond to the 'high culture' categories of *śāstra* and *darśana* that already existed in Indian culture. And Indian cultural-nationalist narratives that drew on premodern literary and religious doxographies also found the trope of the 'classical' strategically useful in relation to yoga to identify a 'pure' and continuous tradition that simultaneously signified the antiquity of Hinduism and the corporeal vigour of the Indian nationalist movement. Finally, the consolidation of 'classical yoga' as Hindu had a corollary in the marginalization of Buddhism, despite Radhakrishnan's keen efforts. This was compounded by the fact that at the point when Radhakrishnan and Keith began to use 'classical yoga' as a synonym for the *Yogasūtra* of Patañjali, there was not even a single critical edition in Sanskrit of one part of the *Yogācārabhūmiśāstra*.

Conclusion: Rethinking 'classical yoga' – a categorical paradigm shift?

Just as Sāṃkhya is called a śāstra, so is Yoga termed a darśana.

(*Mahābhārata*, 12.295.42c)

This book has challenged the scholarly category of 'classical yoga' as one that has been too narrowly defined and understood. Using conceptual metaphor theory, I have argued that the *Pātañjalayogaśāstra* is soteriologically imbricated with Buddhist thought on yoga discipline and that, at the very least, we should consider Asaṅga's *Yogācārabhūmiśāstra* as another potential *yogaśāstra* in our categorical purview. I have also sought to trace the specific historical development of the modern anglophone label 'classical yoga' as a way to problematize its very categorical claim to universality and timelessness. In this closing discussion, I now consider how the research presented in this book can contribute in a more reflexive way to the contemporary academic study of historical yoga in South Asia.

This chapter offers a theoretical reflection on the category of 'classical yoga' within relevant academic disciplines, such as history of religions, world philosophies and philological indology.[1] Drawing on a hermeneutics that incorporates decolonial thought, this approach aims to decentre the Eurocentric and imperialist enterprises of the nineteenth-century 'classical' and to reframe the study of yoga in the cultural setting of the second to fifth century CE using categorical markers from Indic intellectual history. By exploring the value and pitfalls of various alternatives that draw on Indocentric terms and paradigms, this chapter suggests '*śāstra* yoga' or 'śāstric yoga' as a potentially useful way to refer to the accelerated systematic developments in South Asian yoga and meditation during the early first millennium CE.

The continued purchase of 'classical yoga' in contemporary contexts

'Classical yoga' is a category that is still in current use in a range of contexts – from popular culture to health research, from political positioning to academic analysis. Different groups perpetuate an unproblematized and uncritiqued category of classical yoga, including global market sectors that profit from the promotion of classical yoga as rooted in 'timeless tradition' and the present-day public narratives in India that cultivate classical yoga as an essential (and essentialized) component of political ideology.

The purchase of 'classical yoga' as a commodity in today's commercial sectors[2] enfolds some of the meanings imbued in the early twentieth century (discussed in Chapter 5), such as historical continuity, religious purity or cultural authenticity. For example, classical yoga is still used as a synonym for 'Pātañjala yoga' or 'traditional yoga' in religiously oriented yoga trainings offered by transnational organizations.[3] And the label is also used to appeal to secular markets to generate the idea of a basic, original physical practice that is a pared-down form lacking in modern complications and marketing innovations – a notion that somewhat echoes the nineteenth-century oriental emphasis on the neoclassical.[4] Elsewhere, the classical as an equivalent label for Pātañjala yoga is also evident in science-based research on yoga and yogic meditation, where 'classical yoga' is sometimes used as a definitional baseline against which outcomes are measured. One recent positive psychology study in India makes this equivalence clear,[5] aiming to show a link between psycho-emotional 'resilience' and 'classical yoga', even coining a new 'independent variable' titled 'Classical Yoga Intervention' or 'CYI' (Karmalkar and Vaidya 2017: 431). This study shows the continued use of the term 'classical' to mean something like 'ideal', 'perfect' or 'complete/best' type of yoga.[6] In the burgeoning research on public health, 'classical yoga' can reflect the desire for a clear baseline from which to conduct empirical research.[7] One further context for 'classical yoga' is of course the academy, with a growing higher-education economy of global yoga studies and in which an unacknowledged 'premium' can be placed on those scholars who work in ancient languages. This kind of 'classical' cultural capital can create hierarchies in scholarly communities, in which, semantically, the 'classical scholar' can still be a subtle stand-in for 'Western scholar' – apart from the context of Asian scholars of classical South Asia. Scholarship engaged in the 'classical' frame can therefore reinforce or reproduce the problematic oriental mode that is, historically, 'outsider' scholarship. How might this range of contemporary cultural uses of 'classical yoga' intersect with broader questions on the legacy of the classical?

That European classicism has been weaponized politically as a tool of conservatism and fascism has been well documented (e.g. Roche and Demetriou 2017). As Goody points out, the shadow of the European veneration of 'classical' civilization was that in highlighting the 'prestigious attributes' of Greece and Rome, all teleologies pointed to 'Europe's singularity' in the history of civilizations (Goody 2006: 289).[8] The neoclassical attitude (in contrast to the preceding baroque or ensuing Romantic) was

> a mode of thinking more rational, more synthetic, more static, which tends to systematize, to accept what is of proven value, to make use of forms handed down from generation to generation (Secretan 1973: 4).

Such reification of the past has also been evident in contemporary India where majoritarian nationalist discourses have reached back into the distant past for an authentic and continuous Indian culture prior to Muslim 'invasions' and European colonization (van der Veer 2007; Gupta and Copeman 2019). In her deconstruction of the classical in relation to aesthetics and Carnatic music, Vajpeyi unmasks the 'subtexts' of the classical, indicating 'the antiquarianism, Brahminism, patriarchy, sexism, elitism, nationalism, revivalism, and Hindu religious ideology lying buried in the seemingly value-free appellation "classical" ' (Vajpeyi 2017). For Vajpeyi, 'fascist classicism' – with its key strategies of 'hidden violence, othering, and exclusion' – is a main tool in the current Hindutva valorization of the ancient past:

> In the pseudo-history of the Hindu Right, the classical period began once Buddhism had been assimilated into the Hindu fold, and ended as Islam, entering from the outside, came to dominate the subcontinent politically and culturally. (Vajpeyi 2017)

Arguably, however, even the historical value of the classical has been trumped by the cultural 'supremacy' of the Ancient Vedic period, a trend that has been absorbed into Western and globalized yoga and its continued claims for pure origins. McCartney has analysed the unwitting creep of Vedic fundamentalism into commercial Western narratives on yoga (McCartney 2017).[9]

In a range of contexts, then, 'classical yoga' still has cultural capital – from neoliberal consumer culture and branding strategies to 'culture wars' and politically motivated revisionism. It seems timely therefore to propose some constructive approaches to rethinking this category.

Rethinking 'classical yoga'

King states, 'As the age of European imperialism has faded, so increasingly has the belief that European worldviews and epistemologies constitute a normative (and potentially universalizable) way of understanding the world' (King 2011: 38). So how are we to rethink or reposition the category of 'classical yoga' using Indic cultural markers that avoid the epistemic violence of colonialism, but which also resist reifying political Hindu discourses that glorify the past? Let's review some options.

One recent and useful shift in anglophone scholarship has been to designate Patañjali's text as describing 'Pātañjala yoga' rather than 'classical yoga'. The specificity of Pātañjala yoga is more accurate, since the *Pātañjalayogaśāstra* is, after all, just one text and cannot be said to represent the plurality of yoga forms and ideologies that existed from the second century BCE to *c.* the tenth century CE, a stretch of at least one millennium (if we interpret the classical period at its lengthiest characterization). During this long period, Pātañjala yoga existed alongside many other forms of yoga: including the 'epic yoga' of the *Bhagavad Gītā* (Malinar 2007) and the 'Śānti Parvan' (Fitzgerald 2012), the proto-formulations of the late principal *Upaniṣad*s (Killingley 2017), the popular yoga of the *Purāṇa*s (Adluri 2017), the proto-Śaiva yoga of the *Śivadharma* corpus (Mirnig 2019), the Vaiṣṇava yoga of the Pāñcarātrins (Rastelli 2018), the yogācāra of the Buddhist Sarvāstivādins and of the Mahāyanists (Deleanu 2006; Stuart 2015; O'Brien-Kop 2020), the proto-tantra of Hinduism and of Vajrayāna Buddhism (Vasudeva 2017; Serbaeva 2020), the Siddha yoga of the early alchemists (White 1996), an archaic eightfold yoga of the medical āyurvedic treatise *Carakasaṃhitā* (Wujastyk 2012) and the syncretic Jain yoga scheme of Haribhadra's *Yogadṛṣṭisamuccaya* (Chapple 2003). These and many more variations of yoga existed in the so-called classical period – and this is only taking into account the extant textual evidence. So many other records of practice and ideology have been lost. Considering such a plurality of forms, we can no longer justify the synecdochical attribution of Patañjali's text as the part standing in for the whole of the 'classical period' – and 'Pātañjala yoga' appropriately locates the *Pātañjalayogaśāstra* in this complex landscape.

An other approach is to rethink 'classical yoga' as a discourse rather than a cultural or religious entity, a set of texts or a discrete practice. The intertextual approach of this present book has foregrounded concepts (or, more precisely, conceptual metaphors) at the expense of authorial, textual and even religious identities. Investigating the selected texts as intertextual requires accepting the fluidity of technical concepts of liberation, which can be at odds with how the study of religion has assigned particular doctrines to specific traditions (e.g. Yogācāra contains 'x' doctrine whereas Sāṃkhya contains 'y'). Certainly, identity labels were a historical reality in South Asia, and doxography was central to the medieval scholarly enterprise, but labels can nonetheless create the illusion of the exclusive intellectual ownership of bodies of thought. As Buescher states,

> technical concepts (and texts embodying them) are always to be understood within larger units of contextual structures providing their depths of meaningfulness, and within textual frameworks of assimilation and differentiation, both in synchronic and diachronic perspectives. Yet to locate a Yogācāra-Vijñānavāda text within a genre (as a specific horizon circumscribed by identifiable modes of elaboration) entails the task of demarcating it as pertaining to a distinct tradition in some way, and at some point(s?), to develop a specific set of characteristic technical terms for forming the constituents of new reflective models of philosophical understanding. (Buescher 2008: p. x)

Such acknowledgement of 'messy' and 'implicated' philosophies is not always reflected in the ways that Indian religions have been categorized by outsiders. However, whereas in the study of religion the label 'classical' is used to an ever-diminishing extent to describe early developments in Hinduism, Buddhism or Jainism, the term does have an important current valence in the discipline of philosophy; still related to the spirit of Modern Indian Philosophy, the label 'classical Indian philosophy' remains an effective way of asserting the equivalent value of Indian philosophy in the Euro-American paradigms of academic philosophy. In the discipline of history, in comparison, scholarship on South Asia has replaced the Eurocentrism of 'classical' periodization with more emic designations such as the 'Gupta period', used to describe the fourth to sixth century CE by foregrounding the family name of the rulers (see Chapter 5). This has entailed moving away from Eurocentric notions of empire and dynasty and towards translocal political formations that were unique to South Asian culture.

Alternatives to 'classical yoga', then, might include Sanskritic yoga or Gupta-era yoga, but neither of these is specific enough, and Pātañjala yoga, as we have noted, is too singular, not reflecting the broader generation of texts, ideas and practices of yoga and meditation. While taking into account the above historical and aesthetic points, we must arrive back at the only evidence that we have of a shared *discourse* beyond Pātañjala yoga – the texts themselves. The terms *śāstra* (treatise) and *darśana* ('school' of philosophy) are especially relevant here because they do not merely describe types of texts or disciplines but were also key emic indicators of 'high culture' during a period of South Asian history that includes the Gupta era but also precedes it. The fourth to fifth century CE texts that I have examined were produced and finalized at the tail end of the age of *sūtra*s and *śāstra*s, and this textual-cultural marker therefore seems to be the most apt emic designation from this period. The *Pātañjalayogaśāstra*, *Abhidharmakośabhāṣya* and *Yogācārabhūmiśāstra* are designated as *śāstra*s – and so *śāstra* yoga (or śāstric yoga)[10] appears to be a viable alternative to 'classical yoga'. I suggest a style convention of '*śāstra*' in italics (with or without diacritics) to indicate that this is a historical term, and 'yoga' in roman (as a borrowed word in English and many languages) to indicate that we are concerned with an artificial label through a contemporary scholarly lens and not with a solely emic term in historical usage such as *sāṃkhyayoga*, *bhaktiyoga*, *pāśupatayoga*, *haṭhayoga* or any of the other many compounds that appear in texts.

Śāstra yoga: Towards a more emic signifier

So, what new perspectives do we gain if we use the *śāstra* model to inform our thinking on the *Pātañjalayogaśāstra*, the *Abhidharmakośabhāṣya* and the *Yogācārabhūmiśāstra*? Firstly, we must consider what is meant by the context of śāstric culture itself. The first use of the term *śāstra* was *c.* the fourth century BCE in the Sanskrit grammarian Yāska's *Nirukta* (1.2, 14), and *śāstra* subsequently indicated a treatise that explains the Vedas and their ritual practices. (For more on the early development of the genre of *śāstra*, see Witzel 2006.) Centuries later, the *Pātañjalayogaśāstra* was devised as a Sanskrit *śāstra* and hence as an intellectually and culturally privileged form of codified knowledge, an elevated or elite discourse. As Halbfass points out, Indian philosophers identified the *śāstra*s and *darśana*s as systematic thought in contrast to pre-systematic philosophy, valuing 'formal criteria of coherence, the avoidance of contradictions, methods of proof and argumentation, and so on' (Halbfass 1992: 35).[11] Therefore, within the *śāstra* tradition, there was an inherent aesthetic, formal and conceptual basis, which prompts us to shift our vocabulary and understanding on these texts' features to Sanskritic conventions rather than 'neoclassical'. Furthermore, since *śāstra* is a cross-sectarian genre, it transcends any one philosophical or religious canon. *Śāstra* yoga can therefore include Buddhist *śāstra*s and *sutta*s, even if they are formally different to Brahmanic *sūtras*.[12] One advantage of using *śāstra* over *darśana*, then, is that *śāstra* is non-sectarian because it is not divided into *āstika* (adherent) and *nāstika* (non-adherent) positions. Furthermore, acknowledging the role and importance of the Indian doxographies does not mean that we should take those systematic divisions at face value. While it is necessary to highlight the tradition of *darśana* as a motivating factor in the doxographical framing of Pātañjala yoga in South Asia, there are nonetheless problems with oversimplifying this link. Foremost, if we rely on *darśana* to 'justify' the basis of the category of 'the classical', it produces a deadlock because we end up reifying the exclusion of Buddhism from that category.

One of the pitfalls, however, of using an emic signifier such as *śāstra* to denote the yoga/meditation treatises recorded in historical texts is collusion with the 'elite subtexts' that Vajpeyi identifies as the insidious 'classist'[13] drivers of the classical in contemporary Indian culture. We can infer from the address to Brahmins in the commentary[14] that Pātañjala yoga was a socially restricted activity that required training, education, knowledge of Sanskrit and membership of requisite social classes. Furthermore, as a *darśana*, yoga philosophy belonged to the culture of formal debate, with historical records reflecting that many such debates took place in court settings (see Introduction). However, if early yoga discipline was *only* associated with 'high-culture' śāstric specialists, then our view of the social field of yoga practice would be greatly narrowed, excluding other figures such as the forest-dweller on the margins of society, the Buddhist nun, the tantric adept, the antinomian ascetic and so on.[15] In rethinking classical yoga, then, it is necessary to make the distinction between a 'school' of philosophy (*darśana*) and a practice. The two are not identical. The first is a constructed scholarly category[16] based on the conventions of a textual-ideological continuum (the *śāstra* genre) and the second is a social, personal and embodied lifestyle that was materially exercised by individuals in the early centuries of the Common Era.

To critique 'classical yoga' is to interrogate the history of an idea (and its social ramifications), while still acknowledging that we do not have adequate material evidence about the 'on-the-ground' practices from this period. And this is where an extension of the 'classical yoga' bracket to include the *Yogācārabhūmiśāstra* becomes useful: a text as vast as this contains not only systemic thought, but also many marginal descriptions that are interesting and informative in terms of 'depicting' the social and material conditions of yoga discipline. What were the conditions of day-to-day material practice like? The *Śrāvakabhūmi* gives us some quite literal answers to this question in its account of the obstacles for the yogācāra: difficulty in obtaining alms-food, bedding and medicine; trouble in finding a suitable outdoor location for meditation; exposure to the elements at night and fear of spirits; the wearing of clothes made of rough felt or found on the trash heap and so on.[17] Thus *śāstra* yoga can widen our purview from systemic thought to understanding something more about the historical subjects who developed and engaged with this thought – and about their actual, embodied and material practices beyond the ideal prescriptions.

One of the key shifts attained by employing the term *śāstra* is that we can engage in a Gadamerian 'fusion of horizons' in terms of understanding the past on its own terms and diminishing the colonialist ideology of the European classical in relation to the South Asian past. (However, since the hermeneutic approach of Gadamer itself belongs to the Eurocentric episteme, we can employ this critical approach more effectively by incorporating decolonial thought, discussed below.) '*Śāstra* yoga', then, is a categorical attempt to think into and view early yoga from within its own historical frame (while, at the same time, acknowledging that any use of the word 'yoga' in contemporary discussion cannot escape the assumptions of its current semantic domain in anglophone discourse).

What was 'classical yoga' in its own space, time and culture – what do we see when we attempt to step into the shoes of the subjects in this world? If we date the *Pātañjalayogaśāstra* to *c.* 400 CE (Maas 2018), then Patañjali's world was that of the ruling Guptas (*c.* 320–543 CE). As discussed, the addressed subject of the text was a Brahmin male from a relatively privileged stratum of society. This was also the time of the circulation of *Laws of Manu*, a conservative commentary on and codification of Brahmanic social norms. In her early work, Thapar does not reject the application of 'classical' to describe the relatively prosperous and stable Gupta era, but she does point to the connection between the 'classical' and Sanskrit culture which assumes 'certain kinds of social and cultural exclusivity and demarcates social groups' (Thapar 2003: 282). In this context, any notion of 'the classical' therefore only points to 'the upper classes' as described in literature and the arts (Thapar 2003: 282). Here Thapar highlights that 'classical' is, above all, an aesthetic signifier of a historical period and does not accurately reflect anything about life for the majority of society and, indeed, both masks and perpetuates inequalities:

> The existing discrepancy between the level of material culture shown by excavations and that reflected by literature and the arts is in itself a commentary on the social context of classicism. (Thapar 2003: 282)

This is where the main theoretical approach of this book – conceptual metaphor theory – can demonstrate further applications. On one level, I have used conceptual metaphors to try to read 'backwards' into the material conditions in which the texts were produced in order to get a better sense of the real-world environment within which the *śāstra* scholars and yoga practitioners operated (see Chapter 1). The main limitation with metaphors, however, is that they do not offer real-time snapshots of material culture but can circulate in informal discourse for a long time before being incorporated into the formalized discourse of texts. Hence there is the strong possibility that the conceptual metaphors of the texts discussed here were commonplace or 'dead' metaphors that were generated in the distant past from the time of the texts' composition (during the second to fifth century CE).

Another key point is that the Gupta reign is often identified as the period in which Brahmanism was either 'revived' (from the Vedic period) or consolidated its power as a political theology in a new way. Although the Gupta rulers patronized Brahmanism on the whole, at the time when the Guptas assumed power the public religious landscape was still one dominated by Buddhism – which had been patronized on and off from the Maurya to the Kuṣāṇa eras. As Thapar points out,

> there is much in the articulation of these times that evolved from an idiom drawing on the Shramanic tradition, particularly Buddhism. Images of the Buddha were the more impressive icons. Buddhist Sanskrit literature encouraged creative literature, and the philosophic discussions often developed from earlier Buddhist and shramanic questioning of existing thought. (Thapar 2003: 281)

This underscores how Patañjali's text was produced in a cultural, intellectual and public landscape shaped strongly by Buddhism. Therefore, adopting *śāstra* yoga to include the *Yogācārabhūmiśāstra* and acknowledging the imbrication of Patañjali's text with Buddhist *śāstra*s gives a fuller and more accurate picture of what has, to date, been called 'classical yoga'.

In Chapter 5, I laid out three prevailing assumptions as to what constitutes the current scholarly category of 'classical yoga'. I will here revisit those assumptions to mark how this book has attempted to open up discussion about this category.

1. I have shown the artificiality of the first assumption, that the only text in the category of 'classical yoga' is the *Yogasūtra* – be that a sectarian assignation in Indian doxography or the later colonial-orientalist entrenchment of this boundary. The category of 'classical yoga' is itself a

historical-scholarly construct, shaped by complex forces, motivations and ideologies. There is nothing that intrinsically demands that the category be populated by just one text, the *Yogasūtra*.

2. I also hope to have demonstrated that the *Pātañjalayogaśāstra* was not the only or even first systematized treatise on yoga – we have to at least consider the claim that the *Yogācārabhūmiśāstra* contains layers that began to codify a system of yogācāra, yoga discipline, from the second century CE onwards.
3. Finally, this book has challenged the idea that the *Pātañjalayogaśaśtra* is only Hindu – it certainly is Hindu (and the text clearly addresses Brahmins) but not only, since Buddhist soteriology is also integral to understanding this text. Again, such singular characterization reflects traditional Hindu doxography but also later British imperialist agendas that prioritized divisive taxonomies of religions.

Having challenged and reformulated the above assumptions about what should be *in* the category of 'classical yoga', I have also suggested that we update the historical descriptor itself with a label that is less orientalist and better reflects contemporary approaches in the study of religions and philosophies. A starting point has been to suggest *śāstra* yoga (as a more emic signifier) as a way to encapsulate a premodern cultural output in South Asia and an era of remarkable developments in systemic thought in Sanskritic religio-philosophical communities across sectarian lines. It is in this broader cultural context that Pātañjala yoga was formulated.

Ultimately, this book is only a first step towards raising questions and initiating a conversation, and the issue of the academic study of historical yoga must be approached in dialogue with academics working in the South Asian academy where other concerns and parameters arise. However, proposing a Sanskrit term to replace 'classical' is not an invitation to have it infused with Hindutva values or, indeed, the Western search for 'authentic yoga'. How can '*śāstra* yoga' be proposed as a hermeneutic intervention that will not be hijacked by political agendas to substantiate claims that all Western scholars continue to distort yoga in a neo-imperialist mode or that only traditional Indian knowledge offers the truth. I cannot block such moves, apart from to state, emphatically, that this is not the point of this book. Neither is it possible to guarantee that a term like '*śāśtra* yoga' can avoid becoming another cultural commodity. But a critically reformulated label can offer a temporary space of resistance in which to reflect on the valence, violence and value of 'classical yoga' in current scholarship.

Finally, if we change the lens with which we view 'classical yoga', what might a fresh view of *śāstra* yoga show? The *Pātañjalayogaśāstra*, when read without the filter of 'Hindu-only', illuminates the subtle conceptual fabric of the text – an ideologically synthetic composition, framed coherently within a Sāṃkhya worldview but also containing and restitching many Buddhist and Jain ideas. Pātañjala yoga cannot be understood without the concepts of afflictions (*kleśas*), perfected concentration (*samādhi*) and cessative attainment (*nirodhasamāpatti*), ideas and practices that are technically elaborated in the Buddhist literature. A category of *śāstra yoga* makes space for the argument that there were at least two *śāstras* of 'classical yoga': the *Pātañjalayogaśāstra* and the *Yogācārabhūmiśāstra*, as well as a range of Buddhist compendia and Mahāyāna *sūtra* texts that discuss yoga discipline to a greater or lesser extent. And we might include Jain *śāstras* too, such as the fifth-century *Tattvārthasūtra* by Umāsvāti, or the *c.* eighth-century *Yogadṛṣṭisamuccaya*, *Yogaśataka* and *Yogabindu* by Haribhadrasūri – all extensive Jain treatises on '*yoga*' in Sanskrit, albeit with often distinctive and different meanings compared to those discussed in the Brahmanic and Buddhist sources. Furthermore, we see a field of śāstric knowledge in which the *Yogasūtra* cannot be understood in isolation from any of the other Brahmanic *darśana* root texts (e.g. the *Nyāyasūtra* or the *Brahmasūtra* – and not only the *Sāṃkhyakārikā*) and also other relevant contemporaneous literature, such as the Śaiva yogic *Pāsupātasūtra*, the aesthetics and arts treatise *Nātyaśāstra*, or the socially prescriptive *Mānavadharmaśāstra* (*Laws of Manu*).

A hermeneutic intervention: A decolonized fusion of horizons

Drawing further on Gadamer's fusion of horizons – how can we get closer to reaching the meaning of the *Pātañjalayogaśāśtra* on its own historical terms? A fusion of horizons – an attempt to understand the *Pātañjalayogaśāstra* in its own episteme and context of production – can be partly achieved by a synchronic study of textual culture in the northern part of the Indian subcontinent in the third to fifth centuries. Yet, given the colonial provenance of 'classical yoga', Gadamer's fusion of horizons is itself best merged with decolonial thought. Ideally, any fusion of horizons is an ethical commitment in seriously giving up the claim on one's temporal, cultural, regional and linguistic worldview as the only valid one. Here we must investigate two epistemic frames: the premodern South Asian frame and our own contemporary one. The first frame is addressed by the effort to read texts, to compare translations, to learn languages, to study historical and material contexts both broadly and deeply; the second frame is addressed by analysing reception histories and questioning our own cultural positionality and economies of distortion and bias. A historical text's alterity should not, then, be overrun by contemporary meanings:

> this kind of sensitivity requires neither 'neutrality' … nor the extinction of one's self, but the foregrounding and appropriation of one's own fore-meanings and prejudices … The important thing is to be aware of one's own bias, so the text can present itself in all its otherness and thus assert its own truth against one's own fore-meanings. (Gadamer 2004: 271–2)

And yet a decolonized fusion of horizons must go further: it requires a process of 'unsettling' hermeneutics to take into account the colonial frame which Gadamer's work ignores (Kerr 2020) and to take into account ontological-cultural differences, as well as the temporal divide in studying the historic past. As Quijano said of the epistemic violence wreaked on Latin America through the colonialism/modernity matrix,

> the Eurocentric perspective of knowledge is and always has been plainly unable to catch, and even to grasp, such originality and specificity. And the trouble is that most of us keep trying to understand and enact that experience precisely from such a Eurocentric perspective. (Quijano 2000: 215)

By acknowledging the epistemic priorities of South Asian historical subjects in the early Common Era, we may accept that some aspects of *śāśtra* yoga are simply incommensurable with a contemporary Euro-Western worldview, such as the relationship between knowing and being (epistemology and ontology), the adherence to an ontology of karmic causality, a worldview underpinned by a strictly dualist metaphysics, specific theories of temporality, a formulation of the freedom of the subject or even the understanding of the term *yoga* itself. However, through a hermeneutic commitment to epistemic uncertainty, we may reach a more grounded understanding of Pātañjala yoga in its own conceptual and material context.

Appendix 1

A note on the title *Pātañjalayogaśāstra*

Although scholarship has predominantly regarded the *Yogasūtra* and the *Yogasūtrabhāṣya*[1] as separate texts, authored respectively by Patañjali and Vyāsa[2] at least a century apart, this study treats the two texts as part of a single whole, the *Pātañjalayogaśāstra*.[3] This position is in line with Maas's analysis of the text as a unitary composition by one editor (or group of editors). Maas argues that the *sūtra* and *bhāṣya* texts were produced together at the same time and estimates the date range for the *Pātañjalayogaśāstra* as 325–425 CE (Maas 2013: 57–68). Although Maas has provided new and compelling evidence to support this argument, this view has circulated in scholarly circles since the nineteenth century. In the 1883 introduction to his translation of the *Yogasūtra*, Mitra noted that the name Vyāsa rarely appears in the colophons of the manuscripts, and Mitra referred to the combined *sūtra-bhāṣya* text as the *Yogaśāstra* (Mitra 1883: lxx–lxxvi). In 1930, Jacobi proposed the idea that the *Yogasūtra* and *Yogasūtrabhāṣya* comprise a unitary composition (Jacobi 1930: 584). Yet it was Bronkhorst's 1985 article 'Patañjali and the *Yoga Sūtras*' that was instrumental in fleshing out the detail of this argument. It is evident, Bronkhorst argued, that Patañjali was also regarded as the author of the *Bhāṣya* because of the way that subsequent commentators referenced the text – including Śaṅkara, Devapāla, Vācaspatimiśra and Śrīdhara (Bronkhorst 1985: 204). To underline his point, Bronkhorst analysed some grammatical, syntactical and semantic interconnections of the *Yogasūtra* and the *Bhāṣya*. Subsequently, Maas expanded Bronkhorst's analysis and consolidated the evidence for the argument that the text of the *Yogasūtra* forms one unit with its *Bhāṣya* (Maas 2006). Maas synthesized previous arguments and highlighted the following points, among others (Maas 2013):

1. The convention of the *sūtra* genre at the time was to provide an auto-commentary (*svopajñavṛtti*). The *śāstra* structure typically comprised *sūtra*, *bhāṣya* and summary passages to form a whole textual unit.[4]

2. There is no manuscript transmission of the *bhāṣya* independent of the *Yogasūtra*.
3. The first commentary, Śaṅkara's *Vivaraṇa* (*c.* eighth century CE),[5] does not refer to Vyāsa or to a separate author of the *Bhāṣya*.
4. Al-Bīrūnī's eleventh-century translation and Bhoja's *Rājamārtaṇḍa*, an eleventh-century commentary, both refer to the *Yogasūtra* and *Yogasūtrabhāṣya* as a unified text by one author.
5. In places, interconnected grammatical structures may indicate that the *Bhāṣya* author is also the compiler of the *Yogasūtra*.

In this book, I accept that Maas's work has proposed the status of the *Yogasūtra* and *Yogasūtrabhāṣya* to be that of a joint text. I will therefore refer to it as the *Pātañjalayogaśāstra*, redacted, most likely, in the fourth to early fifth century. This is a working hypothesis.

Appendix 2

Classical Indian metaphor theory

Classical Indian poetics had its own theory of metaphor, as part of the classification of linguistic and literary stylistic devices known as *alaṃkāra-śāstra* (precepts of ornamentation). The earliest formal works on Sanskrit poetics were Daṇḍin's *Kāvyādarśa* and Bhāmaha's *Kāvyālaṃkāra*, both *c.* the eighth century (Tzohar 2018: 5 fn. 5). Prior to these systematizations of literary devices was Bharata's treatise on aesthetics, the *c.* fourth-century *Nāṭyaśāstra*. However, as Pollock points out, the *Nāṭyaśāstra* deals primarily with the topic of drama (Pollock 2003: 42 fn. 5). More relevant to the philosophical discourse that I am scrutinizing are accounts of metaphor that we find in the śāstric works of the grammarians. Pāṇinī's *Aṣṭādhyāyī* describes four grammatical aspects of comparison: *upameya* or *upamita* (the subject of comparison), *upamāna* (the comparand), *samānya* or *samānadharma* (the property of similarity) and *sāmānyavacana* or *dyotaka* (the grammatical indicator of comparison) (*Aṣṭādhyāyi* 2.1.55.6, 2.3.72, 3.1.10[1]). Yet there is no extant formal or consistent theory of metaphor (or even of figurative language more generally) in Indian literature – philosophical or otherwise – from the early Common Era (Tzohar 2018: 5; 25). Indeed, any theory of metaphor from poetics is of limited relevance to this study. Since I look at philosophical rather than self-consciously literary texts, I examine metaphors that are often subtly embedded in the texts, rather than being deliberately and showily crafted according the rules of *alaṃkāra-śāstra*.

The challenge of discussing Indian theories of metaphor in the early Common Era is underscored by the lack of a scholarly consensus on a Sanskrit equivalent for the word 'metaphor'. In his study of metaphor as a 'theory of meaning' in Sthiramati's Yogācāra (*c.* sixth century), Tzohar settles on *upacāra* as the best term to denote metaphor in philosophical discourse. However, he acknowledges that this is an uneasy equivalence, since *upacāra* refers to both metaphor and metonomy (Tzohar 2018: 25). He suggests that *upacāra* does not denote metaphor specifically and is better understood generally as 'the referential mechanism' underlying all figurative language (Tzohar 2018: 25).[2] Other scholars have proposed *lakṣaṇā* as an appropriate term for metaphor (e.g. Kunnjuni Raja 1977). Another contender is *rūpaka*, which is discussed as a figure of speech in the *Nāṭyaśāstra*. Sharma translates *rūpaka* as 'metaphor' in his study of the *Mahābhārata* (Sharma 1964). However, Covill suggests that a more accurate translation for *rūpaka* is 'a simile lacking a word indicative of comparison (excluding compound-based similes)' (Covill 2009: 13). Nonetheless, in her study of the Buddhist *mahākāvya Saundarananda* by Aśvaghoṣa (*c.* second century),[3] she groups *rūpaka* (which she reluctantly translates as metaphor) and *upamā* (similes) under the banner 'conceptual metaphor' (Covill 2009: 20).

Conceptual metaphor theory is especially relevant to this study, because the metaphors that I analyse are not employed primarily for ornamental literary effect but are rather used to construct concepts – such as bondage (*saṃsāra*) and liberation (*mokṣa*). These concepts are then combined to create conceptual systems – systems of salvific thought. As a theory of the existential problem of humanity and how to solve that problem (i.e. to become liberated), soteriology is an abstract and conceptual endeavour. Hence analytical tools that help us to apprehend its very conceptuality are useful. Yet despite its potential effectiveness, the application of conceptual metaphor theory to ancient or classical Indian material has, to date, been limited.[4] In his pioneering study of visual metaphors in Mahāyāna Buddhism, McMahan draws on conceptual metaphor theory to decode the way in which knowledge is understood in relation to sight and seeing (McMahan 2002: especially 55–82). Covill's study of a core group of metaphors in Aśvaghoṣa's *Saundarananda* is underpinned by conceptual metaphor theory and supplemented by historical material analysis (Covill 2009). And in her investigation of Aśvaghoṣa's *Buddhacarita*, Patton asserts that 'conceptual metaphor theory is a broader category under which the specifics of metaphorical figures of speech, simile, *upamā*, *rūpaka*, and so on, might be a subset' (Patton 2008: 54).

The necessity of examining both Brahmanic and Buddhist texts together is highlighted by Tzohar's detailed study on metaphor in Yogācāra, in which he concludes that Yogācāra metaphor was produced in a 'cross-sectarian context' (Tzohar 2018: 11). Tzohar found that the earliest self-conscious use of the term *upacāra* was not in the early Mahāyāna sūtras, but in the Abhidharma literature, particularly the *Abhidharmakośabhāṣya* and in the non-Buddhist philosophical texts of Mīmāṃsā and Nyāya.

Appendix 3

Structure of the *Yogācārabhūmiśāstra*

The *Yogācārabhūmiśāstra* consists of the '*Maulī Bhūmih*', which contains fourteen books (detailing seventeen levels of yoga), and the supplementary sections, the '*samgrahaṇī*', of which there are four.

Book	**Title**	***Bhūmi* (Stage)**
The Basic Section (*Maulī Bhūmiḥ*)		
1	*Pañcavijñānakāyasamprayuktā Bhumiḥ*	1
2	*Manobhūmi*	2
3	*Savitarkasavicārādibhūmi:* *Savitarkā Savicārā Bhūmiḥ* *Avitarkā Vicāramātrā Bhūmiḥ* *Avitarkāvicārā Bhūmiḥ*	3–5
4	*Samāhitā Bhūmiḥ*	6
5	*Asamāhitā Bhūmiḥ*	7
6	*Sacittikā Acittikā Bhūmiḥ*	8–9
7	*Śrutamayī Bhūmiḥ*	10
8	*Cintāmayī Bhūmiḥ*	11
9	*Bhāvanāmayī Bhūmiḥ*	12
10	*Śrāvakabhūmi*	13
11	*Pratyekabuddhabhūmi*	14
12	*Bodhisattvabhūmi*	15
13	*Sopadhikā Bhūmih*	16
14	*Nirupadhikā Bhūmiḥ*	17

Book	Title	*Bhūmi* (Stage)
The Supplementary Section (*Saṃgrahaṇī*)		
	Viniścayasaṃgrahaṇī (contains *Saṃdhiniromocanasūtra)*	
	Vyākhyāsaṃgrahaṇī	
	Paryāyasaṃgrahaṇī	
	Vastusaṃgrahaṇī	

Notes

Introduction

1 For just a few of the more recent examples of the hitherto standard identification of classical yoga with the *Yogasūtra*, see Feuerstein (1979: viii–xiii); Potter (1983: 243); and Whicher (2000).

2 Maas has argued that the *Yogasūtra* and its commentary, the *Yogasūtrabhāṣya*, together comprise a single text under the title *Pātañjalayogaśāstra*, compiled and composed by Patañjali around 325–425 CE (Maas 2006, 2008a, 2009, 2010a, 2013: 57–68). Maas argues that the *sūtras* are partly compiled from older sources and partly composed by Patañjali (Maas 2013). His assertion of a single author of the *Yogasūtra* and its *bhāṣya* is in agreement with observations by Jacobi (1930: 584) and Bronkhorst (1985: 203). Maas also considers the argument that Vindhyavāsin may have been the author of the *bhāṣya*, or both the *sūtra* and *bhāṣya* (2013: 62), a view also explored by Bronkhorst (1985: 206) and Larson (1989) among others. Maas's framing of the text provides a compelling working hypothesis with which to evaluate Pātañjali's text. (In discussing secondary scholarship, however, I will reflect how other scholars refer to the text). See also Appendix 1.

3 European colonization in South Asia was not itself a monolithic project. For a distinction and discussion of 'theocolonialism', 'economic colonialism', 'spiritual colonialism' and 'cultural colonialism' (the latter in relation to European Romanticism), see Lussier (2011).

4 I preserve the distinction between the *Yogasūtra* and the *Yogasūtrabhāṣya* in this section, and elsewhere, in order to accurately reflect how other scholars have used these titles in their analysis and approach.

5 Larson agrees with this analysis citing the examples of *śraddhā, vīrya, smṛti, samādhi, prajñā, ṛtambharā, bīja, vāsanā, kleśa, āśaya, nirodha, dharma, lakṣaṇa, avasthā, bhūmi, dharmamegha, samāpatti, pratipakṣabhāvanā* (Larson and Bhattacharya 2008: 42).

6 Deussen identified four core and originally independent texts that were combined in the *Yogasūtra*: YS 1.1–16, 1.17–51, 2.1–27 and 2.28–3.55. All of the other sections, including the fourth *pāda*, were, in his view, newer textual supplements.

7 Although Oberhammer ranks the *aṣṭāṅga* portion as secondary in the four methods he identifies, he concedes that it is still oriented to the goal of Sāṃkhya, the attainment of discerning knowledge (*vivekakhyāti*) (Oberhammer 1977: 210–11).
8 I preserve the spelling Yogācāra with upper-case initial to reflect how previous scholars have spelled this term generally. See note 21 below.
9 A controversial aspect of Bronkhorst's work is his thesis that Buddhism did not evolve out of, or in reaction to, Vedic Brahmanism, but rather had its own distinct origins. See, for example, his denial of any relationship between the Buddhist notion of no-self and the Vedic ideas of *ātman* (Bronkhorst 2007).
10 The *Madhyhāntavibhāga* is attributed to Asaṅga and the *bhāṣya* thereon to Vasubandhu.
11 An earlier version of this article was available as a conference paper since 2014 and sparked my own interest in this topic.
12 See Gelblum (1992) for the argument that the *Vivaraṇa* also unpacks polemical encounter within the Brahmanical tradition – specifically Mīmāṃsā, Nyāya and Vaiśeṣika.
13 Intertextual reading posits that meaning is co-constructed in a dialogic literary network. The theory of intertextuality, as proposed by the literary philosopher Kristeva, is an approach to analysing texts that sees meaning not as fixed or precisely locatable, nor simply reflecting authorial intention. Rather, meaning is discursively and relationally co-constructed between texts by a non-fixed number of authorial agents. Intertextual analysis is typically synchronic and highlights how a lexeme shifts around semantically between texts. Drawing on the work of the philosopher and literary critic Bakhtin on 'dialogism' and 'polyphony' in texts, Kristeva first used the term 'intertextuality' to describe how one or more sets of signs are 'transposed' onto others (Kristeva 1980: 65). Most famously, she described a text as an '*intersection of textual surfaces* rather than a *point* (a fixed meaning)' (author's emphasis) (Kristeva 1980: 65). She also defined a text as a mosaic of citations that dynamically absorbed and transformed other texts (Kristeva 1969: 146).
14 Related to the question of whether yoga existed in any recognizably systematic form before the *Pātañjalayogaśāstra* is the debate as to whether yoga can be counted as a separate school of thought from Sāṃkhya.
15 For a discussion of this distinction in Pāṇini's *Aṣṭādhyāyī*, see Chapter 1, endnote 32. For more on the verbal root √*yuj* in the Vedic context, see Oguibenine (1984) and Oguibenine (1998): 199–222.
16 I discuss Jain soteriological metaphors in brief in Chapter 2.
17 Perhaps the tension between these two definitions can be explained by considering the ancient context of the term *yogakṣema* in the Vedas. *Yogakṣema* was used to describe the pastoralist lifestyle in which there were cycles of mobilization or

activation (*yoga*) of a community followed by periods of rest or cessation (*kṣema*) – thus communities lived in rhythmic cycles of movement and rest (Proferes 2007: 23). *Kṣema* is derived from the root √*kṣi*, meaning 'to possess', which gave rise to the sense of possessing the land and to the terms *kṣema* (settling, rest) and *kṣetra* (field). *Kṣatriya* (indicating 'governing' or 'endowed with sovereignty') is also derived from this root. Oberlies highlighted the fluctuation between mobilization and cessation in pastoralism and asserted that this *yogakṣema* lifestyle shaped not only the social but also the religious life of the Vedic tribes. 'Diese *yóga* + *kṣéma*-Lebensweise prägte das soziale und religiöse Leben der vedischen Stämme' (Oberlies 1998: 337). For a description of this way of life, Oberlies cites RV 7.82.4–5 and RV 4.33.10. According to Oberlies, one major factor that compelled moving on was the competition for pasture between growing numbers of tribes. 'Die Siedlungsweise der vedischen Stämme beschreibt der *Ṛgveda* selbst – darauf wurde bislang in der Diskussion, ob die vedischen Stämme nun *Nomaden*, *Halbnomaden* oder aber seßhafte Viehsüchter waren, nicht geachtet – als *yóga* (+) *kṣéma*, als "Anschirrung" und "Sich-Niederlassen", als eine Fluktuation zwischen Kampf, Weiterzug und friedlicher Seßhaftigkeit' (Oberlies 1998: 334–5). In the two trends of religious life, *yoga* was accompanied by the Indra-Marut religion and *kṣema* by the Āditya religion, the former strand focused on battle and the latter on order (Oberlies 1998: 338–45).

18 For Sāṃkhya in the *Upaniṣads*, see Bakker (1982). For early yoga and Sāṃkhya, see Schreiner (1999). For yoga in the *Mahābhārata*, see Bedekar (1960–1 and 1968); Brockington (2003 and 2005); and White (2009). For yoga in the *Bhagavad Gītā*, see Malinar (2007 and 2012).

19 Respectively, the silent one, the one who has undertaken a vow and the striver.

20 Running in parallel to these developments was the growth of another ascetic religion, Jainism, which shared practices, as well as philosophical and soteriological ideas, with yoga and yogācāra, although not the nomenclature.

21 This book identifies early yogācāras as Buddhist yoga adepts in the first centuries of the Common Era and distinguishes them from the later Yogācāras who by the fifth to sixth centuries had become established as a discrete philosophical school within Mahāyāna Buddhism. I discuss this distinction in Chapter 3 and cite the prior scholarship there.

22 Indeed, given the purported goal and means of Patañjali's method, one can imagine a number of other fitting titles for his text, such as the *Kaivalya-sūtra*, the *Nirbījasamādhi-sūtra* or the *Dharmamegha-sūtra*.

23 This occurs in the fourth *pāda*, considered by some scholars to be an interpolation, at PYŚ 4.15 and 4.21.

24 For example, Potter (1983); Whicher (2000); Burley (2007); Larson and Bhattacharya (2008).

25 It is difficult to decipher which of these sources, starting with Paramārtha's sixth-century biography of Vasubandhu, may be hagiographical and therefore not reliable. Nonetheless, they provide a sense of the issues at stake within the debating communities.

26 It was the [Mūla]Sarvāstivādins who abandoned their Middle Indic vernaculars to take on Sanskrit as their official language (Eltschinger 2017: 310). This was undertaken as part of an attempt to co-opt and disrupt the Brahmins' claims to have a 'monopoly on conceptually and formally well-formed language and eloquence' in order that Buddhists might demonstrate 'self-authorisation, didactic skills and superiority in debate' (Eltschinger 2017: 310).

27 *Asaṃprajñāta samādhi* (non-cognitive *samādhi*), the highest attainment of *samādhi* in the *Pātañjalayogaśāstra*, is conventionally accepted by Buddhist authors as a meditative attainment of non-Buddhist schools (Anacker 1984: 70).

28 E.g. a refutation of the Nyāya-Vaiśeṣikas and the Sāṃkhyas in chapter 9 of the *Abhidharmakośābhāṣya*, 'The Refutation of a Theory of the Self'.

29 This text is not extant in Sanskrit. It rebuts the Sāṃkhyas after the Sāmkhya Vindhyavāsin previously won a debate with Buddhamitra. Indeed, the *Paramārthasaptati* is a refutation in seventy verses of the seventy verses of the *Sāṃkhyakārikā*.

30 That yoga and yogācāra are blended categories is reflected in typical Buddhist references to the 'non-attainer'. For example, Buddhist texts often illustrate the unsurpassability of the Buddhist path by measuring it against the limited surpassibility of the non-Buddhist paths. Thus, ironically, success in the Buddhist path is often measured by considering the non-Buddhist path. For example, Saṅgharakṣa's **Yogācārabhūmi* devotes a whole section to how the non-Buddhists perform the breathing techniques of *śamatha* (Demiéville 1951: 416–17).

31 The *Saṃdhinirmocanasūtra* is an independent work that is quoted in the supplementary section, the *Viniścayasaṃgrahaṇī*, of the *Yogācārabhūmiśāstra* and is dated to the third century CE (Powers 1993: 4; Schmithausen 2007). The *Saṃdhinirmocanasūtra* is often viewed as the first Yogācāra work to outline the key philosophical concepts of the school.

32 The chapter describes how to develop *śamatha* (tranquility) and *vipaśyana* (insight), the two bases of Buddhist meditation.

33 From Lamotte's French translation of the Tibetan, 'Alors, en cette occasion, le Seigneur dit ces stances: L'exposé du Dharma et le Yoga sans négligence sont un grand bien. Ceux qui s'appuient sur le Dharma et qui pratiquent énergiquement le Yoga obtiennent l'Illumination. Ceux qui, en vue de leur intérêt, rejettent le Yoga et qui, pour leur délivrance, scrutent le Dharma, s'écartent du Yoga comme le firmament s'écarte de la terre. … C'est pourquoi, abandonnant toute querelle

et toute parole oiseuse, stimule ton énergie. Pour sauver les dieux et les hommes, consacre-toi au Yoga' (SNS 8. 40; trans. Lamotte 1935: 235).

34 From Lamotte's French translation of the Tibetan, 'Alors le bodhisattva Maitreya dit au Seigneur: Seigneur dans cette prédication de Saṃdhinirmocana, comment appeler cet enseignement? Comment faut-il le prendre? Le Seigneur répondit: Maitreya, c'est l' "Enseignement de sens explicite sur le Yoga"' (SNS 8.41; trans. Lamotte 1935: 236).

35 Notably, Burley does not agree that these *sūtra*s engage with Buddhist ideas: this section of the fourth *pāda* 'exhibits no signs of being directed against Yogācāra or any other form of Buddhism' (Burley 2007: 82). He posits that this attribution of anti-Yogācāra polemicism is merely a mistaken view of the subsequent commentators perpetuated over time and that the passage is entirely concordant with the internal 'non-realist' position of the *Yogasūtra* itself.

36 There is variation in how scholars demarcate this discussion. For example, Woods (1914) identifies the section as YS 4.14–23 and Burley (2007) as YS 4.14–22.

37 There is another, complex discussion of *cittamātra* at PYŚ 4.10.

38 *tad anena cittasārūpyeṇa bhrāntāḥ ke cit tad eva cetanam ity āhuḥ / apare cittamātram evedaṃ sarvaṃ nāsti khalv ayaṃ gavādir ghaṭādiś ca sakāraṇo loka iti. anukampanīyās te / kasmāt / asti hi teṣāṃ bhrāntibījaṃ sarvarūpākāranirbhāsaṃ cittam iti* (PYŚ 4.23; Angot 2012: 712).

39 In the early yogācāra context, *cittamātra* and *vijñaptimātra* were near synonyms (Willis 1979: 33).

40 For background on the term *cittamātra*, see Wayman (1965), Rahula (1972) and Willis (1979: 20–36).

41 In the **Bhadrapālasūtra*, the visualization of the Buddha face to face indicates that the Buddha is nothing but mind (*cittam eva*).

42 Schmithausen points out that the same phrase occurs in the *Lokottara-parivarta* in the 'Buddhāvataṃsaka' (Schmithausen 2009: 141). The *Lokottara-parivarta* is a component of the *Avataṃsakasūtra*, of which the *Daśabhūmikasūtra* is also a chapter.

43 Willis asserts that a proper understanding of the doctrine of *cittamātra* should also include the *Laṅkāvatārasūtra* (Willis 1979: 26).

44 For a history of Sāṃkhya, see Larson (1969: 75–153); Chakravarti (1975); and Larson and Bhattacharya (1987: 3–42).

45 Johnston makes a similar argument, asserting that suffering only comes to the fore in the *Sāṃkhyakārikā*, whereas it is there from the beginning of Buddhism (Johnston 1974: 21–4).

46 For more on categorization and ontology in Indian philosophy, see Frazier (2014).

47 To expand this point, the 'collection of qualities' seems to have existed in accounts of the *tattva*s in pre-classical Sāṃkhya and the classical five subtle elements

(*tanmātras*) 'which in classical Sāṃkhya would seem to make up for the five qualities of preclassical Sāṃkhya and may have undergone a major change in the way they were conceptualized, from atomic to omnipresent' (Bronkhorst 2006: 288).

48 Larson has added detail to this piece of research in the comprehensive *Encyclopedia of Indian Philosophies* volume on yoga (Larson and Bhattacharya 2008), although the core arguments are the same. I will draw on both publications to reproduce his argument.

49 Frauwallner tried to reconstitute passages from the lost *Ṣaṣṭitantra* of Vārṣagaṇya from citations in other works, especially from the sixth to seventh century *Yuktidīpikā*, a commentary on the *Sāṃkhyakārikā* (Frauwallner 1958). See Steinkellner (1999) for an update of Frauwallner's work.

50 The title *Ṣaṣtitantra* refers to the sixty categories, or *padārtha*s, outlined in this branch of Sāṃkhya. As discussed above, Īśvarakṛṣṇa's classical *Sāṃkhyakārikā* purports to be a summary of this lost work. However, a different presentation of the content of the *Ṣaṣṭitantra* appears in the later Pāñcarātra text the *Ahirbudhnyasaṃhitā*.

51 The other candidates whom he rules out are Kapila and Pañcaśikha (Larson 1989: 132).

52 Later on, Larson and Bhattacharya do identify various doctrines as the specifically Buddhist strands of the *Pātāñjalayogaśāstra*: the philosophy of *nirodha-samādhi* with a focus on meditation and altered states of awareness; the principal means of knowing as *pratyakṣa* or perception; a pluralist ontology; a naïve realist epistemology (like Sarvāstivāda) or representationist epistemology (like Sautrāntika and later Yogācāra); and a rejection of any notion of substantive transcendence, unlike Sāṃkhya (Larson and Bhattacharya 2008: 44).

53 Like Larson, Bronkhorst argues for two strands of thought in the early centuries CE, naming them as two epistemes: one is atomistic and the second is onto-linguistic. The first episteme, atomism, was imposed on Buddhism by the Sarvāstivāda school and 'is characterized by the belief that reality is thoroughly atomistic. The second episteme, which succeeds and more or less replaces the first (with some overlaps), is 'the conviction of a close and inseparable connection between language and reality' (Bronkhorst 2006: 291).

54 Larson places these three figures in the date order of Vārṣagaṇya in the second to third centuries CE, Vindhyavāsin in the late fourth century and Īśvarakṛṣṇa 'as a younger contemporary of Vindhyavāsin' (Larson 1989: 135). Vindhyavāsin composed the *Ṣaṣṭitantravṛtti*, of which only fragments survive in other works (Larson 2012: 74).

55 Larson draws on the *Yuktidīpikā* to reconstruct the positions of Vārṣagaṇya or his followers and speculates, along with Chakravarti (1975), that the positions attributed to Pañcaśikha in the *Yogasūtrabhāṣya* should in fact be credited to

Vārṣagaṇya. From one example of misattribution, Larson extrapolates that all of the long quotations attributed to Pañcaśikha were actually from Vārṣagaṇya.

56 Both the *Yuktidīpikā*, the earliest commentary on the *Sāṃkhykārikā*, and the Chinese tradition confirm that there was a debate between Vindhyavāsin and Buddhamitra, a teacher of Vasubandhu (Larson and Bhattacharya 1987: 141; Larson 1989: 134–5).

57 The king was Chandragupta the Second at Ayodhyā who gave Vasbubandhu 300,000 pieces of gold (Anacker 1984: 21).

58 Vindhyavāsin 'conflates' the two types of philosophy to create '*vijñāna*-cum-*nirodha-samādhi* philosophy' which creates 'the hybrid classical yoga philosophy' (Larson 1989: 136).

59 See Burley (2007: 82–90).

60 Burley rejects this common interpretation of the doctrine as referring to material cause and asserts that it makes a metaphysical point: 'It is not a cause in any straightforward sense of the word that is being talked about here. Rather it is the unmanifest ground of the manifest categories ... The part that the *satkāryavāda* seems to be playing in that project is to propose that anything manifest must have an *unmanifest* ground' (Burley 2007: 96). Thus, he reads SKK 9 as 'containing a transcendental argument for the existence of unmanifest *prakṛti*'. On this point, see also Halbfass (1992: 56).

61 According to Mikogami, this is the more general term in Indian philosophy for the assertion that an effect appears from its cause (Mikogami 1969: 443).

62 Unless attributed, translations are my own. *hetuphalasadvādaḥ katamaḥ | yathāpi iha ekatyaḥ śramaṇo brāhmaṇo vā evaṃdṛṣṭir bhavaty evaṃ vādī nityaṃ nityakālaṃ dhruvaṃ dhruvakālaṃ vidyata eva hetau phalamiti tadyathā vārṣagaṇyaḥ* (*Savitarkādibhūmi* VI 38; Bhattacharya 1957: 118–19).

63 *tasmādayamapyahetuḥ / sadālambanatvādvijñānasyeti / yadapyuktaṃ phalāditi / naiva hi sautrāntikā atītāt karmaṇaḥ phalotpatti varṇayanti / kiṃ tarhi / tatpūrvakāt saṃtānaviśeṣād ity ātmavādapratiṣedhe saṃpravedayiṣyāmaḥ / yasya tu atītānāgataṃ dravyato 'sti tasya phalaṃ nityamevāstīti kiṃ tatra karmaṇaḥ sāmarthyam / utpādane sāmarthyam / utpādas tarhy abhūtvā bhavatīti siddham / atha sarvameva cāsti / kasyedānīṃ kva sāmarthyam / vārṣagaṇyavādaś caivaṃ dyotito bhavati / 'yad asty asty eva tat / yan nāsti nasty eva tat / asato nāsti saṃbhavaḥ / sato nāsti vināśa' iti* (AKBh 5.26; Pradhan 1975: 300–1). 'This is also said to be due to fruition. The Sautrāntikas do not describe the production of fruition to be due to past action alone. Why? Because it [production of fruition] is due to the particular sequence [continuum] that comes from the prior [action] – which I will make known as the refutation of the doctrine of self. But for one for whom past and future are substantially real (i.e. the Vaibhāṣikas) the fruit is said to be eternal – how does the action have momentum (*sāmarthya*)? When there

is production, there is momentum. In that case, production (*utpāda*) is resultant (*siddham*), after having been non-existent (*abhūtvā*). Then there would be only existence – in which case where [is the need for] momentum? Thus, one would [adhere to] the doctrine of the Vārṣagaṇyas, as illustrated: "Only what exists, exists; Only what doesn't exist, doesn't exist; What is not real does not arise; What is real does not perish." ' I have here favoured the translation of 'momentum' over 'potential' for *sāmarthya* to illustrate the technical understanding of the potential or capacity as that which propels the entity through time in a sequence. In Buddhism, *ātmavāda* is the mistaken notion of a permanent self; it is also called *satkāyadṛṣṭi*. The false notion of self is often the fourth of the four attachments, the *upādāna*. (*Upādāna* is also the ninth of the twelve links of dependent origination.)

64 The belief that an entity exists simultaneously in the past, present and future.

65 The context of this refutation of the Sarvāstivāda three time periods is discussed fully in Maas (2020).

66 The meaning of *upādāna* is unclear in this passage, as *upādāna* can have different technical meanings in Buddhist and Brahmanic philosophical discourse. There are four *upādāna*s, or forms of grasping, in Buddhism, and the fourth attachment is to a notion of false self, while in both Buddhism and Brahmanism *upādāna* can refer to a material cause. However, the *Mahābhārata* uses *upādāna* to indicate 'the act of taking to oneself; appropriating to oneself' (Monier-Williams 1899), suggesting an overlap with the meaning of 'grasping'. See also endnote 63 above.

67 Literally: 'the doctrine of a cause of it'.

68 I am grateful to Professor Rupert Gethin for his assistance in translating this passage. *tatra duḥkhabahulaḥ saṃsāro heyaḥ. pradhānapuruṣayoḥ saṃyogo heyahetuḥ. saṃyogasyātyantikī nivṛttir hānam. hānopāyaḥ samyagdarśanam. tatra hātuḥ svarūpam upādeyaṃ vā heyaṃ vā na bhavitum arhatīti hāne tasyocchedavādaprasaṅga upādāne ca hetuvādaḥ. ubhayapratyākhyāne śāśvatavāda ity etat samyagdarśanam* (PYŚ 2.15; Angot 2012: 421).

69 The Buddha rejected two extremes. The first was *ucchedavāda*, the doctrine of annihilation, in which there is no fruition of karma or rebirth and in which the individual is completely annihilated at death. The second 'extreme' position rejected by the Buddha was *śāsvatavāda*, the doctrine of eternalism. Patañjali's passage, however, accepts the doctrine of *śāśvatavāda*.

70 Discussed by Maas (2014: 73).

71 An exception is Cleary's title *Buddhist Yoga* for his translation of the third-century *Saṃdhiniromocanasūtra* (which is also embedded in the *Yogācārabhūmiśāstra*); in the introduction he refers to it as 'a complete classical sourcebook of Buddhist yoga' (Cleary 1995: vii). Cleary perhaps overstates the case, because the *Saṃdhiniromocanasūtra* treats the topic of yoga only in part and not in the whole of the text.

72 I discuss the meaning and translation of yogācāra in Chapter 3.
73 'Yoga' refers to Buddhist practice in general 'covering its entire spiritual path, with special emphasis on the practice of meditation' (Kragh 2013b: 30). For his definitions of generic yoga in a Buddhist context, Kragh is drawing on Deleanu (2006: 26) and Schmithausen (2007: 213).
74 In Pāli, Prakrit, Sanskrit.
75 Umāsvāti's *Tattvārthasūtra* was the first Jain work to be written in classical Sanskrit. Balcerowicz assigns this text to 350–400 CE (Balcerowicz 2008: 34 fn. 23). Dundas and Bronkhorst place it *c.* the fourth century (Dundas 1992; Bronkhorst 2006: 290).
76 Additionally, Western scholars have mapped Western categories of religion on to South Asian history, an issue discussed in Chapter 5 and the concluding chapter.

Chapter 1

1 See, for example, Eliade (1958).
2 Materiality here draws on both material culture and material religion as the study of subjects in their embodied and physical environments. Comeau's definition is helpful here: 'New material culture studies provide an approach to religion that centres the material world as the primary condition from which people are motivated to act and a method by which the implied dichotomy of mind and material in South Asian religious studies can be dismantled' (Comeau 2020: 4).
3 Aristotle asserted that a metaphor involves a comparison between a literal object and a metaphoric object with a hidden simile. Thus a simile is 'Achilles is like a lion', while a metaphor is 'Achilles is a lion' with the comparative 'like' removed although nonetheless implied.
4 Cognitive metaphor theory has flourished in recent years and expanded to include definitions of metaphor as not only conceptual but also linguistic, sociocultural, neural and bodily (Kövecses 2006: 126). This book focuses on conceptual metaphors that are expressed linguistically in texts.
5 Lakoff and Johnson's key work *Metaphors We Live By* in 1980 paved the way for conceptual metaphor theory within cognitive linguistics. This theory was further developed in Lakoff (1987) and Lakoff and Turner (1989). Subsequent key scholars include Gibbs (e.g. 2017) and Kövecses (e.g. 2005; 2006; 2015). One of the earliest uses of the label 'conceptual metaphor theory' was by Deignan (2005).
6 Metaphor is closely related to metonomy, in which one thing or term stands in for another. Using metonymy, 'lion' stands in for Achilles entirely, as in the phrase 'Come and speak with the lion'.
7 A recent study that employs contemporary philosophy of language to examine classical Buddhist sources is Bronkhorst (2012). Drawing on Peirce's semiotics and

Deacon's evolutionary linguistics, Bronkhorst utilizes the framework of symbolic representation (understanding how signs relate to each other systematically in order to communicate about the objective world) and also incorporates Freudian psychoanalysis to construct a psychological theory that can be used to analyse Buddhist meditative absorption. Bronkhorst does not, however, discuss concepts – which he acknowledges must be distinguished from symbolic representations (Bronkhorst 2012: 13 fn. 6) – and nor does he discuss metaphors in any detail.

8 'A domain, or frame, is a coherent organization of human experience' (Kövecses 2017: 24).

9 Using the stock example of 'Achilles is a lion', the two domains are 'the specific man called Achilles' and 'a lion'. In the domain-mapping, the qualities of the source domain (the lion) are 'transferred' or 'mapped' to the target domain (Achilles), so that, although it is not explicitly stated, Achilles is understood using the terms of a lion: a hunter, powerful, fierce, a wild creature, with a mane, deadly, etc.

10 For example, in the selective mapping from a lion to Achilles, many inappropriate qualities are edited out, such as possessing a tail or four legs.

11 Following the convention of cognitive metaphor scholars, I will use these schematic phrases in capitals to show when I am referring to a conceptual metaphor.

12 Although I will not examine them in this study, it is worth noting that in recent years the notion of a visceral basis to conceptual metaphor has been extended in emerging neural theories. In other words, neural networks are activated and patterned by everyday experience. 'Metaphor is a natural development of the way that neural systems work with recurring mappings, predictable inference patterns, and emergent properties' (Gibbs 2017: 32–3).

13 Kövecses discusses six prerequisite functions of a human conceptual system (Kövecses 2015: 32–4).

14 The visceral experiences of feeling good or happy include the corners of one's eyes and mouth turning up, while the visceral experiences of feeling bad or unhappy include one's posture slumping downwards.

15 Examples of 'more is up' include 'prices are high', 'their shares skyrocketed' and 'productivity is way up'. Examples of 'down is bad' include 'fallen from grace', 'I feel down', 'the slippery slope to ruin'.

16 For a study of the universality-variation issue in metaphors, see Kövecses (2005). One crosscultural metaphor is KNOWING IS SEEING: 'I see your point', 'clarity of thought', 'gain insight' and 'point of view'. Knowledge is also commonly mapped as physical manipulation – 'grasping' or 'getting' an idea – and as storage – 'filling one's mind' or 'retrieving information' (Egge 2013: 93).

17 Most recently, Fauconnier and Turner have innovated around the theory of orientational metaphor to theorize 'conceptual blending' (Fauconnier and Turner 2003). This proposes a process of conceptual integration by looking at how

metaphoric and metonymic structures are combined and blended to create new structures called blends and, at the largest scale, mega-blends or hyper-blends.

18 For a detailed study of this metaphor, see Lakoff (1987: 380–415).

19 Another key soteriological metaphor in Christianity is 'redemption'.

20 All yoga in the early Common Era is soteriological (although not all soteriology is yogic).

21 E.g. *nirvāṇa* (cessative liberation) in Buddhism, *samādhi* (concentration) in yoga and Buddhism, or *kevala* (isolation) in Jainism and *kaivalya* (isolation) in yoga and Sāṃkhya.

22 The doctrines that lead to the goal of 'liberation' may be very different, resting on concepts of sight, insight, knowledge, vision, discrimination, perception, scriptural reflection, authority, etc and are closely linked to *pramāṇa*, the valid bases of knowledge. Another important soteriological metaphor is that of 'finding the true self', which is derived from the structural metaphor HAPPINESS IS FINDING A HIDDEN (DESIRED) OBJECT.

23 The creative etymologizing of the term *nirodha* (cessation, characterizing the third noble truth) by Buddhist writers highlights the background conceptuality of such metaphors. Breaking the word down, *ni* is said to signify 'absence' and *rodha* to signify 'prison'; *nirodha* therefore means lack of confinement in the prison of *saṃsāra* (Collins 2010: 91–2).

24 See Collins for an investigation of *nirvāṇa*'s expression through four images: quenching of fire, the ocean, dry land and the city. *Nirvāṇa* itself as the extinguished flame contains other notions, such as hot/cool, movement/stillness and presence/absence (Collins 2010: 79–99).

25 *Upāsana* occurs more than two hundred times in the *Upaniṣads*. The vast majority of these references are in *Chāndogya Upaniṣad*, but the term is nonetheless evenly distributed throughout the corpus in that it appears in every text apart from *Kaṭha* and *Īśā*. *Dhyāna*, in contrast, makes its first appearance relatively late in the corpus: in *Śvetāśvatara*, *Muṇḍaka* and *Praśna Upaniṣads*.

26 These terms are widely used in the *Pātañjalayogaśāstra*, *Abhidharmakośabhāṣya* and *Yogācārabhūmiśāstra*.

27 In citations and quotations, the *Yogasūtra* is shown **in bold** and the *Yogasūtrabhāṣya* in non-bold.

28 To date, the most significant studies of cognitive metaphor theory in relation to Brahmanic meditation have been done in the field of tantric studies (see Timalsina 2016; Hayes and Timasina 2017). This is partly due to the important role of visualization in tantric meditation. In the later tantric uses of *bhāvanā*, theories of meditation were directed to the relationship between reality and the imagination. In his examination of Śaiva Siddhānta, Sanderson outlines the binary domains of the imaginative mind and reality and the role of meditation in connecting the two: 'The

thinking which the theorists of the Siddhānta had in mind was not the cognition of a fact but a kind of mental work which produces a result through effort. It is seen as imagination with the power to cross from the imaginary (*kālpanikam*) to the real (*satyam*), so transcending the dichotomy between these domains' (Sanderson 1995: 42). Kiss points to the binary structure of domain-mapping in later tantric *bhāvanā*: 'It is a meditative process during which the yogin visualizes an object, mostly a deity, and usually tries to identify himself with it' (Kiss forthcoming: 65).

29 One example of this can be seen in the 1960s–1970s counterculture in which the lives of a generation of Western youth were so shaped by an intense and amplified cultural expression of the LIFE IS A JOURNEY metaphor that they took up a wandering lifestyle with 'finding the (true) self' as the end destination, be it journeying across the United States or across Asia.

30 For a discussion of the semantic development of the term 'yoga' including *yogakṣema*, see the section 'Defining yoga' in the 'Introduction'.

31 See Witzel (2012: 287) for a discussion of the 'sun horse' in Eurasian myth.

32 In Pāṇini's grammar treatise the *Aṣṭādhyāyī* (*c.* sixth to fourth century BCE), the list of verbal forms contains two for the root '*yuj*': '*yujī*' denotes 'joining' or 'uniting' (cognate with the English 'yoking'), and '*yuja*' denotes 'concentration' in the sense of *samādhi*. Both forms are discussed in the augment rule 7.1.71 (Vasu 1980 II: 1342). The oldest extant commentary on the *Aṣṭādhyāyī*, the *Kāśikāvṛtti* (*c.* seventh century CE), underlines this distinction: 'The KV makes it clear that the verbal base *yuj*- meant in the present rule is not the homonymous base *yuj*- mentioned in the Dhp. 4.68 [*Dhāṭupāṭha*] in the sense of *samādhi* "concentrating the mind". The example quoted is *yujam āpannā ṛṣayah* "the *ṛṣi*s are sunk in contemplation"' (Joshi and Roodbergen 2003: 144). The *Dhātupāṭha* is the list of verbal roots that accompanies the *Aṣṭādhyāyī* – although we cannot be fully certain that it contained all of the verbal roots at the time of Pāṇini or if some were added later (Bronkhorst 1981: 335).

33 For a discussion of the early semantic field of *samādhi*, see Adam (2002: 33–74).

34 The *Oxford Dictionary of English* gives three primary meanings for 'concentration': (1) 'Dealing with one particular thing above all others', (2) 'A close gathering of people or things', (3) 'The relative amount of a particular substance contained within a solution or mixture or in a particular volume of space' (*Oxford Dictionary of English* 2010).

35 These metaphorical traces in the English term 'concentration' provide an interesting starting point for investigating an early semantic field for 'yoga' in relation to ritual, medicine and alchemy, which all featured the applied use of substances and liquids. However, the focus of this present book remains, more narrowly, on the key metaphors of botanical cultivation. For those interested in looking at the broader medical context of Buddhism, Salguero offers an interesting analysis of conceptual

metaphors in Buddhist medicine and highlights the way that five key metaphors were both preserved and strategically revised in Chinese translation to maximize their cultural reach (Salguero 2014: 67–95). As he states, 'each metaphor lies at the foundation of a complex edifice of dependent metaphors, similes, imagery, symbols, and other patterns of language that include many of the most basic and influential Buddhist medical ideas' (Salguero 2014: 68).

36 The term 'root metaphor' was elaborated by Turner (Turner 1974: 25–6), who took the label from Pepper (Pepper 1942: 91–2).

37 For examples of yoga as restraint, reining and tying, see CU 6.8.2, KaU 3.3–4, 5.12–13, 6.10–11 and Sv 2.15.

38 Turner's *A Comparative Dictionary of the Indo-Aryan Languages* gives the Pāli equivalent of the Sanskrit *bhāvayati* as *bhāvēti*, 'produces, begets, cultivates' (Turner 1966: 540). Turner traces the earliest usage of *bhāvayati* to the *Atharva Veda* with the meaning 'causes to be'.

39 Early references cited by Collins are to deepening insight into the doctrine of right view, e.g. *Majjhima Nikāya* i.287, 401 and iii.22, 52, 71; *Dīgha Nikāya* i.55.

40 Mayrhofer (1963: II.486). Mayrhofer here is citing Gonda, who discusses the argument that the 'primary sense of *bhū-* is not "to be, to exist", but "to grow, to thrive, to prosper"' (1956–7: 299). Böhtlingk and Roth also give a primary meaning of causative *bhāvayati* as creative: 'in's Dasein bringen, in's Leben rufen, erzeugen, hervorbringen, bewirken, schaffen' (Böhtlingk and Roth 1865–8: 317).

41 Turner goes further to explain the Pāli meaning of *bhāvanā* as 'applying one's mind to' in contrast to the Sanskrit meaning of 'causing to be' and 'imagination' (Turner 1966: 540). In his view, the Pāli meaning, then, would seem to pertain distinctly to the mental realm or only to non-material realms. On the other hand, Hacker has argued that the difference in understanding between mental cultivation and material production is non-existent: 'mental representations, if reaching a high degree of intensity, are capable of bringing about a reality not only on the psychological level but in the domain of material things' (Hacker 1972: 118). Of course, the supernatural capacities, *ṛddhi*s and *siddhi*s, exist at the threshold of the immaterial and the material worlds. We might also add another strand of meaning related to the production of 'being', broadly referring to the ethical production of virtues and qualities. However, this is a topic for discussion on another occasion.

42 In Vedic sources, *bhūmi* was a synonym for *pṛthivī* (Mayrhofer 1963: II.513).

43 In later periods, *bhāvanā* takes on different nuances but nonetheless stays closely allied to meditation practice. For example, in tantra *bhāvanā* is synonymous with other terms for meditation, such as *bhāva*, *dhyāna* and *smaraṇa* (Kiss forthcoming: 65).

44 In this text, the older canonical doctrine (in the Sūtrapiṭaka) of cankers (*āsravāḥ*) is replaced with a new doctrine of latencies (*anuśayāḥ*), and, as part

of this reformulation, a new distinction is crystallized between *darśana-* and *bhāvanāprahātavayā anuśayāḥ* (Frauwallner 1995: 157–8). I discuss the terms *anuśaya* and *āsrava* in Chapter 2.

45 In Sarvāstivāda Abhidharma, although *bhāvanā* and *darśana mārgas* are paired, they are part of the larger fivefold collection of paths (see Gethin 2007: 336–7).

46 'ou encore, l'apaisement est pareil à l'acte du moissonneur qui saisit les épis de la main gauche, la contemplation à l'acte de les couper à la faucille de la main droite' (SYCB 22, 211c–212a; Demiéville 1951: 409). T606, T607.

47 In a later illustration of this point, Sharf discusses the *mārga* treatises of 'Buddhist modernism', which he relates to three Buddhist texts from the ninth century. One of these, Kamalaśīla's *Bhāvanākrama* proposes the gradualist path and refutes the Chinese Chan doctrine of sudden enlightenment (Sharf 1995: 236).

48 'Ascension' soteriologies include, for example, in the Upaniṣads, travelling beyond the disk of the sun (Āditya) to reach heaven; *yogayukta* in the *Mahābhārata* as ascension to heaven or the episode of Śuka in the 'Sānti Parvan'; visions of cosmic buddhas in the sky in Mahāyāna literature; or the cloud of dharma in Pātañjala yoga and Buddhist texts.

49 For discussions of these regions see Thapar (2003); Olivelle (2006); Samuel (2008); Anacker (1984: 11–16); Cox (1995: 41); Hopkins (1999: 48–52, unpublished typescript cited in Samuel 2008: 50); among others.

50 I am also indebted to Dr Theodore Proferes, who suggested exploring the paradigm of *bhāvanā* more systematically in relation to agriculture.

51 The earliest location for rice cultivation was the Ganga Valley by 3000 BCE (Bellwood 2004: 87).

52 However, Gombrich points to the counterargument that although the Gangetic Plain has ideal fertile soil (an alluvium belt) for rice-farming, the type of profuse vegetation there may also have been harder to clear for farming (Gombrich 1988: 37).

53 For further discussion on this point, see Sharma (2010: 5–6); Bailey and Mabbett (2003: 84); Gombrich (1988: 37); Sattar et al. (2010: 228).

54 I discuss the burnt rice seed in detail in Chapter 2.

55 *ato 'gnidagdhavrīhivad abījībhūte āśraye kleśānāṃ prahīṇakleśa ity ucyate. upahatabījabhāve vā laukikena mārgeṇa* (AKBh 2.36; Pradhan 1975: 63, 20–1).

56 *ko' ayam bījabhāvo nāma. ātmabhāvasya kleśajā kleśotpādanaśaktiḥ yathānubhavajñānajā smṛtyutpādanaśaktir yathācāṅkurādīnāṃ śāliphalajā śāliphalotpādanaśaktir iti* (AKBh 5.1; Pradhan 1975: 278, 22–4).

57 Sanskrit: *nīvāraḥ*. According to Monier-Williams, *nīvāraḥ*, indicating wild rice, is discussed in the Vedas and the *Mahābhārata*.

58 There is a sense in which the theory of rebirth itself is connected to the idea of the self-generating plant.

59 See, for example, *saṃsārasāgara* as the ocean of transmigration at Ja iii.241.

60 *bhavacakkam aviditādīni idaṃ, kārakavedakarahitaṃ, dvādasavidhasuññatā suññaṃ. Sātataṃ samitaṃ pavattatī ti veditabbaṃ* (Vism. XVII; Rhys Davids 1975: 576, 19–21).

61 *Yañ c'etaṃ avijjābhavataṇhāmayanābhi puññādi-abhisankhārāraṃ jarāmaraṇanemi āsavasamudayamayena akkhena vijjhitvā ti bhavarathe samāyojitaṃ anādikālappavattaṃ saṃsāracakkaṃ, tassānena Bodhimaṇḍe viriyapādehi sīlapathaviyaṃ patiṭṭhāya saddhāhatthena kammakkhayakaraṃñāṇapharasuṃ gahetvā sabbe arā hatā ti arānaṃ hatattā pi ARAHAṂ. Atha vā saṃsāracakkan ti anamataggaṃ saṃsāravaṭṭaṃ vuccati; tassa ca avijjā nābhi mūlattā, jarāmaraṇaṃ nemi pariyosānattā, sesā dasadhammā arā avijjāmūlakattā, jarāmaraṇapariyantattā ca* (Vism. VII; Rhys Davids 1975: 198, 15–30).

62 For typical examples, see *dhammacakka* at Vin i 11f and Vv-a 249, 5; see *cakkavatti* at Ja i 252 and ii 268, 269; and *Brahmacakka* at MN i 69; AN ii 24, iii 9,417. Wiltshire argues that the concept of *dhammacakka* is overlaid on the older Brahmanic notion of *brahmacakra*, the cycle of creation, in an act of discursive appropriation (Wiltshire 1990: 265).

63 The potter's wheel is also a common metaphor, although the qualitative connotations are somewhat different.

64 *Yathā nāma rathacakkaṃ pavattamānam pi eken' eva nemippadesena pavattati, tiṭṭhamānam pi eken' eva tiṭṭhati, evam eva ekacittakkhaṇikam sattānam jīvitam, tasmiṃ citte niruddhamatte satto niruddho ti vuccati* (Vism. VIII; Rhys Davids 1975: 238, 14–18).

65 *Ettakā yeva te loke ye dhammā bodhipācanā, tat' uddhaṁ n' atthi aññatra, daḷhaṁ tattha patiṭṭhaha'. Ime dhamme sammasato sabhāvasarasalakkhaṇe dhammatejena vasudhā dasasahassī pakampatha. Calatī ravatī puthavī uchhuyantaṁ va pīḷitaṁ; telayante yathā cakkaṁ evaṁ kampati medinîti* (Ja i.25, 339; Fausbøll 2000: 25, 175–7).

66 For another reference to the sugar mill, see Mil 166, and for *yantracakra* see *Laṅkāvatārasūtra* 2, 132.

67 For discussions of the *saṃyojana* in Pāli texts, see: Vin i.183; SN i.23, v.241, 251; AN i.264, iii.443, iv.7; MN i.483; Sn 62, 74, 621; Ja i.275; ii.22; Nett 49.

68 For a discussion of the fetters as a subset of the influxes (*āsravas*), alongside the afflictions (*kleśas*), see Chapter 2 of this book.

69 The metaphor MIND IS A MACHINE is also evident in this conceptual system in the notions of cognition and cogitation as the 'turning' of the mind or in Patañjali's description of *cittavṛtti nirodha*, the cessation of the 'turnings' of the mind.

70 This metaphorical complex is not necessarily referred to as *bhāvanā*, but rather contains the key markers of agriculture: planting, ripening, maturing, harvesting, etc.

71 I rely here on the important references laid out by Collins in his discussion of 'vegetation imagery' in early Buddhist texts (Collins 1982: 218–24).

72 *karotaṃ opadhikaṃ saṅghe dinnaṃ mahāphalan iti.*

73 See an extended version of this in AN iv, 237.

74 For this epithet in relation to the Buddha, see SN i 167; Sn 486; It 98; in relation to advanced monks, see MN i 446; AN i 244, ii 113, iii 158, 248, 279, 387, iv 10, 292; Mil 416; Pv iv I; in relation to the institution of monkhood, see DN iii, 5, 227; MN iii 80; S i 220, v 343, 363, 382; AN ii 34, 56; It 88.

75 For further references to metaphors of botanical cultivation in Pāli texts, see Chapter 2, note 37 of this study.

76 In a Sutta entitled 'City' in the *Saṃyutta Nikāyā*, the Buddha describes a person who wanders through a jungle forest and sees an ancient road. At the end of the road, he sees an old royal city that is somewhat dilapidated. The city is then rebuilt so that it becomes rich and prosperous and crowded with people (Collins 2010: 89).

77 See also Shaw's discussion of rice in relation to the virtue of *dāna* and the 'passive' versus 'active' models of Buddhism (Shaw 2007: 33).

78 There is also a story in which the Elder Sammuñjani sees the forest ascetic Revata sitting in solitude, cross-legged and thinks that he is an idler. Revata reads his thoughts and reproaches him (*Dhammapadaṭṭhakathā* iii.168 f; cited in Malalasekera 1938 II: 754; 1065).

79 This internalization of labour is also reflected in the internalization of the ritual as discussed in Upaniṣadic contexts. In the internalization of yogic ritual, the public domain of priestly work, the ritual, is appropriated at an individual level via mind/body practices perceived to generate power (Heesterman 1993). Collins discusses how 'Buddhism drew on Brahmanical ideas of "constructive activity" … and on the renouncers' introjection of sacrificial motifs into individual consciousness' (Collins 1982: 223). I would add that the introjection occurred not just at the level of action or ritual action but also in the terms of communal work and labour.

80 There are also numerous examples in the early Buddhist canon. The tree of desire grows unless it is chopped at the roots (*Saṃyutta Nikāyā* 2.87–9). Birth, old age and death are like weeds and creepers that cannot be stopped (*Vishuddimagga* 15.58). A related image, though not one that advocates cessation of growth, is: just as sap flows when someone cuts a tree, so when the sense objects enter the mind, one becomes obsessed with the three *kleśas* (*Saṃyutta Nikāya* 4.60). The three primary *kleśas* are weeds (*Dhammapada* 24.356–9).

81 Other, related ways of framing this division include Larson's two systems of philosophy: the *ṣaṣṭitantra* tradition of knowledge and the Abhidharma tradition of cessation (Larson 1989: 134). I am also indebted here to Sarbacker's analysis of two currents in Indo-Tibetan yoga as the 'numinous' and the 'cessative' (Sarbacker 2005). See also in this present book 'Introduction' endnotes 54 and 59.

Chapter 2

1 An earlier version of this chapter was published as O'Brien-Kop 2018.
2 This is the standard formatting in conceptual metaphor theory – see Chapter 1.
3 Abhidharma is characterized as a scholastic tradition centred on ontology, but the importance of insight meditation to Abhidharma should not be overlooked (Cousins 1996: 51; Stuart 2015, 1: 245). Although in the early centuries of the Common Era, Sarvāstivāda Abhidharma expounded dharma theory in the context of philosophical enquiry, the tradition is also marked by insight meditation practices upon the nature of those dharmas. The production of the early Mahāyāna meditation *sūtras* and the Abhidharma treatises is contemporaneous in the early centuries and it is reasonable to presuppose some degree of mutual influence (Stuart 2015, 1: 244).
4 The Abhidharmapiṭaka forms one of the three *piṭakas* or 'baskets' of the Buddhist canon. Mahāyāna tradition sometimes refers to this basket as the Śāstrapiṭaka. The other two *piṭakas* are the Sūtra and the Vinaya.
5 Some scholars believe that each of the schools of early Buddhism had its own Abhidharma texts, but only three Abhidharma collections are extant: the Theravāda Abhidharma, the Sarvāstivāda Abhidharma and the Dharmaguptaka Abhidharma.
6 The seven books are the *Prakaraṇapāda*, *Vijñānakāya*, *Dharmaskandha*, *Prajñaptiśāstra*, *Dhātukāya*, *Saṅgītaparyāya* and *Jñānaprasthāna*. They are all extant in Chinese, apart from the *Prajñaptiśāstra*, which is partially extant in Chinese and fully extant in Tibetan. Although each book was attributed to an individual author, the Vaibhāṣikas claimed that, ultimately, these texts contained the words of the Buddha, a point that the Sautrāntikas disagreed with. The central text of the group was the *Jñānaprasthāna*, while the other six books were satellites. The *Jñānaprasthāna* introduces soteriological schema, together with a detailed description of the afflictions (*kleśas*). See Willemen et al. (1997: 177–229).
7 Although the name *Mahāvibhāṣā* is not actually attested in the literature, this is how it is most commonly referred to (Kritzer 2005: xxi, fn. 23).
8 Kritzer gives a useful account of the controversy over the texts that can be attributed to Vasubandhu (Kritzer 2005: xxiv–xxvi). For a summary of the scholarship that has successfully resolved date discrepancies of Vasubandhu's lifespan, as well as further historical context, see Anacker (1984: 7–24). Skilling traces a tentative chronology from a Sautrāntika phase in Vasubandhu's output, namely the *Abhidharmakośabhāṣya*, to a later Mahāyāna phase (Skilling 2000: 309–10). Kritzer's conclusion is that the *Abhidharmakośabhāṣya* is not a Sarvāstivāda work at all but constituted a covert Yogācāra work that disguises itself as a Sautrāntika production (Kritzer 2005).
9 After Vasubandhu, there were no further Sarvāstivāda Abhidharma treatises, only commentaries on those treatises. Although the AKBh purports to be a

summary of the commentarial *Mahāvibhāṣā*, scholars now think that it drew on the *Abhidharmasāra* (also called *Abhidharmahṛdayaśāstra*) by Dharmaśrī. See Kritzer (2005: xxi) for more detail on where the AKBh fits into the broader scheme of Abhidharma literature. For more on the *Abhidharmasāra*, see Frauwallner (1995: 137–40) and Willemen, Dessein and Cox (1998: 255–69).

10 In total, there were eight Sanskrit commentaries on the *Abhidharmakośabhāṣya*, now preserved in the Tibetan Bstan-'gyur, the collection of commentaries to the Buddhist teachings, including Sthiramati's *Tattvārtha* (Kritzer 2005: xxii).

11 Some later Vaibhāṣika commentators rejected the *bhāṣya* since, in their view, it contained philosophical positions that were incompatible with orthodox Sarvāstivāda. Gold argues that within the textual conventions of *kārikā* and auto-commentary, this is an 'extremely unusual disjunction' (Gold 2015: 3).

12 The *Abhidharmakośabhāṣya* is divided into nine chapters in total: the first eight contain *kārikā*s and commentary, and the ninth is a prose chapter.

13 Kritzer gives a useful account of the controversy over the texts that can be attributed to Vasubandhu (Kritzer 2005: xxiv–xxvi).

14 Gold argues that the only evidence for identifying multiple Vasubandhus is the ascription of the name 'Vasubandhu' to three half-brothers, Vasubandhu, Asaṅga and Viriñcivatsa (Gold 2015: 11, 18). They shared the same father but had different mothers, and *vasubandhu* means 'good kin' (Gold 2015: 20).

15 For more on the identity and affiliation of Vasubandhu and the likelihood of the *bhāṣya* as an auto-commentary, see Kritzer (2005: xx–xxii); Park (2014: 1–29); and Gold (2015: 1–20).

16 For Gold, '"Sautrāntika" was not definitely attested as a doctrinal school before Vasubandhu, and "Yogācāra" definitely postdated him' (Gold 2015: 5). However, Gold cautions us to maintain the difference between Yogācāra and Mahāyāna, as a broader scholastic classification: 'Paramārtha's Chinese biography mentions Mahāyāna, but not Yogācāra, as Vasubandhu's final scholastic identity' (Gold 2015: 3). Gold further asserts that 'it is a mistake to set up a teleological directionality for Vasubandhu's works, with the Yogācāra system as its ultimate end' (Gold 2015: 19).

17 For more on the scholastic affiliations of Vasubandhu's output, see Anacker (1984).

18 Other names for the Sautrāntikas include Saṁkrāntivādin, Sūtrāntavādin, Sauryodayika, Dārṣṭāntika and Sūtraprāmāṇika (Lamotte 1988: 25).

19 Sanderson claims that the rivalry between the Vaibhāṣikas and the Sautrāntikas goes back at least to the second century CE when Nāgārjuna presented the current Buddhist theories on karma and retribution in the *Karmaphalaparīkṣa* (*Mūlamadhyamakakārikā* 17.2–20) (Sanderson 1994: 41).

20 See Kritzer (2005: xxvii–xxx) for a review of numerous scholarly views on the affinity between the Sautrāntika positions in the *Abhidharmakośabhāṣya* and later Yogācāra texts.

21 Deleanu suggests that one could be a Sautrāntika in terms of scholastic views and hermeneutical approaches, but still be an orthodox Sarvāstivādin in the sense of adopting different perspectives from the Vaibhāṣika establishment and authority (Deleanu 2006: 159). Hwang (2006: 86–102) gives a detailed account of the Sautrāntika theories that we know about.

22 There are two references to the Sautrāntikas in the *Mahāvibhāṣā*, but this is thought to be a retrospective label applied by the Chinese translator (Cox 1995: 38). See also Gold (2015: 3) and Kritzer (2005: xxvii). Stuart argues that in the *Saddharmasmṛtyupasthānasūtra* (second to fourth century CE) 'a number of philosophical concepts in the text seem to correlate with a putative "Sautrāntika position". Thus, the text may be one of the few historical documents extant that presents an actual work of masters connected to the somewhat elusive Sautrāntika school' (Stuart 2015, 1: 6 fn. 6).

23 Unless we equate Sautrāntika with Dārṣṭāntika whose founder is traditionally revered as Kumāralāta.

24 The *Nyāyānusāra* and other sources state an identity between Śrīlāta and Sthavira.

25 The name Dārṣṭāntika is derived from √*dṛś*, to see, and *tānta*, an example or simile.

26 Deleanu, for example, argues that the Dārṣṭāntikas and the Sautrāntikas basically propose the same philosophical positions (Deleanu 2006: 214 fn. 69). See also Park (2014: 1–42 and 59–64) for an overview of recent theories on the Dārṣṭāntikas and Sautrāntikas, as well as more about Vasubandhu's representation of these groups.

27 See also Gold (2015: 3).

28 It is important to note that some of the Sautrāntika ideas in the *Abhidharmakośabhāṣya* appear in 'a less developed form' as Dārṣṭāntika ideas in the *Vibhāṣā* (Kritzer 2005: xxviii). Park asserts that many of the passages in the *Abhidharmakośabhāṣya* which are said to have been influenced by the *Yogācārabhūmiśāstra* are, in fact, derived from the Mainstream (Śrāvakayāna) Buddhist Dārṣṭāntika-Sautrāntika tradition that preceded Vasubandhu (Park 2014).

29 Gold argues that Vasubandhu coined the label Sautrāntika to name his own philosophical positions. Subsequently, according to Gold, the name Sautrāntika took on a separate life and came to denote other positions (Gold 2015: 25). Gold argues that this divergence is not illogical and constitutes the detail of a total 'worldview' which is unique to Vasubandhu (Gold 2015: 25). This argument, however, has been critiqued by Franco (2017).

30 In the manner typical of commentaries, the *bhāṣya* includes an objection, *pūrvapakṣa*, before returning to establish the *siddhānta*, the accepted position. However, 'what distinguishes [Vasubandhu's] commentary is that the *siddhānta*

position from the root verses quite often appears to *lose* the debate. Even when the *siddhānta* is restated as though proven at the end of a given line of argument, the best arguments with unmet objections have often been those put forward as a *pūrvapakṣa*' (Gold 2015: 24).

31 Anacker discusses this term in Buddhist studies: 'The Sanskrit root "*kliś*" means "to be afflicted, to be tormented, to suffer," and a *kleśa* is accordingly "an affliction, pain, anguish, suffering"' (Anacker 1984: 146–7). He also challenges the appropriateness of the translation of 'defilement' for this term: '*kleśa* has never meant, either in Sanskrit or for any people in direct contact with Indian masters, "defilement", as it is usually translated' (Anacker 1984: 146–7).

32 *yas tv ekāgre cetasi sadbhūtam arthaṃ dyotayati, kṣiṇoti kleśān, karmabandhanāni ślathayati, nirodham āmukhīkaroti, sa saṃprajñāto yoga ity ākhyāyate* (PYŚ 1.1; Maas 2006: 4–5, 8–11).

33 Anacker suggests that in Buddhist discourse the *kleśa*s are linked to knowledge and not to ethics. For example, he argues that although the *kleśa*s are 'bad' in that they entail suffering, they are 'not necessarily unbeneficial' and thus not 'ethically reprehensible' (Anacker 1984: 147). Thus, there is 'an entire category of factors which are categorized as afflicted, but which are ethically beneficial (the *kuśalasāsravas*), and another which is similarly afflicted, but ethically indeterminate (the *nivṛtāvyākṛta*s, "obstructed but indeterminate events") … So "attachment may sometimes be beneficial, and doubts, remorse, and aversion, though afflicted, may have good results" ' (Anacker 1984: 147).

34 The image of the tree is also used to describe a person who is still standing if the roots have not been properly cut (*Dhammapada* 3.56 and *Saṃyutta Nikāya* 4.60). The *Abhidharmakośabhāṣya* also contains a discourse about the 'good' or wholesome roots. There are four wholesome roots of spiritual penetration (*nirvedabhāgīyakuśalamūla*). These are the four aspects of the direct path of preparation, *prayogamārga*: heat (*ūṣman*), summit (*mūrdhan*), receptivity (*kṣānti*) and highest worldly dharma (*laukikāgradharma*). The *nirvedabhāgīya*s open access to the path of sight (*darśana*). This model is part of the larger Vaibhāṣika scheme of *kuśalamūla* which contains other models, such as the tenfold formations associated with the mind (*cittasaṃprayuktasaṃskāra*). Jaini argues that the Sautrāntika theory of seed is partly formulated in response to the Vaibhāṣika root theory (Jaini 1992: 101–2).

35 The generative context of this metaphor may be botanical in that some undesirable (i.e. 'bad') plants yield poisons, but it may also indicate poison in other contexts such as medical (e.g. snake/insect poison) or even alchemical, in the sense of ingestion. In the Vedic texts, *viṣa*, indicating 'poison', can refer to a range of situations, such as virus, impurity or venom (Monier-Williams 1899: 995), thereby indicating an early discursive context relating to medical healing. In the Pāli texts,

viṣa as poison of various sorts is discussed at, for example, MN I 316; Sn 1; AN ii 110; Mil 302.

36 As Salguero explains, the 'textual core' of the *Suvarṇabhāsottamasūtra* is thought to have been composed in Sanskrit during the first centuries CE, although Dharmakṣema's Chinese translation is the earliest surviving version (Salguero 2017: 30).

37 *Dosa* (Skt. *doṣa*) is common in the Pāli sources, e.g. *snehadosa* at Sn 66. *Dosa* also stands in for one of the three *mahākleśas*, *dveṣa* 'aversion' (P. *disa*) (see SN i 98; MN i 47, 489; AN i 134, 201, ii 191, iii 338). Interestingly, to bring the concept of *doṣa* out of the medical context and back to botanical cultivation, we find *khettadosa* in *Milindapañha* 360 as 'the blight of the field', and the *Dhammapada* elucidates that the three *doṣas* are the 'roots' of what is bad and that they are 'weeds' in the 'field' of mankind (*Dhammapada* 3, 56–9). The Buddha is referred to as *tridoṣāpaha* (destroying the three *doṣas*) in *MahāVyutpatti* 71. The *tridosā* are described at *Milindapañha* 43 and 172; DA i.133.

38 See Chapter 4 for a further outline of the complex relationship between *doṣa* and *kleśa*.

39 Different traditions invented different schemata for the *kleśas*. In Sarvāstivāda Abhidharma, for example, the Vaibhāṣikas counted ten *kleśas* and regarded them as identical to the *anuśayas*, which Willemen et al. translate as 'contaminant': *āhrikya*, *anapatrāpya*, *styāna*, *kaukṛtya*, *mātsarya*, *īrṣyā*, *auddhatya*, *middha*, *krodha* and *mrakṣya*. The Sautrāntikas, however, separated the two concepts and numbered the *anuśayas* as only eight (Willemen et al. 1997: 31). For the Sautrāntikas, the *anuśaya* was the seed of the affliction and the *āsraya* was the seedbed. I will unpack this distinction later on in this chapter.

40 As discussed above, although Gombrich refers to the 'three poisons' in English, the Sanskrit equivalent that he cites is *doṣa*, 'fault', specifically *tri-doṣa*.

41 In this act of metaphoric revision, Gombrich claims, *upādāna*, which literally meant 'fuel' in the original metaphor of the three fires, now became understood in the abstract sense as 'attachment' or 'grasping'.

42 See the section on *bhāvanā* in Chapter 1 for more detail.

43 Discussed in Chapter 1 in the introduction to conceptual metaphor theory.

44 In his analysis of conceptual metaphor theory in relation to the *Dhammapada*, Egge notes that 'passions' or *āsravas* are configured by different metaphors: *āsravas* are 'plants that may quickly become overgrown, currents that threaten to carry people away, and fetters that may ensnare' (Egge 2013: 97 fn. 33). What is entailed in all three metaphors, however, is that *āsravas* are dangerous. This underlying concept of 'danger' is derived from the sensorimotor experience of being caught in overgrown thicket, or being in a strong current, or being physically trapped. Egge concludes, 'Therefore, metaphors are motivated not by the perceived similarity

between the inherent structures of source and target domains, but by the perceived similarity between our pragmatic relationships with source and target domains' (Egge 2013: 98).

45 *jñātvā devaṃ sarvapāśāpahāniḥ kṣīṇaiḥ kleśairjanmamṛtyuprahāṇiḥ / tasyābhidhyānāttṛtīyam dehabhede viśvaiśvaryaṃ kevala āprakāmaḥ* (ŚvetUp 1.11). 'When one has known God, all the fetters fall off; by the eradication of the blemishes, birth and death come to an end; by meditating on him, one obtains, at the dissolution of the body, a third – sovereignty over all; and in the absolute one's desires are fulfilled' (verse and translation Olivelle 1998: 416–17).

46 In the *Bhagavad Gītā*, the term *kliṣṭa* appears in a general context: *dīyate ca parikliṣṭaṃ tad dānaṃ rājasaṃ smṛtam* (BG 17.21; Bolle 1979: 190). And *kleśa* appears twice in apparently generic contexts: *kleśodhikataras teṣāṃ avyaktāsaktacetasām / avyaktā hi gatir duḥkhaṃ dehavadbhir avāpyate* (BG 12.5; Bolle 1979: 146). And *niyatasya tu saṃnyāsaḥ karmaṇo nopapadyate / mohāt tasya parityāgas tāmasaḥ parikīrtitaḥ / duḥkham ity eva yat karma kāyakleśabhayāt tyajet / sa kṛtvā rājasaṃ tyāgaṃ naiva tyāgaphalaṃ labhet* (BG 18.7–8; Bolle 1979: 196).

47 The *Nyāyasūtrabhāṣya* also discusses the *kleśa*s in relation to the PYŚ: *tadarthaṃ yamaniyamābhyām ātmasaṃskāro yogāc cādhyātmavidhyupāyaiḥ || tasyāpavargasyādhigamāya yamaniyamābhyām ātmasaṃskāraḥ / yamaḥ samānam āśramiṇāṃ dharmasādhanam, niyamas tu viśiṣṭam / ātmasaṃskāraḥ punar adharmahānaṃ dharmopacayaś ca / yogaśāstrāc cādhyātmavidhiḥ pratipattavyaḥ / sa punas tapaḥ prāṇāyāmaḥ pratyāhāro dhyānaṃ dhāraṇeti / indriyaviṣayeṣu prasaṃkhyānābhyāso rāgadveṣaprahāṇārthaḥ / upāyas tu yogācāravidhānam iti* (NySBh 4.2.46; Sastri 1984: 239). This passage refers to *prasaṃkhyāna* as a practice and explains it as contemplation on the sense objects, which leads to the abandonment of the two major *kleśas*: *rāga* and *dveṣa*. The dating for Vātsyāyana's *Nyāyasūtrabhāṣya* (the first *bhāṣya* on the *Nyāyāsūtra*) is debated, but as we must place it after the *Pātañjalayogaśāstra*, Potter's estimation of 425–500 CE seems appropriate (Potter 1977: 239).

48 Here is the list of forms of confusion (perplexity) from the *Sāṃkhyakārikā*: *bhedas tamaso 'ṣṭavidho mohasya ca daśavidho mahāmohaḥ / tāmisro 'ṣṭādaśadhā tathā bhavaty andhatāmisraḥ*. 'There are eight kinds of dullness, and also of perplexity, ten kinds of great perplexity; depression is eighteenfold, as is intense depression' (SK 48; trans. Burley 2007: 174). And here is Patañjali's closely concordant list: *seyaṃ pañcaparvā bhavaty avidyā. avidyāsmitārāgadveṣābhiniveśāḥ kleśā iti. eta eva svasaṃjñābhis tamo moho mahāmohas tāmisro 'ndhatāmisra iti. ete cittamalaprasaṅgenābhidhāsyante* (PYŚ 1.8). 'Of this there are five varieties: ignorance (*avidyā*), egoism (*asmitā*), attachment (*rāga*), aversion (*dveṣa*) and fear of death (*abhiniveśaḥ*) are the *kleśas*. These are also given their own

names: darkness, delusion, great confusion, great darkness, and total darkness. These will be named by means of their connection to the impurity of the mind.'

49 For more on the evolution of *doṣa* as a medical paradigm in relation to Pātañjala yoga, see Maas 2008b.

50 In his Buddhist-Hybrid dictionary, Edgerton translates *visaṃyoga* as 'dissociation' or 'severance'. It is a synonym for *nisṛjā*, which is '(religious) abandonment (of worldly things)' (Edgerton 1953).

51 Esler defines *pratisaṃkhyānirodha* as 'cessation due to deliberation ... the definitive eradication through deliberation (*pratisaṃkhyā*) of the latencies (*anuśaya*) producing new existences' (Esler 2016: 341). Edgerton's Buddhist-Hybrid dictionary gives the meaning of *pratisaṃkhyā* as 'careful (point by point) consideration'. This translation refers to both an analytical component ('careful consideration') and an enumerative aspect ('point by point') (Edgerton 1953). But it is somewhat unwieldy, and so I will use the translation 'analysis' to translate *pratisaṃkhyā* as many Buddhist scholars do and also because I wish to differentiate it from Patañjali's *prasaṃkhyāna*. In his list of the *lakṣaṇas* that pertain to the seven *saṃbodhi-aṅgas*, Gethin includes *paṭisaṃkhāna*, which he translates as 'judgement' and which corresponds to the *bodhi-aṅga* of *upekṣā* (equanimity) (Gethin 2007: 161). Gethin points out that the term is used occasionally in the Nikāyas in the context of 'insight or wisdom' but concludes, 'What precisely is intended by *paṭisaṃkhāna* in the context of *upekkasambojjhaṅga* is unclear; "reviewing" or "balanced judgement" might be appropriate' (Gethin 2007: 162). I have been unable to ascertain whether this Pāli term is the equivalent of *pratisaṃkhyā* or *pratisaṃkhyāna* but it appears closely related. See endnote 53 below.

52 From the explanation, we are to understand 'by *pratisaṃkhyā* cessation can be attained' (AKBh 1.5; Pradhan 1975: 4, 1–2). To expand the description, it is cessation due to analysis in meditation of the real nature of phenomena. *Pratisaṃkhyānirodha* applies specifically to the elimination of each of the *kleśas* that is associated with the three *dhātus*, or realms of existence: *kāmadhātu* (sensuous realm), *rūpadhātu* (material realm) and *ārūpyadhātu* (immaterial realm).

53 *duḥkhādīnām āryasatyānāṃ pratisaṃkhyānaṃ pratisaṃkhyā prajñāviśeṣas tena prāpyo nirodhaḥ* (AKBh 1.5; Pradhan 1975: 4, 1–2). '*Pratisaṃkhyāna* of the four noble truths of suffering, etc. is *pratisaṃkhyā* (analysis), i.e. a special kind of *prajñā* (insight). By means of that, *nirodha* can be attained.' In Buddhism *prajñā* is 'practical knowledge' (Lusthaus 2002: 164). It is the breakdown of the factors of sensation and experience, and these factors are called *dharmas* (Lusthaus 2002: 164).

54 The mind, in this context, is a series of aggregates.

55 *ity etad ākāśādi trividham asaṃskṛtaṃ mārgasatyaṃ ca anāsravā dharmāḥ / kiṃ kāraṇam / na hi teṣv āsravā anuśerata iti.* 'The three unconditioned [things] of

akāśa etc. and the truth of the path are pure dharmas because the afflictions do not stick to them' (AKBh 1.4; Pradhan 1975: 3, 19–20).

56 Even in the earlier canonical *Prakaraṇapāda* – one of the seven texts of the Sarvāstivāda Abhidharma Piṭaka, composed by Vasumitra *c.* second century CE – *pratisaṃkhyānirodha* is the means to the ultimate goal of *saṃyojanaprahāna* (abandonment of fetters), the *saṃyojanas* (fetters) being another subcategory of *kleśa* in Buddhism (PP 7 T 26 (1542) 719a55ff, cited in Cox 1992: 95 fn. 24.)

57 This assertion is made repeatedly from the first chapter of the *Abhidharmakośabhāṣya*: *pratisaṃkhyānirodho yo visaṃyogaḥ / yaḥ sāsravair dharmair visaṃyogaḥ sa pratisaṃkhyānirodhaḥ* (AKBh 1.5; Pradhan 1975: 3–4). 'Cessation via analysis is disjunction. Disjunction from the defiled *dharmas* is cessation via analysis.'

58 The four noble truths are the truth of suffering, the truth of the cause of suffering, the truth of cessation and the truth of the path of cessation. *Pratisaṃkhyānirodha* is particularly identified with the third noble truth, the truth of cessation: '*pratisaṃkhyānirodho yo visaṃyoga' iti nirodhasatyaṃ*. 'Saying "cessation via analysis is disjunction", indicates the truth of cessation' (AKBh 6.1; Pradhan 1975: 327, 14).

59 The theory of *visaṃyoga* as the disjunction of the *kleśas* from *citta* also recurs in the *Yogācārabhūmiśāstra*. See, for example, the *Bodhisattvabhūmi*, which explains that the fruit of disjunction is the cessation of affliction: *āryāṣṭāṅgasya mārgasya kleśanirodho visaṃyogaphalam* (BoBh 1.8; Wogihara 1930–6: 102, 24–5). See another example of this theory at SamāBh 2.4.4.2.1.4.2; Delhey (2009: 154).

60 *yo dharmaṃ śaraṇaṃ gacchati asau nirvāṇaṃ śaraṇaṃ gacchati pratisaṃkhyānirodham* (AKBh 4.32; Pradhan 1975: 216, 28–9).

61 See AKBh 4.32: *svaparasaṃtānakleśānāṃ duḥkhasya ca śāntyekalakṣaṇātvāt* (Pradhan 1975: 216, 29–30). 'Because [*nirvāṇa* and *pratisaṃkhyānirodha*] have for their sole characteristic the pacifying of the continuous afflictions and suffering of oneself and others.'

62 *visaṃyogalābhas teṣāṃ punaḥ punaḥ* (AKBh 5.62; Pradhan 1975: 321).

63 For the Vaibhāṣikas no *kleśa* could be truly destroyed because of their unique ontology of a dharma existing simultaneously in the past, present and future.

64 The *Abhidharmakośabhāṣya* adheres to the late Sarvāstivāda path-structure and delineates four graded paths: preparatory, successive, liberating and special (*prayogamārga*, *ānantaryamārga*, *vimuktimārga* and *viśeṣamārga*) (AKK 6.65; Pradhan 1975: 381). *Visaṃyoga* is instrumental to *ānantaryamārga*, but also provides a bridge to *vimuktimārga*. *Vimukti* is the attained state of liberation from the afflictions (*visaṃyogaprāpti*). Additionally, two overarching paths of knowledge and cultivation, *darśana* and *bhāvanā* – which were characteristic of late Sarvāstivāda (Cox 1992: 75) – are integrated with the basic fourfold path-structure

so that, at a certain level of attainment, *bhāvanā* has disjunction (*visaṃyoga*) as its result: *svargāya śīlaṃ prādhānyāt visaṃyogāya bhāvanā* (AKK 4.123; Pradhan 1975: 274, 4). 'Essentially, the precepts have heaven for their result; meditation has disconnection for its result' (trans. Pruden 1988–90, 2: 705).

65 In Buddhist texts of this period, *pratisaṃkhyāna* can also appear as a more general term for contemplation, as in contemplating one's food while one eats.

66 See discussions of *prasaṃkhyāna* pertaining to seven different *sūtra*s, albeit primarily located in the *bhāṣya*: PYŚ 1.2, 1.15, 2.2, 2.4, 2.11, 2.12, 4.29.

67 *yas tv ekāgre cetasi sadbhūtam arthaṃ dyotayati, kṣiṇoti kleśān, karmabandhanāni ślathayati, nirodham āmukhīkaroti, sa saṃprajñāto yoga ity ākhyāyate* (PYŚ 1.1; Maas 2006: 4–5, 8–11). 'But when the mind is one-pointed, that [*samādhi*] which illuminates an existing (real) object destroys the *kleśas* [and] loosens the bonds of karma; it conduces towards cessation. That *saṃprajñāta [samādhi]* is called yoga.'

68 ***samādhibhāvanārthaḥ kleśatanūkaraṇārthaś ca*** (YS 2.2; Angot 2012: 379). 'It [*kriyā yoga*] has the purpose of cultivating *samādhi* and the purpose of attenuating the *kleśas*.'

69 *tad eva rajoleśamalāpetaṃ svarūpapratiṣṭhaṃ sattvapuruṣānyatākhyātimātraṃ dharmameghadhyānopagaṃ bhavati. tat prasaṃkhyānam ity ācakṣate dhyāyinaḥ* (PYŚ 1.2; Maas 2006: 5–6, 6–8).

70 Additionally, destruction of the *kleśa*s is categorized as part of *saṃprajñāta samādhi* at PYŚ 1.2 (Maas 2006: 3, 5–7), and if *prasaṃkhyāna* is a specific meditational technique to destroy the *kleśa*s, then that, too, must be part of *saṃprajñāta samādhi*. Furthermore, *dhyāna* belongs to *saṃprajñāta samādhi:* YS 1.39 includes *dhyāna* at the end of a list of object-centred methods, and the four *samāpatti*s of *dhyāna* take gross or subtle objects (PYŚ 1.44; Maas 2006: 76, 11–12).

71 For the view that *prasaṃkhyāna* and *vivekakhyāti* are synonyms, see Sundaresan (1998: 67) and Endo (2000: 79). However, I argue that the two terms are distinct in meaning. In the cited passage above (PYŚ 1.2), *sattvapuruṣānyatākhyātimātraṃ* (only discernment of the difference between *sattva* and *puruṣa*) is a description of *prasaṃkhyāna*. This is not identical to *vivekakhyāti* (discriminating discernment), because although both terms indicate the same perceptive state, one is provisional (*sattva* from *puruṣa*) and one is ultimate (*prakṛti* from *puruṣa*).

72 In the Brahmanical tradition, there is another related term: *parisaṃkhyāna*. For more detail on this point, and a fuller discussion of the meaning of *prasaṃkhyāna*, see O'Brien-Kop 2018.

73 From early Sarvāstivāda texts, e.g. the *Vijñānakāya*, the path of vision (*darśanamārga*) can take the four noble truths as its object (Cox 1992: 75–6).

74 *vivekadarśanābhyāsena kalyāṇasrota udghāṭyate, ity ubhayādhīnaś cittavṛttinirodhaḥ* (PYŚ 1.12; Maas 2006: 22, 6–7). 'It (the stream towards evil) is cut off; the stream

towards what is wholesome is produced by the practice of the knowledge (*darśana*) of discrimination.'

75 I acknowledge here that *vivekakhyāti* is an epistemological state and not ontological, while *kaivalya* is ultimately ontological.

76 See, for example, *Saṃyutta Nikāya* 1.1.27: 'Like the seed that is sown, so is the fruit that is harvested. The doer of good (plants and reaps) good, and the doer of bad, bad. When the seed is sown and planted, you shall experience the appropriate fruit' (trans. Collins 1982: 220). The canonical Jain *Uttarādhyana* 7.20 states that all beings will reap the fruit of their actions.

77 There is commonly a positive context for the image of the seed in Brahmanical sources, connoting the rewards of good actions: 'the objects given to Brahmins become treasures in the next world, and there is no end to the fruits produced by the seed-like gifts sown in the land-like Brahmins and cultivated with the plough of the Vedas' (*Viṣṇudharmottara Purāṇa* 2.32.2f; cited in Gonda 1965: 225). Generally, within Brahmanical literature, the metaphor of the seed is used to illustrate the theory of birth and rebirth, as well as the nature of the true self in invisible potential form. See, for example, BU 3.9.28 for the analogy of a human life to that of a tree, which comes from a seed. The seed image also appears in CU 6.11.12 in the analogy of how tiny the essence of the self (*ātman*) is. For the image of the manifest springing from the unmanifest, see MB 12.211.1 (in Wynne 2009: 336). See also three contrasting meanings of the term *bīja*, collected together in one passage: to indicate 'soul' (*jīva*), karmic seed that prompts the sense faculty into action, and procreative seed i.e. semen (MB 12.213.10–15 in Wynne 2009: 351–3). For seed meaning 'divine source of all lifeforms', see BhG 7.10, 9.18, 10.39, 14.4 (Bolle 1979). The 'Śānti Parvan' also contains references to *prakṛti* as 'the great receptacle of seed properties' (*bīja dharmāṇāṃ mahāgrāha*) (MB 12.308 appendix I: 29A line 22; Belvalkar 1954, 16: 2075, 22) and to *prakṛti* as being *bījadharma* or 'having the quality of seed' (MB 12.308 appendix I: 29B line 303; Belvalkar 1954, 16: 2083, 303). There are many other similar examples in the *Mahābhārata*.

78 Although this chapter deals with *bīja* in relation to karma and *kleśa*, it must be noted that the image of the seed was also employed to challenge the Sarvāstivāda theory of dharma. Both the Sautrāntika positions of the *Abhidharmakośabhāṣya* and the *Yogācārabhūmiśāstra* broadly refute the key Sarvāstivāda doctrine – the idea that past, present and future dharmas all really exist. Specifically, the *Yogācārabhūmiśāstra* denies the real existence of the Sarvāstivāda concepts of *cittaviprayuktasaṃskāra* and *avijñaptirūpa* and refers instead to the operations of the *bīja*s to explain phenomena (Kritzer 2005: xix).

79 Within Buddhist Studies, prior research has been done on the role of the seed in soteriology and I will draw on these. Collins analysed the image of the seed in 'Theravāda Buddhism' under the rubric of 'vegetation imagery' in relation to

'conditioning, consciousness, and time' and particularly in relation to notions of selfhood (Collins 1982: 187–8, 218–24). Hwang (2006) usefully theorizes metaphor and literalism in the doctrinal history of *nirvāṇa*, and, most recently, Park has produced an important study that elucidates how the Dārṣṭāntika-Sautrāntikas elaborated their unique theory of the seed (Park 2014).

80 Yet there are two specific technical uses of the burnt seed image in the 'Mokṣadharma' section of the 'Śānti Parvan' (Book 12 of the *Mahābhārata*) that are worth noting: *bījāny agnyupadaghdhāni na rohanti yathā punaḥ, jñānadagdhais tathā kleśair n'ātmā saṃpadyate punaḥ*. 'Just as seeds burned by fire will not sprout again, so too will the self not be reborn when its defilements are burned by gnosis' (MB 12.211.15, trans. Wynne 2009: 341). In this passage, the seeds of *kleśa* are burnt by *jñāna*, which is redolent of the *jñānāgni* of PYŚ 4.28 (Angot 2012: 721, line 1), where it appears as a synonym for *prasaṃkhyāna*. Yet in this second passage from the 'Śānti Parvan', the specific technical function of the seed as a residue of *karma* is identified as a Buddhist theory: *avidyākarmatṛṣṇānāṃ ke cid āhuḥ punarbhave, kāraṇaṃ lobhamohau tu doṣānāṃ tu niṣevaṇam. avidyāṃ kṣetraṃ āhur hi, karma bījaṃ tathā kṛtam. tṛṣṇāsaṃjananaṃ sneha: eṣa teṣāṃ punarbhavaḥ. tasmin vyūḍhe ca dagdhe ca, citte maraṇadharmiṇi, anyo 'nyāj jāyate tam āhuḥ sattva saṃkṣāyam.* 'Some say that greed, delusion, and the habitual tendency towards other vices are the cause of the rebirth of ignorance, *karma* and thirst. These – the Buddhists – say that ignorance is the field, the act committed is the seed and the arising of thirst is the moisture necessary for its germination: this, for them, accounts for rebirth. When the seed that causes an existence develops and is burned away, and since the mind is characterised by death, another body is born from another seed: that, they say, constitutes the dissolution of a living thing' (MB 12.218.30, trans. Wynne 2009: 391–3) (Wynne's translation is from the Vulgate). The author of the 'Śānti Parvan' goes on to critique and refute this Buddhist position. Although the passage does not refer to the Buddhists by name, this passage occurs in a longer section of polemical attacks on other schools of thought. This section can be understood to attack the Buddhist position on non-self and non-continuity of consciousness after death. Later texts such the *Nyāyasūtrabhāṣya* refer to *nirbījam* (without seed) and *bījaprarohá* (the germination of the seed). But this text is, as we have seen, directly picking up on the discourse of the *Pātañjalayogaśāstra*: *tadabhāvaś cāpavarge / tasya buddhinimittāśrayasya śarīrendriyasya dharmādharmābhāvād abhāvo 'pavarge/ tatra yad uktam apavarge 'py evaṃ prasaṅga iti, tad ayuktam/ tasmāt sarvaduḥkhavimokṣo 'pavargaḥ/ yasmāt sarvaduḥkhabījaṃ sarvaduḥkhāyatanaṃ cāpavarge vicchidyate tasmāt sarveṇa duḥkhena vimuktir apavargaḥ/ na nirbījaṃ nirāyatanaṃ ca duḥkham utpadyata iti* (NySBh 4.2.45; Thakur 1997: 279). And *svapakṣarāgeṇa caike nyāyam ativartante, tatra: tattvādhyavasāyasaṃrakṣaṇārthaṃ jalpavitaṇḍe bījaprarohasaṃrakṣaṇārthaṃ kaṇṭakaśākhāvaraṇavat / anutpannatat*

tvajñānānām aprahīṇadoṣāṇāṃ tadarthaṃ ghaṭamānānām etad iti (NySBh 4.2.50; Thakur 1997: 281).

81 *pratanūkṛtān kleśān prasaṃkhyānāgninā dagdhabījakalpān aprasavadharmiṇaḥ kariṣyati iti* (PYŚ 2.2; Angot 2012: 379). For the same image, see PYŚ 2.4 and 2.13.

82 Noting the long history of *tapas* in the *Mahābhārata*, in which it is 'believed to bring about a magical power symbolized by heat' (Endo 2000: 78), Endo concludes of the *Yogabḥāṣya*: 'it seems reasonable to suppose that the author of the *YBh* had in mind that *prasaṃkhyāna* has a magical power similar to that of *tapas*' (Endo 2000: 78).

83 Endo also glosses over the primary nature of *tapas* as physical asceticism in contrast to *prasaṃkhyāna* as mental discipline. Furthermore, *tapas* is austere practice that leads to heat, while *prasaṃkhyāna* is described as fire itself.

84 Kritzer notes the central role of seed theory in Vasubandhu's rejection of orthodox Vaibhāṣika positions: in several contexts 'statements by Vasubandhu explicitly or implicitly rely on the idea of *bīja* in giving explanations that deviate from Vaibhāṣika orthodoxy' (Kritzer 2005: xxxv).

85 The image of the burnt seed also appears in the commentarial section of the *Yogācārabhūmiśāstra*. As Kritzer states, 'the *Viniścayasaṃgrahaṇī* on the *Pañcavijñānakāyamanobhūmi* compares seeds burned by fire, which are permanently rendered unproductive, with the seeds of internal dharmas that have been destroyed by the *ārya*' (paraphrase in translation of original Tibetan, Kritzer 2005: 53).

86 *āśrayo hi sa āryāṇāṃ darśanabhāvanāmārgasāmarthyāt tathā parāvṛtto bhavati yathā na punas tatpraheyāṇāṃ kleśānāṃ prarohasamartho bhavati / ato 'gnidagdhavrīhivad abījībhūte āśraye kleśānāṃ prahīṇakleśa ity ucyate / upahatabījabhāve vā laukikena mārgeṇa / viparyayād aprahīṇakleśaḥ* (AKBh 2.36 c–d; Pradhan 1975: 63, 20–1).

87 See PYŚ 1.2, 3.50 and 4.29 for clarification that even the *vivekakhyāti* produced by *prajñā* must be abandoned.

88 PYŚ 4.28–29 also clearly states that all *saṃskāras* must be completely eliminated.

89 ***tasyāpi nirodhe sarvanirodhān nirbījaḥ samādhiḥ*** (YS 1.51; Maas 2006: 158).

90 For examples of scholars who translate the *nirbīja* of 1.51 as 'objectless', see Āraṇya (1983: 116) and Raveh (2012: 130). Larson translates *nirbīja* as 'without content' in Larson and Bhattacharya (2008: 167) and as either 'seedless or objectless' in Larson (2012: 96). Bryant translates *nirbīja* as 'seedless' but in his commentary on the *sūtra* interprets this as meaning 'not focused on any aspect of an object' (Bryant 2009:164). For a different discussion of *nirbīja* see Maas (2009: 274 fn. 32).

91 For example, see Larson and Bhattacharya (2008: 27).

92 Although PYŚ 1.2 and 1.18 argue for an equivalence of *nirbīja* and *asaṃprajñāta* and PYŚ 1.46 relates *sabīja* to external object, it does not give us free licence to

interpret *nirbīja* as 'objectless'. 'Seed' meaning 'object' occurs in only two passages of the *Pātañjalayogaśāstra* out of some forty occurrences of *bīja*. See the next endnote.

93 Apart from its primary technical context as the seed of *kleśa*, there are, additionally, other contexts in which the term *bīja* is employed generically in the *Pātañjalayogaśāstra*: the seed of omniscience (YS 1.25), direct perception as the seed of inference and testimony (PYŚ 1.42; Maas 2006: 70, 9–10), the external object of meditation (PYŚ 1.46; Maas 2006: 78, 2–4; PYŚ 2.23; Angot 2012: 460, line 11), the origin of life as semen (PYŚ 2.5; Angot 2012: 384, line 5), the seed of error (PYŚ 4.23; Angot 2012: 712, line 8).

94 See Saṅkara's *Vivaraṇa* (*c.* eighth century CE) on PYŚ 1.2: 'The *samādhi* in this state of inhibition is the seedless. The meaning is, that here the seed is gone; in this all the seeds of taint and so on are gone' (trans. Leggett 1990: 63).

95 *Adhikāra* is here understood as 'appointed role'.

96 *tasmād avasitādhikāraṃ saha kaivalyabhāgīyaiḥ saṃskāraiś cittaṃ nivartate* (PYŚ 1.51; Maas 2006: 160–1, 11–12).

97 Maas points to a further relevant passage that occurs in PYŚ 1.2: 9–13, where the cessation of *vivekakhyāti* leads to a state in which only *saṃskāras* remain in the *citta* (*tadavasthaṃ saṃskāropagaṃ bhavati. sa nīrbījaḥ samādhiḥ*) and to PYŚ 2.10: *te pañca kleśā dagdhabījakalpā yoginaś caritādhikāre cetasi pralīne saha tenaivāstaṃ gacchanti* (personal communication, 7 December 2016). In my view, both of these instances underline the link between *prasaṃkhyāna* and *vivekakhyāti*: when *prasaṃkhyāna* burns the seed of *kleśa*, the function of the mind is brought to an end, a process which creates the condition for *vivekakhyāti* to arise and to produce the *kaivalya saṃskāras* (the karmic impressions that are conducive to *kaivalya*).

98 In the early canon, the theory of the two *nirvāṇas* was characterized as the *nirvāṇa* of the afflictions (*kleśas*), which still contained a remnant of attachment and the *nirvāṇa* of the aggregates (*skandhas*), which had no remnant of detachment (Collins 2010: 41). In what is regarded as the Buddha's first sermon after enlightenment, he explains the third noble truth, the cessation of suffering, as 'fading away without remainder' and 'cessation' as synonyms for nirvāṇa (Collins 2010: 65).

99 To be clear on the development of *bīja* as a Sautrāntika idea, we also need to clarify the chronology of the *Abhidharmakośabhāṣya* and the *Yogācārabhūmiśāstra*. This is because the *Yogācārabhūmiśāstra* predates the *Abhidharmakośabhāṣya* and although credited as a Mahāyāna work is in the majority a Sarvāstivādin treatise with newly emerging Mahāyāna ideas. Thus, when Kritzer identifies the concept of *bīja* as important to the *Yogācārabhūmiśāstra* he is right in asserting that the first textual developments of *bīja* occur in a Yogācāra text in relation to *ālayavijñāna*, i.e. the *Yogācārabhūmiśāstra*, although not yet in a systematic way; that would come later in the *Abhidharmakośabhāṣya* (Kritzer 2010: xix). Although their texts are not extant, the Sautrāntikas had a unique elaboration of the theory of the

seed, and Vasubandhu clearly attributes this theory to them (AKBh 5.3; Pradhan 1975: 278). Kritzer's study highlights how the *Abhidharmakośabhāṣya* utilizes arguments from the *Yogācārabhūmiśāstra* to reject Vaibhāṣika ideas: 'In Chapter Two, Vasubandhu relies on the *Śrāvakabhūmi* and on the *Viniścayasaṃgrahaṇī* on the *Pañcavijñānakāyamanobhūmi* for his statement that *bīja*s are nothing other than *nāmarūpa* or the *āśraya* … He explains many of the *cittaviprayuktasaṃskāra*s in terms of *bīja*s, and in almost every case, a similar explanation can be found in the *Viniścayasaṃgrahaṇī* on the *Pañcavijñānakāyamanobhūmi*' (Kritzer 2010: xxxv). We cannot therefore overlook the importance of *bīja* in the *Yogācārabhūmiśāstra*; it is, rather like the concept it denotes, there in latent form. It emerges in a more fully developed way in the later *Abhidharmakośabhāṣya*. Although this present study concentrates on the development of seed theory by the Sautrāntikas in the *Abhidharmakośabhāṣya*, other scholars have pointed to the importance of seed theory in the *Yogācārabhūmiśāstra*. See Schmithausen (1987: 21) for detail on the seed theory in the commentarial *Viniścayasaṃgrahaṇī* of the *Yogācārabhūmiśāstra*. See also Yamabe (2017b) for agreement with Kritzer that Mahāyāna seed theory evolved in the *Yogācārabhūmiśāstra*; although this seed theory is cited in a summarized form in the *Abhidharmakośabhāṣya*, it is not derived from the Sautrāntikas.

100 In other schools, the remainder can also refer to *skandha*s or to conventional reality.

101 Other Buddhist groups such as the Vibhajyavādins (a northern Indian Abhidharma school) also developed and innovated the theory of the seed of karma and *kleśa* in slightly different ways (Park 2014: 456).

102 See Park (2014: 433 fn. 896) for a summary of the main positions in this debate.

103 Collins notes that the 'idea of consciousness as seeded or seedless is important in all Buddhist thought' (Collins 1982: 223). He cites the *Milindapañha* 146: *abījam viññāṇam kataṃ* 'consciousness rendered seedless'.

104 Although legend relates that Vasubandhu went to Kashmir to study the *Mahāvibhāṣā*, more precisely the *Abhidharmakośabhāṣya* is now thought to have been composed partly on the basis of the **Saṃyuktābhidharmahṛdaya*, attributed to Dharmatrāta, early fourth century CE (Willemen et al. 1997: 271).

105 The key doctrinal difference between this Vibhajyavāda position and that of the Sautrāntikas is that for the Sautrāntikas the *anuśaya*s, as seeds, are not real, existent entities or *dravya*, but are potentialities.

106 Cox also translates this passage: 'Contaminants [*anuśaya*] are the seeds of manifestly active defilements. Contaminants are, by nature, not associated with thought; manifestly active defilements are, by nature, associated with thought. Manifestly active defilements are produced from contaminants. [Even if it were said that] one retrogresses from arhatship due to the present operation

(*saṃmukhībhāva*) of manifestly active defilements, since manifestly active defilements would not arise when the contaminants have been abandoned, how could one be said to have retrogression?' (*Mahāvibhāṣā* 60 T 27.313a1ff; cited in Cox 1992: 70). Cox also invites comparison with a passage from the *Nyāyānusāra* by Saṁghabhadra (NAS 45 T 29.598c16ff). Both works are extant only in Chinese, and so I have been unable to access them directly.

107 See also the Dārṣṭāntika passage in the same *Vibhāṣā*. They assert the difference between latent and manifest *kleśa*s. The Dārṣṭāntikas say, 'Wordlings are not able to cut off latent dispositions (**anuśāya*). They are merely able to subdue their outbursts or manifest activity (... *paryavasthāna*)' (*Vibhāṣā* T1545.264b; trans. Park 2014: 427 fn. 888).

108 This passage of the *Viniścayasaṃgrahaṇī* is commenting on the *Savitarkādibhūmi*.

109 Park's translation is based on the Tibetan of Yamabe (2003: 233). See Yamabe (2003) and Kritzer (2005: 273) for the argument that this passage is the forerunner of Vasubandhu's *Abhidharmakośa* passage. Kritzer outlines a series of other passages in the *Yogācārabhūmiśāstra* that describe the manifest and latent form of *kleśa* in relation to the seed (Kritzer 2005: 272–7).

110 The remaining *kleśa*s here could refer to the other four *kleśa*s that 'grow' in the field of the master *kleśa*, ignorance (*avidyā*). Like the Sautrāntikas, Patañjali posits that the *kleśa*s must be tackled one by one and are not eliminated at once (see the rest of PYŚ 2.4).

111 This notion of *bījabhāva* was used to explain karma in relation to ontology: *ko 'yam bījabhāva nāma. ātmabhāvasya kleśajākleśotpādanaśaktiḥ yathānubhavajñānajā smṛtyutpādanaśaktir yathācāṅkurādīnāṃ śāliphalajā śāliphalotpādanaśaktiriti* (AKBh 5.1; Pradhan 1975: 278, 22–4). The *Saṃdhinirmocanasūtra* of the *Yogācārabhūmiśāstra* presents a different way of understanding the accumulation of the seed as *āśraya*, which accounts for the continuation of a personality through time: *ādānavijñāna gabhīrasūkṣmo ogho yathā vartati sarvabījo / bālana eṣo mayi na prakāśi mā haiva ātmā parikalpayeyuḥ* (SNS 5.7; quoted in Sthiramati's commentary on *kārikā* 15 of Vasubandhu's *Triṃśikā*; cited in Aramaki 2013: 421). 'Then, at this occasion, the Bhagavān spoke the following verse: The pursuing subconsciousness – deep and subtle, and having been cumulative of all seeds [of evolution] – transmigrates like a flood. This I do not teach to the uninitiated, because they should not conceptualise it as a self' (trans. Aramaki 2013: 421).

112 The transformation of the series (*saṃtānapariṇāmaviśeṣa*) of the seed replaces the Vaibhāṣika notion of *prāpti*, or acquisition, the idea that *visaṃyoga* (disjunction) is a *dharma* to be possessed like any other. Instead, the Sautrāntikas posited a series of momentary karmic seeds that reproduce themselves over time. This idea is also essential to the notion of the continuity of the *ālayavijñāna* (store consciousness)

that first appears in the *Saṃdhinirmocanasūtra* of the *Yogācārabhūmiśāstra*. We cannot, of course, speak of an entirely unified theory of *bīja* in a text as stratified as the *Yogācārabhūmiśāstra*. Deleanu points out that after the most refined presentation of *ālayavijñāna*, there is a different passage that describes a theory of seeds 'which holds that the mind and body contain their own seeds (*bīja*) as well as the seeds of each other' (Deleanu 2006: 177). This body/mind frame does not refer to *ālayavijñāna*, and the text goes on to say that the theory was devised before *ālayavijñāna* had been taught. And so Deleanu concludes that this must be 'a redactional remark which attempts to harmonise the old (but apparently still influential) *bīja* concept with the new *ālayavijñāna* theory' (Deleanu 2006: 177). This older theory of the mind and body containing seeds of each other is similar to the doctrine presented in the *Abhidharmakośabhāṣya*, where it is attributed to the 'old masters' (*pūrvācārya*) and later considered to be a Sautrāntika view (Deleanu 2006: 227 fn. 169). For a related discussion, see Schmithausen (1987: 271–2, fn. 131, 353 fn. 495). Yamabe argues for seven distinct uses of the term *bīja* in the YĀBh: (1) seeds of future life, (2) seeds of *kleśa*s, (3) seeds of *karma*, (4) seeds of good *dharma*s, (5) seeds of the *pravṛttivijñāna*s, (6) seeds of *rūpa*, (7) seeds of all *dharma*s (Yamabe 2018).

113 These understandings of *āśraya* might shed further light on the notion of *saṃtāna* in YS 2.5 as an unbroken series of moments in relation to *karmāśaya*: *eṣā catuṣpadā bhavaty avidyā mūlam asya kleśasaṃtānasya karmāśayasya ca savipākasyeti* (PYŚ 2.5; Angot 2012: 384, 20–1). 'This *avidyā* is fourfold and is the root of the flow (*saṃtāna*) of *kleśa*s, the karmic substratum, and retribution.'

114 As Sanderson puts it, 'the action is to the effect as the seed is to the fruit: between the two lie processes of gradual transformation [*pariṇāma*]' (Sanderson 1994: 42).

115 Waldron suggests that the 'very suggestive' metaphor of *bīja* leads to the development of the model of mind centred on *ālayavijñāna* (Waldron 2003: 73).

116 *kleśatimiravināśī yogapradīpaḥ* (Angot 2012: 653, 13).

117 *na hi dagdhakleśabījasya jñāne punar apekṣā kācid asti* (Angot 2012: 663, 4–5).

118 On the basis of what I have presented so far, it is possible to argue that *nirbīja samādhi* and *dharmameghasamādhi* are synonyms for the same state: (1) *prasaṃkhyānadhyāna* is a synonym for *dharmameghadhyāna*, (2) *dharmameghadhyānā* and *dharmameghasamādhi* cannot be synonyms because in both the *aṣṭāṅga* yoga method and within Buddhist schemes of meditation, *dhyāna* and *samādhi* are treated as different stages, (3) *dharmameghadhyāna (= prasaṃkhyānadhyāna)* logically leads to *dharmameghasamādhi* and not to another type of *samādhi*, (4) *dharmameghadhyāna (= prasaṃkhyānadhyāna)* leads to the *samādhi* that is seedless, (5) Therefore, the *samādhi* that is seedless (*nirbīja samādhi*) is *dharmameghasamādhi*.

119 Collins argues that in the Mainstream discussions of continuity of mind, the preferred metaphor was that of a stream or river and not that of a seed (Collins 1982: 225–61).

120 As part of his overall thesis that the *Abhidharmakośabhāṣya* draws on the *Yogācārabhūmiśāstra*, Kritzer argues that the *bīja* innovation in Buddhism occurs in early yogācāra. Vasubandhu only borrows ideas like *bīja* from the *Yogācārabhūmi* which are not radically at odds with the Abhidharma content but leaves aside radically contradictory ideas such as *ālayavijñāna* (Kritzer 2005). This argument cannot be overlooked, and I will address the role of early yogācāra in the next chapter.

121 In the Sautrāntika school, the term *āśraya* was used to refer to the substratum of existence that exists independently of momentary existence and which provides the physical support for *citta* (thought) and *caitta* (function of mind). This idea was critiqued within Buddhism for being dangerously close to idea of *ātman*. *Āśraya* was also used in the *Yogācārabhūmiśāstra* to refer to *āśrayaparāvṛtti*, the transformation of the basis (which is the mind, the path and the proclivities) and which transforms an ordinary person, a *pṛthagjana* into an *ārya*, a noble person. The key transformation in *āśrayaparāvṛtti* is the abandoning of the *kleśa*s (*kliṣṭamanas*).

122 As follows: *ā-√śri* (*ā* + 'to resort') for *āśraya*, and *ā-√śī* (*ā* + 'to lie') for *āśaya*.

123 See *A Critical Pāli Dictionary* (Trenckner et al. 1924–48; 1960). In Pāli, the Sanskrit *āśaya* is *āsaya*, while *āśraya* is *assaya*. The Pāli *āsaya* is defined as '1. abode, lair, dwelling place; seat; place of origin; (metaphorically) basis, support, refuge; receptacle' (Trenckner et al. 1960, 2: 237). The Dictionary entry states that both *āsaya* and *assaya* are 'semantically related' (as are the Sanskrit *āśaya* and *āśraya*). The meaning of *āśraya/āsaya* therefore overlaps with *āśraya/assaya*; *A Critical Pāli Dictionary* gives the meaning of *assaya* as 'support' (Trenckner et al. 1924–48, 1: 522).

124 Frauwallner traces the inception of *anuśaya* as a doctrine to the development of the distinctive pairing of *darśanamārga* and *bhāvanāmārga* in the *Abhidharmasāra* (Frauwallner 1995: 154). He argues that the concept of *anuśaya* underpins the two new paths of *darśana* and *bhāvanā* and is a reworking of the older canonical concept of *āsrava* (Frauwallner 1995: 155). In the older canon (*Sūtrapiṭaka*), *anuśaya* represents something like 'bad inclination', but in the *Abhidharmasāra* Dharmaśrī reformulates *anuśaya* to have a more flexible meaning (Frauwallner 1995: 155). The new *anuśaya*s are increased in number, now include the five *dṛṣṭayāḥ*, and are assigned as states to be abandoned on the *bhāvanāmārga* and the *darśanamārga*.

125 This may partly explain the creative etymology used to define the word *anuśaya* as 'subtle' – because it comes from *aṇu*, meaning 'atom'. This definition is offered

in the *Abhidharmahṛdayaśāstra*, in the *Abhidharmakośabhāṣya* and in Yaśomitra's *Vyākhyā* (Cox 1992: 96 fn. 32). The *Mahāvibhāṣā* describes several etymologies for the term *anuśaya*: *aṇu* as atom and *anuśerate* to mean 'adhering closely' and later 'growing'. These both were used to reason that *anuśaya* is intrinsic with thought. But a third etymology was *anubadhnanti* (binding), used 'to refer to those contaminants that are dissociated from thought' (Cox 1992: 71).

126 *Anuśaya* is identified as the cause of *kleśa* in the *Abhidharmakośabhāṣya*: *aprahīṇād anuśayād viṣayāt pratyupasthitāt ayoniśo manaskārāt kleśaḥ* (AKK 5.33; Pradhan 1975: 305, 17–18). 'A *kleśa* arises due to non-abandoning of the *anuśaya*, from the encounter with an object, and from non-thorough focus.'

127 Nagao notes that in Vasubandhu's *Triṃśikā*, *āśraya* is explained as *ālayavijñāna*, which has the characteristics of *vipāka* (maturation) and *sarvabījaka* (universality of seeds). 'The word *ālaya* here has meanings similar to those of *āśraya* … Thus *ālaya* is a "basis" where the effects (*vipāka*) of all the past are stored and from which the future originates. Accordingly, *ālaya* is *āśraya*' (Nagao 1991: 79).

128 Potter argues that the Sautrāntika use of seed comes first and is elaborated afterwards by the Yogācāra school, who 'retain the agricultural analogy of seeds and sprouts, fleshing out talk of a "dependent" nature in terms of seeds laid down by our awarenesses; a seed, perfumed by the trace created in the awareness which caused it, conditions a subsequent act in the future' (Potter et al. 1996: 61). From recognizing that the seed theory was analogical and by grappling with the many questions that seed theory threw up, the Yogācāras arrived at the idea that there must be a place where the seeds are stored: storehouse-consciousness (*ālayavijñāna*).

129 *Āśaya* appears four times as frequently as *āśraya* in the *Pātañjalayogaśāstra*, around forty times, usually in the compound *karmāśaya* but also as *saṃskārāśaya*.

130 In the context of *sukhānuśayī rāgaḥ. duḥkhānuśayī dveṣaḥ* (PYŚ 1.11; 2.6, 2.8). *Rāga* and *dveṣa* are two of the primary *kleśa*s in Brahmanical and Buddhist discourse.

131 Cox notes that *anuśaya* is the word used least frequently for affliction in the Buddhist *sūtra*s (Cox 1992: 96 fn. 30). She points to Frauwallner's argument: because *anuśaya* was 'loose in meaning and infrequently used in the *sūtra* … it became the convenient focus of Abhidharma elaboration' (Cox 1992: 96 fn. 30, citing Frauwallner 1971: 75ff).

132 For recent research on the distinctively Buddhist terminology of parts of the *Pātañjalayogaśāstra* see, for example, Angot (2012), Squarcini (2016), Wujastyk (2018), Gokhale (2020) and Maas (2020).

133 *kleśahetukāḥ karmāśayapracaye kṣetrībhūtāḥ kliṣṭāḥ* (PYŚ 1.5) (Maas 2006: 16–17, 4–5). However, *sūtra* 2.12 describes the causal link as the other way round, from *kleśa* to *āśaya*: ***kleśamūlaḥ karmāśayo dṛṣṭādṛṣṭajanmavedanīyaḥ*** (YS 2.12)

(Āgāśe 1904: 67). 'Having *kleśa*s as its root, the *karmāsaya* is to be experienced in the present birth as well as future ones.'

134 Nagao terms *āśraya* 'one of the most important terms in the Yogācāra Vijñānavāda School of Mahāyāna Buddhism' (Nagao 1991: 75) and suggests the translations of 'basis', 'support or 'substratum'. The reasons for its importance are its close association with the terms *ālayavijñāna* and *paratantra-svabhāva* as well as its appearance in *āśraya-parāvṛtti*, the reversal of the basis (Nagao 1991: 75). He analyses a cluster of technical uses of the term *āśraya* in Asaṅga's *Mahāyānasūtrālaṃkara*: namely, '(1) substratum, support, (2) basis, (3) seeking shelter, (4) origin, source, (5) agent or subject, in the grammatical sense, (6) physical body, sometimes the six sense organs, (7) the total of (human) existence, (8) *dharma-dhātu* (sphere of dharma), (9) basis of existence (*āśraya*) which is to be turned around (*āśraya-parāvṛtti*)' (Nagao 1991: 75).

135 In the *Laṅkāvatāra Sūtra*, dated to the fourth to fifth centuries, *āśraya* is used to stand in for *ālayavijñāna* (Forsten 2006: 56 fn. 124). Schmithausen also argues for correspondence between the term *āśraya* and *ālayavijñāna* (Schmithausen 2007), and he defines *ālayavijñāna* thus, 'The container or storehouse of the latent residues or impressions of previous actions (*karman*) and mind process, or ... the basic layer of mind processes or even the very basic constituent of the whole living being' (Schmithausen 1987: 1). That the two concepts are linked is also reflected in the sixth book of the *Yogācārabhūmiśāstra*, the *Sacittikā Acittikā Bhūmiḥ*, in which *nirvāṇa* is without remainder of an existential substratum (*nirupadhiśeṣa nirvāṇadhātu*) because the *ālayavijñāna*, the latent consciousness has ceased. In fact, it is important to acknowledge a distinction between the ways in which the concept of *āśraya* is treated in the *Abhidharmakośabhāṣya* and in the *Yogācārabhūmiśāstra*. For example, in the *Abhidharmakośabhāṣya* there is reference to an individual who attains abandonment without remainder in the *darśanamārga*: *darśanamārga-vyutthitasyāśeṣa-darśana-prahātavyaprahāṇāt / pratyagrāśraya-parivṛtti-nirmalā saṃtatir* (AKBh 4.56; Pradhan 1975: 232). The *darśanamārga* is the way of intuiting the truths, and the transformation that occurs brings about a new version of consciousness that is pure via the reversal/transformation of the *āśraya*, the existential basis. The process of liberation is when the *kleśa*s have been totally eliminated in both the *darśanamārga* and the *bhāvanāmārga* and when the *kleśa*s cannot rearise: *āśrayo hi sa āryāṇām darśanabhāvanā-mārgāsāmarthyāt tathā parāvṛtto bhavati yathā na punas tatpraheyāṇāṃ kleśānāṃ praroha-samartho bhavati / ato 'gnidagdhavrīhivadavījībhūte āśraye kleśānāṃ prahīṇakleśa ityucyate* (AKBh 2.36; Pradhan 1975: 63).

136 *tallābhād avidyādayaḥ kleśāḥ samūlakāṣaṃ kaṣitā bhavanti kuśalākuśalāś ca karmāśayāḥ samūlaghātaṃ hatā bhavanti* (PYŚ 4.30; Angot 2012: 723, 1–2). See

also, for example, ***tatra dhyānajam anāśayam***. 'For those [minds with powers] that are born of *dhyāna* are without *āśaya*' (YS 4.6). And the statement that, along with absence of *kleśa*, *karma* and *vipāka*, absence of *āśaya* is a condition of *īśvara*: ***kleśakarmavipākāśayair aparāmṛṣṭaḥ puruṣaviśeṣa īśvaraḥ*** (YS 1.24).

137 Whereas *karmāśaya* is the seedbed that fructifies in this lifetime, *vāsanā*s are more subtle traces of karmic action that will fructify at an unknown point in the future (PYŚ 2.13).

138 *manas tu sādhikāram āśrayo vāsanānām / na hy avasitādhikāre manasi nirāśrayā vāsanāḥ sthātum utsahante* (PYŚ 4.11; Angot 2012: 687, 6–7).

139 As with other key soteriological terms, *āśraya* is not found to have the same technical meaning in the *Sāṃkhyakārikā*. Rather it appears in a general sense to denote support, but in a metaphysical context: as a function of the *guṇa*s (SKK 12); the unmanifest (*avyaktam*) is a support of the *guṇa*s (SKK 16); the specific is a support of the liṅga (SKK 42); or the support/abode of *prakṛti* (SKK 62). This is a quite specific and consistent use of *āśraya* in a metaphysical sense, and different to *āśraya* as a physical or psychological function in the *Pātañjalayogaśāstra*, which is more aligned to Buddhist denotation of this term.

140 It is important to note that the *āśraya* of the *Bodhisattvabhūmi*, for example, is not just psychological but also an aspect of the real in that it forms part of the twofold *vastu* theory: 'One is that of entity which exists objectively but is incorrectly reflected in or distorted by our ordinary linguistic conventions or designations (*prajñapti*). The other is the objective basis (*āśraya*) which remains (*avaśiṣṭa*) after all conceptual constructions have been eliminated' (Deleanu 2006: 218). In this second sense, *vastu* is a synonym of 'suchness' or *tathatā*.

141 Nonetheless, *vāsanā* is not absent from the *Abhidharmakośabhāṣya*, and Waldron points outs the ways in which *vāsanā* (perfuming or after-effect) and *bhāvanā* come to be closely related in the *Abhidharmakośabhāṣya* so that *bhāvanā* in relation to the mind can also mean 'infusing' or 'steeping' (Waldron 2003: 213 fn. 103). When *bhāvanā* is used in connection to *vāsanā* as the after-effect, it is being used within a theory of causality.

142 Later Yogācāra further develops the notion of the seed in relation to karma to differentiate between inner seeds (personal conditioning) and outer seeds (external influences), as well as debating the relationship of *bīja* to *vāsanā* (perfuming) (Lusthaus 2015).

143 Yamabe argues that there is a specific technical context to *bīja* and *āśraya* in the *Bodhisattvabhūmi* – i.e. it has a different ontological function. He views it as equivalent to *prakṛti*, *gotra* and *dhātu* (Yamabe 2017a); the development of *bīja* theory in the *Yogācārabhūmiśāstra* has two distinct phases: an earlier traditional model in which *bīja* is synonymous with *dhātu* (element) and *gotra* (spiritual disposition) and a later model in which *bīja* is equal to *āśraya*, which he describes

as a 'distinct state of the totality of one's existence' (Yamabe 2018). Along with Kritzer, Yamabe views the Sautrāntika model of the seed as a concealed reworking of the Yogācāra model. He also makes a distinction between the seed/sprout metaphor, which illustrates successive causality theory and two other metaphors that illustrate simultaneous causality, namely the flame and wick and the bundle of reeds (Yamabe 2017b: 11).

144 More specifically, the *kaṣāyas* operate in relation to karma, which is understood as a very subtle form of matter. The actions of body, speech and mind attract this karma to the soul and the *kaṣāyas* act as active bonding agents to make karma 'stick' (Wiley 2002: 90). Different types of *karman* give rise to different effects: thus *āyus-karmans* determine lifespan while *nāma-karmans* determine the formation of the body (Wiley 2002: 90).

145 *Mohanīya-karmans* create false views of reality (*mithyātva*) and produce the four *kaṣāyas* (Wiley 2002: 90).

146 For example, see *Sūtrakṛtāṅga* i.2.26–8, ii.2.29, i.6.17; *Ācārāṅga Sūtra* i.9.512, 520; *Bhagavati Sūtra* 25.8.802; *Thāṇaṃga Sūtra* 4.1.308.

147 In the progressive formula of the four *dhyānas*, only the last two steps of *śukla dhyāna*, or pure meditation (i.e. steps fifteen and sixteen), can lead to *mokṣa* because they constitute *tapas*, which in Jainism is privileged over *dhyāna* as the means to attain liberation. The sixteen steps are resonant of the sixteen moments of consciousness in the Sarvāstivāda Abhidharma path scheme.

148 Incidentally, this ladder scheme of upward ascension affirms the metaphorical direction of liberation as 'up' (see Chapter 1 for a discussion of orientational metaphors and image-schemas).

149 There are four 'doors', respectively: initial study, assignment by name, exposition, exposition from specific standpoints (Petrocchi 2016: 237).

150 Buddhism conveys the metaphor of the doors of liberation, but this is not schematized in the same way that botanical cultivation is as the framework for an elaborate soteriology, e.g. *anāsravās tv ete trayaḥ samādhayas trīṇi vimokṣamukhāny ucyante | śūnyatā vimokṣamukham apraṇihitam ānimittaṃvimokṣamukham iti | mokṣadvāratvāt* (AKBh 450.7–8). 'But these untainted concentrations are called the three entrances to liberation: emptiness is an entrance to liberation, as are the wishless, and the signless, because of their being doors to liberation.'

151 Another way to destroy the *kleśa* is to cut its roots completely.

152 A notable divergence, for example, between the Buddhist discourse of *kleśas* is that of *upakleśa*, or secondary affliction, a notion that is absent from Pātañjala yoga. The *upakleśas* stand in distinction to the *mūlakleśas* (root or primary *kleśas*) and are variously schematized as 10, 16 or 20 in number according to different schools.

153 As Lopez notes, the Buddhist scholastic sees 'the very function of the path as the destruction of the *kleśas* and the prevention of their recurrence' (Lopez 2001: 182). Cox argues, 'Abandoning defilements is indeed the goal of Abhidharma religious praxis and the organizing principle of its construction of the path' (Cox 1992: 66). Furthermore, within Buddhism, it is Sarvāstivāda Abhidharma that develops the taxonomic classification of *kleśa*s to 'an apex' (Cox 1992: 74).

154 Discussed further in Chapter 4.

Chapter 3

1 Buescher suggests the title Yogācāra to refer to the earliest strands of this school of thought and the compound Yogācāra-Vijñānavāda to differentiate a later, more developed strand (Buescher 2008: 2).

2 These are the translations used by Kragh (2013b).

3 A topic (*sthāna*) signifies a division containing a series of doctrinal points (Kragh 2013b: 103).

4 For a detailed breakdown of the four *Saṃgrahaṇī* sections, see Delhey (2013).

5 See Deleanu (2006: 154) for a summary of scholarly positions in concord with this view.

6 Indeed, if Asaṅga is to be credited as the author/compiler, then the *Yogācārabhūmiśāstra* must be dated to Asaṅga's lifetime, which spanned from the late fourth to the early fifth century (Kritzer 2005: xviii).

7 Deleanu dates the *Bodhisattvabhūmi* to *c.*230–300 CE (Deleanu 2006: 195).

8 Among the first scholars to identify the chronological formation of the *Yogācārabhūmiśāstra* was Schmithausen, who used the absence of any reference to the innovative Mahāyāna concept of store consciousness (*ālayavijñāna*) to identify the earliest parts of the text (Schmithausen 1987). In Schmithausen's view, the absence of *ālayavijñāna* and other core Mahāyāna concepts demonstrates that these three layers of the *Yogācārabhūmiśāstra* precede the advent of Mahāyāna proper. Accordingly, Schmithausen identified the next chronological layer of text as the rest of the *Maulī Bhūmi* combined, because it contains a smattering of references to *ālayavijñāna* but no reference to the *Saṃdhinirmocanasūtra*, an independent text that discusses *ālayavijñāna* and which became a key text of Mahāyāna Buddhism. The third and newest layer, in Schmithausen's analysis, is the *Viniścayasaṃgrahaṇī*, which contains the *Saṃdhinirmocanasūtra*. More recently, Aramaki put forward a revised hypothesis about the structure of the *Yogācārabhūmiśāstra*, arguing that while books ten to fourteen (including the *Bodhisattvabhūmi* and the *Śrāvakabhūmi*) constitute the oldest layers of the *Yogācārabhūmiśāstra*, the first six books represent the newest layers, and

the threefold complex of *Śrutamayī-*, *Cintāmayī-* and *Bhāvanāmayī Bhūmiḥ*s represents a bridge between the 'old' and 'new' blocks (Aramaki 2013: 427–8). See also Kritzer for a view of the possible chronologies of the layers (Kritzer 2005: xviii). In contrast, Wayman attributed the whole text to Asaṅga and built up the layers as chronological events in Asaṅga's life (375–430 CE, starting at 395 CE) (Wayman 1960).

9 The *Saṃdhinirmocanasūtra* is quoted in the *Viniścayasaṃgrahaṇī* apart from its prologue and its colophons (Powers 1993: 4). Powers (1993: 4) and Schmithausen (1976) date the *Saṃdhinirmocanasūtra* to no earlier than the late third century because it refers to the *Prajñāpāramitāsūtra* (*The Perfection of Wisdom Sūtra*s). Deleanu dates *Saṃdhinirmocanasūtra* to 300–50 CE (Deleanu 2006: 195).

10 For more on the dating of the *Yogācārabhūmiśāstra*, see Deleanu (2006: 183–96) and Delhey (2013).

11 The six *aṅgas* are *prāṇāyāma*, *pratyāhāra*, *dhyāna*, *dhāraṇā*, *tarka* and *samādhi*.

12 The asterisk conventionally indicates that the title is a hypothetical reconstruction of the text's name, which is not apparent from surviving manuscripts. The following contextualization of the **Yogācārabhūmi* is indebted to Deleanu (2006).

13 For more on the **Yogācārabhūmi*, see Demiéville (1951), Deleanu (2006) and Yamabe (2013).

14 This is Stuart's translation of the title (Stuart 2015, 1: 15). T606.

15 This is Deleanu's translation of the title (Deleanu 2006: 157). T618. This text is also referred to as the *Dharmatrāta Dhyānasūtra* (DDS).

16 Demiéville dated An Shigao's partial Chinese translation of the **Yogācārabhūmi* to around the second century CE (Demiéville 1951: 343–7). For a discussion of the influence of the **Yogācārabhūmi* and the *Dao di jing* on another portion of the *Yogācārabhūmiśāstra*, the *Manobhūmi*, see Yamabe (2013).

17 Hence it is also sometimes called the *Dharmatrātadhyānasūtra*. According to Lamotte, Dharmatrāta wrote a *Yogasamasanasūtra* that has been lost (Lamotte 1988: 696).

18 Stuart dates the *Damoduoluo chan jing* to the fourth century CE (Stuart 1, 2015, 1: 15).

19 Stuart dates the *Saddharmasmṛtyupasthānasūtra* to between 150 and 400 CE but adds that parts of the second chapter could be older.

20 The *Damoduoluo chan jing* refers to the ten stages, the *daśabhūmi* (DDS 11.8; trans. Chan 2013: 383).

21 The stories of these masters were recorded by Dao-An, a Chinese master (Demiéville 1951: 364–6; Lamotte 1988: 696–8).

22 See Kritzer (2005).

23 There are three narrative frames; the middle frame focuses on a master yogācāra and reflects on how an ordinary monk becomes a yogācāra.

24 See Silk (1997 and 2000). For further discussions on the term '*yogācāra*' and its expression in early sources, see Demiéville (1951); Buescher (2008 10–15); and Deleanu (2012).

25 The discussions about the word *yogācāra* must also consider the related Pāli word *yogāvacāra*. The second-century *Milindapañha*, for example, contains 207 occurrences of this Pāli term (Seton 2009: 35). For more on *yogāvacāra*, see Silk (2000).

26 The term *yoggācariya* also appears in the Second Minor Rock Edict of Aśoka in the form of *yūg*[y]*ācāriyāni*. Stuart comments that this reference is to non-Buddhist religious practitioners (Stuart 2015, 1: 233).

27 This passage from the *Śrāvakabhūmi* shows how yogācāras were also referred to as yogins: *tatra labdhamanaskārasya yoginaḥ / evaṃ parīttaprahāṇaratipraviṣṭasya tadūrdhvaṃ dve gatī bhavataḥ / ananye / katame dve tadyathā / laukikī ca lokottarā ca / tatrāyam lokottarayā veti* (ŚBh S 14A.3–7b; Wayman 1960: 125).

28 Although Stuart has translated *yogī* as 'practitioner', I would venture that it means yoga practitioner more specifically: *yo nādatte 'śubhaṃ karma śubhakarmarataḥ sadā candrāṃśunirmalaratir yogī bhavati tādṛśaḥ* (*Saddhsu* 4.2.24.3).

29 Nonetheless as Deleanu points out, 'the ŚrBh does not, however, seem to make a doctrinally relevant distinction between these two words' (Deleanu 2006: 35 fn. 4). Silk agrees with this point, discounting any sectarian limits on the term 'yogācāra' (Silk 1997: 233).

30 This study will use the term Śrāvakayāna to refer to the school of Buddhism formerly called Hīnayāna but also referred to by contemporary scholars as Mainstream. This school includes the Sarvāstivāda Abhidharma tradition.

31 As noted above, the two translations of the **Yogācārabhūmi* into Chinese still have a recognizable 'Śrāvakayānika core' with some Mahāyānist elements (Deleanu 2006: 158).

32 Early Mahāyāna is conventionally divided into two schools, Nāgārjuna's 'nihilistic' Madhyamaka school with its doctrine of *śūnyatā* (emptiness) and Asaṅga's and Vasubandhu's 'idealist' Yogācāra school with its doctrine of *ālayavijñāna* (store consciousness). Recent and contemporary scholarship has problematized the neat divisions of schools, founders and doctrines, and we must accept that the emergence and interaction of the 'schools' was more dynamic, messy and complicated than this.

33 Deleanu clarifies this point, 'If we exclude the *Bodhisattvabhūmi* and the *Bodhisattvabhūmiviniścaya* as well as the few sporadic Mahāyāna accretions and elements, the rest of the *Yogācārabhūmi* could have evolved and remained a *śāstra* within the "Lesser Vehicle" spectrum … The *Yogācārabhūmi* became a fundamental treatise of one of India's major Mahāyāna traditions in spite of the fact that a large part of it contains or presupposes no teachings peculiar to the Great Vehicle'

(Deleanu 2006: 182). Kragh agrees that the *Yogācārabhūmiśāstra* became 'in its final redacted form, a virtual Mainstream Buddhist discourse with an imperative Mahāyāna slant'. See also Kritzer (2005: xix–xx), who concurs with this analysis. However, Stuart suggests that Deleanu, in characterizing the *Yogācārabhūmiśāstra* as predominantly Śrāvakayāna in tone, 'may very well have overlooked the incipient *vijñānavāda* ideas that are present in texts such as the **Yogācārabhūmi* of Buddhasena' (Stuart 2015, 1: 280), i.e. the *Damoduoluo chan jing* or *Dharmatrāta Dhyānasūtra*.

34 Although *yogācāra* was initiated in Sarvāstivāda circles, when we take into account the self-representation of the *Yogācārabhūmiśāstra*, the highest system of yoga depicted is ultimately characterized as Mahāyāna yoga. This is because the ultimate attainment in the path structure is that of the *bodhisattva*, the quintessential Mahāyāna ideal and the figure who embodies fully realized and compassionate Buddhahood. The *Yogācārabhūmiśāstra* focuses on the mainstream practices of *śrāvaka* and *pratyekabuddha*, but 'its overall objective seems to be to present a coherent structure of Buddhist *yoga* practice with the Mahāyāna path of the *bodhisattva* placed at the pinnacle of the system' (Kragh 2013b: 25).

35 We must also acknowledge that the term yogācāra began to appear in both Śrāvakāyana and Mahāyāna sources from the first century CE onwards (Deleanu 2006: 224 fn. 142). As Kragh points out, the *Yogācārabhūmiśāstra* seeks to strike a balance between Śrāvakayāna and Mahāyāna Buddhist practice and 'endeavours to juxtapose and align these meditational systems of *yoga*' (Kragh 2013b: 29)

36 The Chinese pilgrim Xuanzang, who visited India between 629 and 645 CE, observed that Sarvāstivādin monasteries only existed in the northwest region and the upper north Ganges Valley. Another Chinese pilgrim Yijing, who was a Sarvāstivādin and visited between 671 and 695 CE, noted that this sect was dominant only in the northwest and in the region now called Indonesia.

37 As Deleanu points out, 'it is impossible to ascertain how these *yogācāra*s were organized. They may have been one single unitary group or loosely connected groups' (Deleanu 2006: 217 fn. 92).

38 See also Davidson (1985: 126ff) for the analysis that Hsüang-tsang's (Xuanzang's) translation of the *Mahāvibhāṣā* contains sixty instances of the word *yogācāra* and that almost all bar three refer to 'master meditator'.

39 AMVibh T27.704b27-cl.

40 Dating from Buescher (2008).

41 See also Ruegg (1967: 157) and Demiéville (1951), in which he discusses *buddhānusmṛti* as a characteristic feature of yogācāra in relation to Saṅgharakṣa and Buddhasena.

42 There are complex taxonomies of practitioner in the *Yogācārabhūmiśāstra*, including hierarchical rankings in terms of social status (householder, ascetic, solitary disciple, monk/nun), ability (novice, intermediate, advanced) and overarching path affiliation (*śrāvaka*, *pratyekabuddha*, *bodhisattva*). The goal of yogācāra depends on which path structure one takes: the path of the *śrāvaka*, the *pratyekabuddha* or the *bodhisattva*.

43 'Définition de yogācāra: "Pratiquer la culture et les exercices." Définition de yogācārabhūmi: "Ce que pratique le pratiquant, c'est la la terre du pratiquant" (trans. from Chinese, Demiéville 1951: 398).

44 The second *yogasthāna* of the *Śrāvakabhūmi* contains an exposition of the word 'person' or *pudgala* in relation to practice, listing labels used by the Buddha. The types of practitioner include renunciant (*śramaṇa*), Brahmin (*brāhmaṇa*), one who is celibate (*brahmacārin*), monk (*bhikṣu*), ascetic/striver (*yati)* and itinerant mendicant (*parivrājaka*). On the whole, however, the context of the yogācāra is specifically that of a monk. For the contrary view, that a *yogācāra* is not necessarily a monk, see Silk (2000: 304–5).

45 See also this example, from the *Saddharmapuṇḍarīkasūtra* (early centuries CE): *bhikṣubhikṣuṇyupāsakopāsikā yogino yogācārā* (SDhPu 6,12 cited in Buescher 2008: 11).

46 There is not space here to fully address the range of scholarly positions regarding the 'origins' of Yogācāra doctrine. Buescher usefully maps out three important theses, setting his own research on the *Saṃdhinirmocanasūtra* against Lindtner's on the proto-*Laṅkāvatārasūtra* and against Schmithausen's theories (Buescher 2008: 4–6). For other recent in-depth discussions, see Boucher (2008) and Drewes (2010 and 2018), who have respectively argued for and against the forest hypothesis to account for early Mahāyāna.

47 This is explained in the seventh segment of the *Bhāvanāmayī Bhūmiḥ*, which describes the path of cultivation (*bhāvanāmārga*) as part of the higher path of practice (*lokottaramārga*). One 'lives in a remote and secluded place' (*prāntāni ca śayanāsanāni pratiniṣevate*) (Sugawara 2013: 806).

48 *vanāraṇyavihāreṣu śmaśānatṛṇasaṃstare | ramate yasya tu mano bhikṣur bhavati tādṛśaḥ.*

49 *dhyānādhyayanakarmaṇyaḥ kausīdyaṃ yasya dūrataḥ | hitakārī ca sattvānām āraṇyo bhikṣur ucyate.*

50 There are three references to *yogācāra* in the *Abhidharmakośabhāṣya*: AKBh 3.15, 4.4 and 6.10.

51 For a summary of scholarship on this issue, see Park (2014).

52 The crediting of Asaṅga as the founder of Yogācāra can be traced to sixth-century commentaries on the *Abhidharmakośakārikā*, such as the *Sphuṭārtha Abhidharmakośavyākhyā* by Yaśomitra. Other doxographical uses of the label

yogācāra occur in the sixth-century commentaries of Sthiramati and Bhavya (Buescher 2008: 14).

53 One of the challenges in working with the *Yogācārabhūmiśāstra* is its sheer size. The number of components that make up this overall text (fourteen books and four supplementary sections) mean that the nature of the scholarship on this text is still somewhat fragmented, with gaps in critical editions and translations (discussed in Chapter 5). Although completely extant in Chinese and Tibetan, not all parts of the *Yogācārabhūmiśāstra* have been preserved in Sanskrit. For an overview of the state of *Yogācārabhūmiśāstra* philology in Sanskrit, see Delhey (2013).

54 Although the **Yogācārabhūmi* of Saṅgharakṣa is 'not a direct textual prototype of the *Śrāvakabhūmi*', it is nonetheless 'one of its distant "forefathers"' and 'probably represents the same ascetic current which led to the birth of the *Śrāvakabhūmi*' (Deleanu 2006: 158). We do not know if *Śrāvakabhūmi* was the original title of the text, and Deleanu suggests that it may even have been called *Yogācārabhūmi* 'in the sense of "levels or ground of spiritual praxis" ... and as new related texts and parts kept on being compiled the title of *Yogācārabhūmi* was employed for the whole corpus' (Deleanu 2006: 221–2 fn. 126).

55 However, the Vaibhāṣika Sarvāstivādins in the *Abhidharmakośabhāṣya* and some works by Asaṅga also judge the *śrāvaka* path as inferior and the *pratyekabuddha* path as middling in comparison to the *bodhisattva* path, although both produce personal liberation.

56 Literally: 'He knows it as it is.'

57 *katamā śikṣā / katame śikṣānulomikā dharmāḥ katamo yogabhraṃśaḥ katame yogāḥ katamo manaskāraḥ kati yogācārāḥ / katamad yogakaraṇīyaṃ katamā yogabhāvanā katamad bhāvanāphalam* (Śbh 7A.9–2a; Wayman 1960: 83).

58 ... *dāne 'pi prayujyate śīle kṣāntau vīryem dhyāne prajñāyām api prayujyate iti* (BoBh 1.1).

59 Von Rospatt reminds us that there are no traces of the *bodhisattva* ideal in this book, no substantial treatment of *śūnyatā* nor of the concept of *ālayavijñāna* (von Rospatt 2013: 854). However, this does not mean that the book is unaware of the Māhayāna context; indeed, it cites the *Bodhisattvabhūmi*.

60 The *Bhāvanāmayī Bhūmiḥ* is not yet available in a critical edition, and I therefore base my reading on the detailed summary of contents provided by Sugawara and on the extracts from the critical edition published therein (Sugawara 2013 in Kragh 2013).

61 The titles of these seven segments are, respectively, *abhinivṛtti saṃpat, saddharma-śravaṇa saṃpat, nirvāṇa pramukhatā, vimukti paripācinyāḥ prajnāyāḥ paripākaḥ, pratipakṣabhāvanā, sarvākāra laukikī viśuddhiḥ*, and *sarvākāra lokottarā viśuddhiḥ*.

62 Five conditions pertain to the self: being born human, in a good country, with healthy body and mind, free of the five obstacles (*pañcāntarāyaṇi karmāṇi*) and not believing in bad teachings (*adhimuktyanāvaraṇasaṃpat*). And five pertain to the external: finding a good teacher, receiving instructions from that teacher, receiving teaching on the highest meaning, attaining permanent understanding and sustaining oneself with donations (Sugawara 2013).

63 Here, the *pañcāntarāyaṇi karmāṇi* refer to the five standard *nivaraṇas*.

64 Theodore Proferes has pointed out that this threefold structure of soteriology is also present in Vedānta. This topic deserves further investigation.

65 Not all of the obstacles are explained, however. Only three are unpacked in detail (the first, third and seventh): the awareness of foul things, the awareness of misery and the awareness of splendour.

66 This same list is also found in the ŚrBh 268 (12)–270 (14).

67 The segment that concentrates on the counterstates is itself titled '*Bhāvanāmayī Bhūmiḥ*'. It is, as Sugawara puts it, 'the core part of the entire book' (Sugawara 2013: 800).

68 *Yogabhāvanā* is also presented in the *Śrāvakabhūmi* as step four of the twelfth segment of the second topic of yoga (*yogasthāna*). There are two types of cultivation: (1) cultivation of notions (*saṃjñābhāvanā*) and (2) the cultivation of the thirty-seven factors of awakening (*bodhipakṣyā bhāvanā*). For more on the thirty-seven factors, see Gethin (2007).

69 *Satyābhisamaya* is the 'realization of the four noble truths'.

70 The *Saṃdhinirmocanasūtra* is considered to be stratified, either with clusters of chapters representing older and newer layers or with individual chapters representing prior independent texts (Matsuda 2013: 938). Aramaki suggest that chapters 5–8 constitute the oldest layer and a conscious attempt to form 'a new *Mahāyānasūtra*' (Aramaki 2013: 411).

71 Matsuda has edited two fragments, written in Buddhist-Hybrid Sanskrit and in Sanskrit (Matsuda 2013). Other Sanskrit sections are available as quoted in Buddhist works such as Kamalaśīla's *Third Bhāvanākrāma* and Sthiramati's *Triṃśikābhāṣya*.

72 Maas has recently narrowed down this date range to *c.*400 CE (Maas 2018).

73 Although both the *Śrāvakabhūmi* and the *Bhāvanāmayī Bhūmiḥ* deal with the obstacles to the path (*mārga*), the treatment in the *Śrāvakabhūmi* is more ideal, while the *Bhāvanāmayī Bhūmiḥ* appears to be more gounded in real-life examples.

Chapter 4

1 I use the neutral terms 'state' and 'counterstate' to denote the binary of problem/ solution (which in Indic soteriology reflects the ultimate binary of captivity/liberation).

2 There is also a fourth structural metaphor, YOGA IS PURIFICATION (= *KLEŚA* IS A DEFILEMENT), which constructs yoga as a purifying force that eliminates pollution, illness or toxicity. However, given the complex contexts of ritual, medicine and alchemy from which it derives, I must reserve that discussion for another occasion and focus the analysis here more specifically on the context of botanical cultivation. (For a preliminary consideration of this topic, see note 5 below.) As the discussion in this present chapter shows, the contexts of the path (on the earth), (the field of) vision and the (plant) antidote are all closely interwoven with metaphors of cultivation.

3 For the translation of *pratipakṣa* as 'antidote', see, for example, Hanson (1998: 241); Mejor (1999: 114); Kragh (2013b: 99); von Rospatt (2013: 789, 791–2, 794, 801); Woo (2014: 501).

4 Of course, *kleśa*s are not the only spiritual problems that require counterstates; in Buddhist discourse, the problem can also be framed as obscurant (*āvaraṇa*) or hindrance (*nivaraṇa*) and in Patañjali's text as an obstacle (*antarāya*).

5 *Kleśa* is not a prevalent term in Brahmanism, but we do find the related term *doṣa*, a 'fault' that can be remedied by a counterstate. (See also my discussion in Chapter 2 in the section 'The metaphor of affliction'.) The term *doṣa* itself is mapped from āyurvedic discourse, where the 'doctrine of the three humours, or *tridoṣa-vidyā*, teaches that the three semi-fluid substances are present in the body and regulate its state' (Wujastyk 2003: xvii). The three humours are wind (*vāta*), bile (*pitta*) and phlegm (*kapha* or *śleṣman*). The term *doṣa* migrated from medical discourse to soteriology – for further discussion, see Wujastyk (2012). See also Maas (2014) for an analysis of the paradigm of medicine in relation to soteriology in the *Pātañjalayogaśāstra*, focusing on PYŚ 2.14, 45–9. Furthermore, in the *Mānavadharmaśāstra* (second to third century CE) the section on yogic meditation describes the stages of yoga as counterstates: *dahyante dhmāyamānānāṃ dhātūnāṃ hi yathā malāḥ | tathendriyāṇāṃ dahyante doṣāḥ prāṇasya nigrahāt | prāṇāyāmaidaheddōṣān dhāraṇābhiśca kilbiṣam | pratyāhāreṇa saṃsargān dhyānenānīśvarān gūṇān* (MDh 6.72; Olivelle 2005: 608). 'He should burn away his faults by suppressing the breath, his taints by concentration, his attachments by the withdrawal of senses, and his base qualities by meditation' (MDh 6.72; trans. Olivelle 2005: 152). Being linked to defects of the body and their remedies, this metaphor maps qualities from the medical domain. Interestingly, however, the counterstate for eliminating the *doṣa*s in the *Mānavadharmaśāstra* is not a remedy or antidote but rather the application of intense heat to destroy impurity. This image of intense heat to remove a problematic factor in the self is one we examined in

Chapter 2 as the fire necessary to remove the germinating impulse of the seed. The image of heat or fire in the body itself is linked to *tapas*, but also to the medical context of fever, as a potentially healing force.

6 The Mīmāṃsā school also utilized the concept of the counterstate, specifically in relation to the notion of *śakti* (force, power or efficacy). The Mīmāṃsakas conceived of a counterforce to *śakti*, which they termed a *pratibandhaka*. Matilal translates *pratibandhaka* as 'antidote' although it generally refers to an opposing force (Matilal 1985: 289).

7 In compound with *pratipakṣa*, Patañjali's text uses the neuter form *bhāvana* while the Buddhist sources employ the feminine form *bhāvanā*. I have been unable to identify a clear difference in meaning between the two from the Monier-Williams or Edgerton dictionaries (Monier-Williams 1899; Edgerton 1953). In translated passages of the *Pātañjalayogaśāstra*, I retain the neuter noun, but in general discussion I use the feminine noun.

8 *pratipakṣabhāvanād dhetor heyā vitarkā / yadāsya syur aprasavadharmāṇas tadā tatkṛtam aiśvaryaṃ yoginaḥ siddhisūcakaṃ bhavati* (PYŚ 2.35; Angot 2012: 498).

9 For accounts of the historical 'isolation' of *aṣṭāṅga yoga* from Pātañjala yoga as a whole, see De Michelis (2005) and White (2014).

10 Although Pātañjala yoga is often conflated with *aṣṭāṅga yoga* as its only path structure, the *Pātañjalayogaśāstra* contains several path structures with their own stages. In addition to the well-known *aṣṭāṅga* path of eight stages, Patañjali expounds *kriyā yoga* path and a complex *nirbīja samādhi*. The *kriyā yoga* path has only three components (austerity, recitation, contemplation of the lord – *tapas, svadhyāya, īśvarapraṇidhāna*), but the opening chapter on concentration (*samādhipāda*) outlines a complex scheme with several branching, paired and non-consecutive stages including concentration with and without seed (*nirbīja/sabīja samādhi*), cognitive and non-cognitive concentration (*saṃprajñāta/asaṃprajñāta samādhi*) and the four attainments (*samāpatti*s). Hence Pātañjala yoga appears to entail a syncretic path structure that combines aspects of other path structures, and it cannot therefore necessarily be reduced into a single conceptual frame.

11 *tanutvam ucyate pratipakṣabhāvanopahatāḥ kleśās tanavo bhavanti* (PYŚ 2.4; Angot 2012: 381, line 12–13).

12 *yathaiva pratipakṣabhāvanāto nivṛttas tathaiva svavyañjakāñjanenābhivyakta iti* (PYŚ 2.4; Angot 2012: 381, lines 20–1). 'Just as cultivation of the counterstate produces cessation (*nivṛtta*), so do they (the *kleśa*s) become manifest by revealing their character.' I discuss manifest and unmanifest *kleśa*s in relation to the seed of *kleśa* in Chapter 2.

13 Furthermore, the paradigm of state/counterstate is also present in more implicit ways. At the end of Patañjali's *samādhipāda*, seedless *samādhi* itself (i.e. *nirbīja samādhi*, the ultimate *samādhi*) is explained using the binary paradigm of state/

counterstate. Certain types of mental imprints (*saṃskāras*) act like counteragents that cancel or sublate the active mind (*vyuthāna-citta*) (PYŚ 1.51, lines 6–7; Maas 2006: 86). 'By means of the *saṃskāras* conducive to isolation (*kaivalyam*) along with those produced by the concentration (*samādhi*) of ceased activity (*vyutthānanirodha*), the mind becomes dissolved in the ground of materiality (*prakṛti)* herself.'

14 The metaphor of counterstates for the *kleśa*s is also present in Buddhasena's **Yogācārabhūmi*: 'In fact, the five desires are also five destructions. Each of them should be properly treated by administering the right antidote.' (DDS 11.13; trans. Chan 2013: 381).

15 This refers to the contemplation of the three marks of existence, which together with contemplation of emptiness (*śūnyatā*) make up the paradigm of the four forms or *ākāras*.

16 *tatrāvaraṇaviśuddhiḥ katamā | āha | caturbhiḥ kāraṇair evaṃ samyakprayukto yogī āvaraṇe svañcittaṃ pariśodhayati | svabhāvaparijñānena, nidānenādīnavaparijñānena, pratipakṣabhāvanayā ca* (ŚBh 3.12A.2.4–5; Shukla 1973: 398).

17 See Sugawara for the thesis that the *Bhāvanāmayī Bhūmiḥ* is an independent work that is modified to fit with the *Śrāvakabhūmi* (Sugawara 2013).

18 Chapter eight of the *Saṃdhinirmocana Sūtra*, the chapter on yoga, describes the ten counterstates that eliminate the bondage of the afflictions (*kleśa*s): 'Bhagavan, when [Bodhisattvas] eliminate the ten kinds of signs, what are the signs that they eliminate? From what signs of bondage are they liberated?' 'Maitreya, eliminating the sign of the image, the focus of *samādhi*, one is liberated from the signs that are the signs of the afflictions; these [signs] are also eliminated. Maitreya, know that the emptinesses are, in actuality, antidotes to the signs. Each [emptiness] is also an antidote to any of the signs' (SNS 8; Powers 1995: 191).

19 *Bhāvanāmayī Bhūmiḥ* section 5 summarized in Sugawara (2013: 800–2). This list also appears in the second *yogasthāna* of the *Śrāvakabhūmi* (Śbh 2.9B–6.3; Shukla 1973: 270).

20 Von Rospatt is using Sugawara's unpublished edition of the Sanskrit text of the *Yogācārabhūmi* manuscript microfilmed by R. Sāṃkṛtyāyana in Tibet in 1938 (von Rospatt 2013: 871).

21 *Pratipakṣa* literally means 'the opposite side, opposition' and in this sense can even mean 'obstacle' (Monier-Williams 1899). Its synonym *vipakṣa* literally means 'an opponent, counter-statement, counter-instance' (Monier-Williams 1899).

22 I discuss root metaphors in Chapter 1.

23 In general, the binary opposition of state and counterstate is vital to the theory of karma: *yatredam uktam 'dve dve ha vai karmaṇī veditavye pāpakasyaiko rāśiḥ puṇyakṛto 'pahanti tad icchasva karmāṇi sukṛtāni kartum ihaiva te karma kavayo*

vedayante' (PYŚ 2.13). 'In which case (*yatra*) it is said, "Deeds are to be known as twofold; one heap of good deeds destroys one by [one of] evil deeds; so choose to do good acts alone in this life; the poets have instructed this as karma."' Yoga and yogācāra also share understandings of state/counterstate as the colours black/white. For example, Patañjali references white karma shortly after his list of the nine obstacles (*antarāyas*) (PYŚ 1.3), and the *Śrāvakabhūmi* also frames the *pratipakṣas* in terms of black and white karma – there are nine types of practice that produce white karma, while their opposites produce black karma: *tatra navavidhaḥ śuklapakṣasaṃgrītaḥ / prayogas tadviparyayeṇa ca navavidhaḥ / kṛṣṇapakṣasaṃgṛhīto yoginā veditavyaḥ* (ŚBh 13.B.1-3c; Wayman 1960: 116). The nine types of 'white' practice produce *samādhi* while their opposites hinder *samādhi*.

24 In yogācāra, and in early Buddhism generally, the precepts for ethical behaviour (*śīla*) are also presented as counterstates (*pratipakṣas*) to ethical failings. See, for example, the five precepts (*pañcaśīla*) undertaken by Buddhist laity: refraining from killing, stealing, sexual misconduct, false speech, consuming intoxicants.

25 *yatredam uktaṃ tataḥ pratyakcetanādhigamo 'py antarāyābhāvaś ceti / eteṣāṃ yamaniyamānām* (PYŚ 2.32) ***vitarkabādhane pratipakṣabhāvanam*** (YS 2.33; Āgāśe 1904: 105).

26 *Vitarka* in this instance means 'opposite' or 'contrary' idea, rather than 'discursive thought' or 'apprehension' of an object as it does elsewhere in the *Pātañjalayogaśāstra*.

27 Philipp Maas has suggested that this may refer to transgressive ascetics who behaved in the manner of dogs (personal communication, 12 July 2018).

28 *evam unmārgapravaṇavitarkajvareṇātidīptena bādhyamānas tatpratipakṣān bhāvayet. ghoreṣu saṃsārāṅgāreṣu pacyamānena mayā śaraṇam upāgataḥ sarvabhūtābhayapradānena yogadharmaḥ. sa khalv ahaṃ tyaktvā vitarkān punas tān ādadānas tulyaḥ śvavṛtteneti bhāvayet. yathā śvā vāntāvalehī tathā tyaktasya punar ādadāna iti* (PYŚ 2.33; Angot 2012: 489).

29 ***vitarkā hiṃsādayaḥ kṛtakāritānumoditā lobhakrodhamohapūrvakā mṛdumadhyādhimātrā duḥkhājñānānantaphalā iti pratipakṣabhāvanam*** (YS 2.34; Angot 2012: 491). 'The contrary ideas, violence and so on, done or caused to be done or condoned, preceded by greed, anger or delusion – mild, medium, or intense – all result in endless suffering and ignorance. This is the cultivation of the counterstate (*pratipakṣabhāvanā*).'

30 See endnote 3 of this chapter.

31 We also witness similar techniques in the yogācāra *Saddharmasmṛtyupasthānasūtra*, in which the three basic meditation techniques are the contemplations of the unattractive (*aśubha*), friendliness (*maitrī*) and the twelve steps of dependent origination (*pratītyasamutpāda*), respectively designed to counter the three *kleśas* of

craving, hatred and ignorance (Stuart 2015, 1: 74 fn 111). One of the contemplations prescribed by the *Saddhsu* to overcome ignorance is visualizing a greedy dog eating its own tongue, not dissimilar to Patañjali's image of the dog consuming its own vomit.

32 One of the forerunners of Asaṅga's *Yogācārabhūmiśāstra*, the *Damoduluo chan jing* (Buddhasena's **Yogācārabhūmi*) reflects this paradigm of the counterstate: 'Therefore, from the initial practice of the mindfulness of the body to the ultimate stage, this meditation of impurity taught by the Buddha is of paramount importance. All the seeds of greed and desires can be eradicated from the bottom by applying the right antidotes. It is also essential to be disgusted with the world which will cure, in a split second, all the remaining defilements of the world' (DDS 11.22; trans. Chan 2013: 387).

33 'The meditations on conditional causation involve the contemplations on the link of ignorance (*avidyā*) and sensation (*vedanā*). The purpose is to eradicate ignorance (*avidyā*) and replace it by wisdom (*prājñā*). As regards the two links of craving (*tṛṣṇā*) and grasping (*upādāna*), which are, indeed, the contamination caused by the attachment to purity, the meditations on impurity definitely provide the perfect antidote for that' (Chan 2013: 114).

34 The seventh segment of the *Bhāvanāmayī Bhūmiḥ* describes the supramundane path and advocates two techniques for attaining concentration (*samādhi*); agitating the mind (*cittasaṃvigna*) and steadying the mind (*cittasthiti*). Agitating the mind is necessary in order to be freed from *saṃkleśa*.

35 See Chapter 1 for an introduction to conceptual metaphors.

36 *sa punar yogam āsthāya mokṣamārgopalabdhaye.*

37 Gethin also highlights two understandings of the path in the *Abhidharmakośabhāṣya* in which it either (1) culminates in the thirty-seven factors of awakening (*bodhi-pakkhiyā dhammā*) or (2) is composed of the thirty-seven factors as successive stages (Gethin 2007: 23). However, he also points out that scholars can place too much emphasis on definitions of Buddhist path structures as successive, which results in the exclusion of other possible interpretations, such as simultaneity of attainments on the path (Gethin 2007: 210–12).

38 *Aṅga* is traditionally translated as 'limb' of yoga, but scholars such as Sanderson (e.g. 1999: 7 fn 25) and Birch (e.g. 2011: 540) have respectively argued for a technical translation of 'auxiliary' or 'ancillary', in order to convey the concept of support or means to an overall process, as opposed to a spatial metaphor of locatable parts that make up a bigger structure. However, it is debatable as to whether this interpretation of yoga as 'means' within a process can be justified without distorting the content of the *aṅga* metaphor, which in the Brahmanic context often indicates a spatial or bodily domain. It should be noted that *aṅga* is not exclusive to Brahmanic schemes of yoga; alongside the seven *bodhy-aṅgas* (Pāli: *bojjhaṅgas*), or 'factors

of awakening', Buddhism also proposes the eight *margāṅgas* or 'auxiliaries of the path' that make up the Noble Eightfold Path (Gethin 2007: 146–89). I suggest that the early Buddhist *aṭṭhaṅgika-magga* / *aṣṭāṅgika-mārga* is *already* an accretion or blend of two different concepts: *aṅga* as part of a whole and *mārga* as path with stages. When these two concepts are combined into one, however, there are internal contradictions in the entailments.

39 The concept of *bhūmi* is first elaborated in the Abhidharma sources, such as Kātyāyanīputra's *Jñānaprasthāna*, one of Abhidharma's seven canonical treatises. In this text, there are ten stages (*bhūmis*) of practice divided into a lower and a higher level: the first four *bhūmis* comprise the lower path of *bhāvanābhūmi* and the upper path is called *darśanabhūmi* (Potter et al. 1996: 117). In this Abhidharma scheme, the tenth level is *aśaikṣabhūmi* (*aśaikṣa* here refers to the adept who is no longer a pupil), and *nirvāṇa* is the fruit of the ten *bhūmis*. Additionally, in the Abhidharma commentarial tradition, Ghoṣaka's *Mahāvibhāṣā* (*c.* second century) has a tenfold scheme with the attainment of fruition (*prāptaphala*) as its tenth stage. A ten-*bhūmi* scheme also appeared in the *Mahāvastu*, a late canonical work of the Mahāsaṅgikha school that recounts legends of the Buddha. As discussed in Chapter 3, the ten stages (*daśabhūmis*) are associated with the path of cultivation (*bhāvanā*) rather than seeing (*darśana*).

40 For example, the *Abhidharmakośabhāṣya* (AKBh 2.26–8) lists the following *kleśas* (which are congruent with those in the older *Vibhāṣā*): delusion or ignorance (*moha* or *avidyā*), heedlessness (*pramāda*), sloth (*kauśīdya*), lack of confidence (*aśrabdhi*), lethargy (*styāna*) and excitedness (*auddhatya*). These afflicting factors are countered by the ten great stages (of attainment) (*mahābhūmika*): *vedanā, cetanā, saṃjñā, chanda, sparśa, mati, smṛti, manaskāra, adhimokṣa, samādhi/dhyāna* and also the ten *kuśalamahābhūmikas*, the ten great stages of virtue (*śraddhā, vīrya, upekṣā, hrī, anapatrāpya, alobha, adveṣa, ahiṃsā, praśrabhdhi, apramāda*). The ten *kleśamahābhaumikāḥ* are also listed in the *Saddharmasmṛtyupasthānasūtra* (Stuart 2015, 2: 310–11) and are followed by the 'limited mental states' (*parīttabhaumikā*) which act as antidotes (Stuart 2015, 2: 310–12). These terms are distinct from other related sets of factors, such as the *akuśalabhūmika* or the ten *upakleśabhūmikas*, which refer to different qualities and affects: anger (*krodha*), hypocrisy (*mrakṣa*), selfishness (*mātsarya*), envy (*īrṣyā*), spite (*pradāsa*), violence (*vihiṃsā*), vengefulness (*upanāha*), deceit (*māyā*), craftiness (*śāṭhya*) and arrogance (*mada*). In Vasubandhu's *Madhyāntavibhāgabhāṣya*, he lists nine *kleśas*: 2.2–3a (and later in this text he also accepts six, as he does in the *Pañcaskandhaprakaraṇa*). Potter offers a useful overview in 'The Buddhist Way to Liberation' in Potter et al. (1996: 59–72).

41 I am not referring to the term *pratipakṣa* here, but to the structural function of the perfections (*pāramitās*) within the tenfold scheme of the *bodhisattva* path to act as

the requisite counterstates to the obstacles. Even if not explicitly termed *pratipakṣas*, the *pāramitās* fulfil this soteriological function.

42 *sā vivekakhyātir aviplavā hānopāyaḥ. tato mithyājñānasya dagdhabījabhāvopagamaḥ punaś cāprasava ity eṣa mokṣasya mārgo hānasyopāya iti* (PYŚ 2.26; Angot 2012: 467). 'Discriminating discernment, being unwavering, is the means to cessation. From that (discriminating discernment) comes the acquisition of the state of burnt seed of false knowledge and furthermore of non-propagation. This path of liberation is the means of cessation.'

43 Here, *mokṣamārga* appears to be comprised of distinct stages: (1) the bristling of the hairs on the body and the eyes fill with tears, (2) accompaniment by the seed of perception of the difference, (3) investigation of the nature of self-existence, (4) rejection of the self, (5) perception of the difference and of the self as *puruṣa*, accompanied by cessation of investigation of the self.

44 This fourth stage entails (1) realization of the four noble truths (*satyābhisamaya*), (2) removing obstacles hindering the aforesaid realization of truths (*abhisamitasatyasya antarāyavivarjanam*), (3) focusing the mind on pleasant objects in order to gain clairvoyance (*kṣiprābhijñātāyai prāmodyavastumanasikāraḥ*), (4) practising the path of contemplative cultivation (*bhāvanāmārganiṣevaṇā*), (5) attaining the path of complete purification plus its fruits/results and benefits (*saphalānuśaṃsā suviśuddhamārgaprāptiḥ*) (BhāvBh 7; Sugawara 2013: 804–5).

45 This third example, framed in the negative as *alabdha* (non-attainment) rather than *labdha* (attainment) of *samādhi*, occurs in the commentary on the nine obstacles (*antarāya*).

46 As a result of this devotion, the obstacles are eliminated: ***kiṃ cāsya bhavati tataḥ pratyakcetanādhigamo 'py antarāyābhāvaś ca*** (YS 1.29; Angot 2012: 312) 'And what else occurs to him? Then [there is] acquirement of thoughts turned inwards [upon one's self] and also the obstacles disappear.' Devotion to *īśvara* is also noteworthy here as one of the three stages of *kriyā yoga*.

47 This next *sūtra* lists a set of physical symptoms that accompany the obstacles, namely, pain and dejection, trembling limbs and irregular breathing cycles (YS 1.31). The commentary to this *sūtra* concludes, 'These are the distractions, the opposites (counterstates) to *samādhi*, which are to be ceased by practice and dispassion alone.' The context of the obstacles thus shifts somewhat from YS 1.29–31. The obstacles are introduced at 1.29 as a phenomenon that disappears upon practice of *īśvarapraṇidhāna*, but in 1.31 the distractions (by-products of the obstacles) are said to disappear as a result of practice (*abhyāsa*) and dispassion (*vairāgya*). Although *īśvaraprāṇidhāṇa* can be said to be a component of practice, it is not particularly associated with dispassion and, indeed, may even be said to be its opposite (because the cultivation of devotion to a lord is not a state of dispassion).

48 Patañjali does not use the term *brahmavihāra* (abode of Brahma), as the Buddhists do, to refer to the projections of friendliness, compassion, joy and equanimity (*maitrī, karuṇā, muditā, upekṣā*), but Patañjali does refer to them as the *vihāras*: *tathā coktam – ye caite maitryādayo dhyāyinām vihārās te bāhyasādhananiranugrahātmānaḥ prakṛṣṭaṃ dharmam abhinirvartayanti* (PYŚ 4.10; Angot 2012: 685). See also PYŚ 3.23. These projections are also called the four immeasurables (*catvāry apramāṇāni*) in Buddhism, but given that the term *brahmavihāra* also has an early context in Brahmanism, this term seems more appropriate in relation to Patañjali's text. For a full-length study of this topic see Maithrimurthi (1999).

49 Most of these practices also appear in the *Yogācārabhūmiśāstra* in a comparable context of counterstates to the obstacles. For example, in early Buddhist formulations, *ekāgratā* is a counterstate to the three poisons (*triviṣa*) or *kleśa*s (to *rāga* in particular); the *brāhmavihāra*s (see previous endnote) – either in full or in part – appear as counterstates to aversion (*dveṣa*) or malice (*vyāpāda*) in the *Śrāvakabhūmi*, the *Bodhisattvabhūmi* and the *Bhāvanāmayī Bhūmiḥ*; mindfulness of breathing (*ānāpānasmṛti*) appears as an antidote to *vitarka*. See Table 4.1.

50 See PYŚ 3.41 and 3.45 where *anāvaraṇa* appears to describe space (*ākāśa*) that is unobstructed and thus allows the free expression of the *siddhis*. In the *Bodhisattvabhūmi*, *anāvaraṇam* appears in particular as the counterstate to the obstacle to knowledge (*jñeyāvaraṇam*).

51 Two short first-person narrations are presented. The first is the narration of the gods who are jealous of the yogin's accomplishments and who try to lure the yogin with temptations of beautiful women, a wish-fulfilling tree and immortality (PYŚ 3.51). The second narration is the voice of the yogin, who counters the temptations of the gods with opposite images. The gods present alluring, sensual delights of heaven; the yogin's counter-narration presents the scorching fires of *saṃsāra* and the virtues of asceticism. As in the previous example of self-narrated contemplation to create a counterstate (the *yama* of *ahiṃsā* at PYŚ 2.33, see above), the primary image here is, once again, fire.

52 *catvāraḥ khalv amī yoginaḥ prāthamakalpiko madhubhūmikaḥ prajñājyotir atikrāntabhāvanīyaś ceti / tatrābhyāsī pravṛttamātrajyotiḥ prathamaḥ / ṛtaṃbharaprajño dvitīyaḥ / bhūtendriyajayī tṛtīyaḥ sarveṣu bhāviteṣu bhāvanīyeṣu kṛtarakṣābandhaḥ kṛtakartavyasādhanādimān. caturtho yas tv atikrāntabhāvanīyaḥ / tasya cittapratisarga eko 'rthaḥ / saptavidhāsya prāntabhūmiprajñā* (PYŚ 3.51; Angot 2012: 653).

53 The paradigm in each case being problem, cause, cessation, means of cessation.

54 There are also four types of person on the mundane path, but they are less relevant here: the person outside of Buddhism, one who follows doctrine but has weak aptitude due to previous practice of calm, one who has keen aptitude but whose

roots of virtue are not mature, a bodhisattva who desires to attain *nirvāṇa* in a future life but not in this present one: *catvāras tadyathā / sarva itobāhyakaḥ / iha dhārmiko 'pi mṛduḥ / pūrvaśamathacaritas tathā tīkṣṇo 'py aparipakvakuśalamūlaḥ / bodhisar(t)vaś cāyatyāṃ bodhim anuprāptukāmaḥ* (ŚBh 12A.3–7b; Wayman 1960: 125).

55 Somewhat puzzlingly, however, in the *Pātañjalayogaśāstra* the focus is not on the *atikrānta* stage; the gods are only jealous of the Brahmin in the honeyed stage, the *madhubhūmi*, and thus the narrated contemplation (a counterstate) takes place at the honeyed stage, which is explained as equivalent to the state of YS 1.48 in which *ṛtambharaprajñā* (truth-bearing wisdom) is produced.

56 For example, the Theravādin path structure has seven levels of purification, which culminate in *prajñā*: (1) purification of morals, (2) purification of mind, including pure meditations and realization of the eight *samāpatti*s (attainments), (3) purifying views, (4) transcending doubt, (5) knowledge and vision of the correct path over the incorrect, (6) knowledge and vision of the correct method of salvation and (7) purification of wisdom (Hirakawa 1990: 205–6). Sarvāstivāda interprets these seven stages as three degrees of the wise and four degrees of favourable roots (Hirakawa 1990: 208), while adding on three paths: the path of insight (*darśana mārga*), the path of meditation (*bhāvanā mārga*) and the path in which there is nothing left to be learned (*aśaikṣa*). These last three stages are called the 'three degrees of the worthy' but cannot be approached unless the practitioner has undertaken practices to purify his body (Akira 1998: 208–9). Together the seven stages make up the *prayoga*, or preparatory steps, for the path of insight. For a summary account of the Sarvāstivāda path structure, see Gethin (2007: 335–7).

57 ***anityāśuciduḥkhānātmasu nityaśucisukhātmakhyātir avidyā*** (YS 2.5; Āgāśe 1904: 61).

58 These four errors also appear in Dharmaśrī's *Abhidharmasāra* as part of the four recollections (*smṛthyupasthānāni*): 'The disciple at first contemplates the body (*kāyāḥ*) according to its characteristics as impure, impermanent, suffering, and non-self' (Frauwallner 1995: 162). Contemplation on the body is followed by the same formulaic consideration applied to sensation, mind and elements.

59 For example, see BhāvBh 142a3; von Rospatt (2013: 858) and BhāvBh 7-1-B-1; Sugawara (2013: 830).

60 In Buddhist contexts, *bhāvanā* (meditation/cultivation) is often split into *śamatha* and *vipaśyana*. *Vipaśyana* is direct apprehension of the three marks of existence. *Vipaśyana* leads to *prajñā*, insight, while *śamatha* leads to *samādhi* and then to *dhyāna* (absorption) and to special powers, *abhijñā*. In practice, however, the two approaches were combined. *Śamatha* produces *dhyāna*, but *dhyāna* is then made the object of *vipaśyana* meditation by reflecting on how *dhyāna* contains the three marks of existence of the phenomenal world: *anitya*, *duḥkha* and *anātman*.

(However, less commonly, *vipaśyana* can also be used alone, without *śamatha*, by analysing the three marks of existence in ordinary mental phenomena.) Together with the four noble truths, the three marks of existence form the doctrinal basis of early Buddhism.

61 These four errors appear in the earlier * *Yogācārabhūmi* of Saṅgharakṣa in its tenth chapter called 'Avoiding Mistakes'. The text explains the four mistakes as taking the impermanent for permanent, suffering for pleasure, the non-self for self and the empty for the real. The yogācāra guards oneself against these and meditates upon their opposites, the fundamental inexistence (of all permanence etc.). Then one recognizes that one is capable of obtaining these, as well as the four fruits and the quality of the Buddha. 'Bref exposé, agrémenté de comparaisons, des quatre méprises: prendre l'impermanent pour le permanent, la douleur pour le plaisir, l'impersonnel pour le personnel, le vide pour le réel (litt. "le plein"). Le *yogācāra* s'en gardera et méditera au contraire sur l'inexistence foncière (de toute permanence, etc.); il se reconnaître alors capable d'obtenir lui aussi les quatre fruits et la qualité de Buddha' (SYCB 10.198b–199c: Demiéville 1951: 405–6). See also the BoBh: *tathā sarvasaṃskāreṣvanityasaṃjñāmanitye duḥkhasaṃjñāṃ duḥkhe 'nātmasaṃjñāṃ nirvāṇe cānuśaṃsasaṃjñāṃ bhāvayati* (BoBh 1.16; Wogihara 1930–6; 236, lines 8–12).

62 *Caturbhir ākārair duḥkhasatyasya lakṣaṇaṁ pratisaṁvedayate/ tadyathā 'nityākāreṇa duḥkhākareṇa śūnyākareṇa anātmākareṇa ca* (ŚBh 3.29.1.1.1; Deleanu 2006 1: 31).

63 It is also worth noting that the Mahāyāna *tathāgatagarbha* traditions reclaimed the four qualities as those of transcendent Buddha-nature (the *guṇapāramitās*). Both the *Śrīmālādevī Siṃhanāda Sūtra* and the *Ratnagotravibhāgavyākhyā* contain the idea that buddha-nature is possessed of four transcendental qualities: permanence, bliss, self, purity – the identical formula to Patañjali's.

64 "*sthānād bījād upaṣṭambhān niḥsyandān nidhanād api / kāyam ādheyaśaucatvāt paṇḍitā hy aśuciṃ viduḥ*" (PYŚ 2.5).

65 Above, we saw how *aśubha* meditation also utilizes the metaphor YOGA IS AN ANTIDOTE. Such is the visual experience of bodily disease/decay that it can be used to map qualities from both the domain of medicine (antidote) and of vision (visual horror).

Chapter 5

1 In this book, I refer to the 'classical period' as covering the era of the production of the *sūtras* and *śāstras* of Indian philosophy and religion, approximately third century BCE to fifth century CE.

2 Colebrooke is discussed below and we see that his view persists for at least a century, e.g. Garbe (1897: 50); Deussen (1914: 21).

3 The Haṭha Yoga Project was a five-year ERC research initiative, based at SOAS, University of London from 2015 to 2020: http://hyp.soas.ac.uk (last accessed 14 January 2021). Another largescale and concurrent ERC-funded project AyurYog, ran from 2015 to 2020 and sought to problematize the yoga canon by demonstrating the porous boundaries with āyurvedic medical texts: www.ayuryog.org (last accessed 14 January 2021).

4 To be clear: Mallinson's assessment is not that the techniques are devised by Buddhists but simply that the first known record is in a Buddhist text.

5 A plethora of studies on classical yoga focus on this one text alone, e.g. Feuerstein (1979: viii–xiii); Potter (1983: 243); Whicher (2000); Larson and Bhattacharya (2008: 23) and many other studies, too numerous to list.

6 I will use the title *Yogasūtra* rather than *Pātañjalayogaśāstra* when it is necessary to convey that a particular scholar treats the *Yogasūtra* and the *Yogasūtrabhāṣya* as separately authored.

7 White (2014) examines the reception history of this text, and its canonical status, but not its status as a categorically 'classical' text.

8 As an alternative to teleology, Goody offers 'an anthropo-archaeological approach' (Goody 2006: 287).

9 Hellwig's online database the Digital Corpus of Sanskrit is interesting in terms of what it designates as belonging to 'timeslots'. The *Yogasūtra* is classified as 'epic' while the *Yogabhāṣya* is 'classical'. This demonstrates that the question of authorship plays a key role in periodization; if the date of the *Yogaśūtra* is moved back in time to coincide with the dates of the grammarian Patañjali (*c.* second century BCE), it becomes an early classical or even 'epic' text, while the *bhāṣya*, if believed to be separately authored by Vyāsa, stays in the 'golden age' of Indian classicism. Equally interesting is how texts are assigned to 'subjects' – which seems to combine religious labels such as 'Buddhist' alongside genre labels, such as '*kāvya*' and corpus labels such as '*Upaniṣads*'. The *Yogasūtra* and *Yogabhāṣya* are both designated as 'yoga' texts, alongside others such as the *Gorakṣaśataka*, *Gheraṇḍasaṃhitā*, *Haṭhayogapradīpikā*, the *Tattvavaiśāradī* and the *Rājamārtaṇḍa* – the latter two of which are commentaries on the *Yogasūtra*. http://www.sanskrit-linguistics.org/dcs/index.php?contents=corpus (last accessed 30 June 2020).

10 For critiques of the category of religion as a construction of the European Enlightenment, see, for example, Asad (1993); Smith (1998); and King (1999).

11 See also, for example, Mehta (1985); Schwab (1984); Lussier (2006); App (2011).

12 However, as Clarke and many other postcolonial scholars have argued, the knowledge production on the ground of empire was nuanced, and motivations for informing and representing were more complex, leading to 'a conceptual framework

that allows much fertile cross-referencing, the discovery of similarities, analogies, and models; in other words, the underpinning of a productive hermeneutical relationship' (Clarke 1997: 27). See also Strube 2020.

13 This translation was later printed by the Theosophical Society.

14 Herder translated passages from the *Bhagavad Gītā* into German in 1792 in his *Zerstreute Blätter*. Halbfass (1988), Singleton (2008), and White (2014) have all outlined the intense dialogues that occurred in Europe in the eighteenth to nineteenth centuries between Romantic thinkers such as Humboldt and Schlegel who held the *Yogasūtra* in high esteem and philosophers such as Hegel, who did not. For specific discussions of the *Yogasūtra* in this context, see Singleton on Weber (Singleton 2008: 85–7) and White on the Romantics and Hegel (White 2014: 81–91). Davis also outlines these debates but only in relation to the *Bhagavad Gītā* (Davis 2015).

15 Schlegel made a direct comparison with the way in which studying Greco-Roman culture and language had inspired the European renaissance and predicted that a new wave of studying Sanskrit would create a new European Renaissance, one in which 'the Orient' figured prominently (Schlegel 1849: 427).

16 The first translation of parts of the Upaniṣads into a European language was in 1801–2 by French scholar Anquetil-Duperron, who translated from Persian. Schlegel studied Sanskrit and published *On the Language and Wisdom of the Indians* in 1808.

17 His lectures were published as 'Proceedings of the Historical-Philological Section of the Berlin Royal Academy'.

18 Humboldt: *Works* ed. 1841 ff vol I p11 (cited in Herring 1995: xv).

19 The beginnings of oriental scholarship are typically located in the establishment of the Asiatic Society of Bengal by William Jones in 1784, helped by Hastings. By this time there was already a significant community of Sanskrit scholars in the British East India Company as well as the removal of Sanskrit manuscripts to European libraries.

20 Clarke paraphrases the attitude to Asia more broadly: 'Confucius is the equal of Aristotle, the Bhagavad Gītā on a par with the Bible, the Upaniṣads comparable to Kant, Buddha to Christ, Taoist naturalism to Greek science' (Clarke 1997: 27).

21 Colebrooke was the head of the Department of Sanskrit at the College of Fort William set up by Wellesley in 1800. The first European academic chairs in Sanskrit studies were established in France in 1814 and Germany in 1816, with a British chair following at Oxford in 1831.

22 These lectures were published as 'On the Religion and Philosophy of the Hindus' in *Transactions of the Royal Asiatic Society*.

23 'PATANJALI'S *Yóga-śástra* is occupied with devotional exercise and mental abstraction, subduing body and mind: CAPILA is more engaged with investigation of principles and reasoning upon them. One is more mystic and fanatical. The other

makes a nearer approach to philosophical disquisition, however mistaken in its conclusions' (Colebrooke 1858: 160).

24 Colebrooke aligned Pātañjala yoga with 'religious observances' and 'ritual' and not with philosophy (Colebrooke 1858: 232). In his discussion of the Pāśupatas, he, again, translates yoga as 'abstraction' (263) 'perseverance in meditation', 'profound contemplation' (262) and, for the Jains, 'profound abstraction' (245). However, the only reference to 'classical' in this volume is to the language of 'classical Sanskrit' (69).

25 Although the 1827 essays are generally perceived as taking a dim view of Indian philosophy, Staiano-Daniels defends Hegel's treatment of the *Bhagavad Gītā* in this essay as reflecting 'an unexpectedly positive view of Indian thought' (Staiano-Daniels 2011–12: 75).

26 Echoing Colebrooke again, Hegel notes, 'Even Sāṅkhya, which is essentially different from the Patañjali doctrine, agrees with it as to the final and only aim and is in this respect Yoga. Only the way is different; whereas Saṅkhya clearly gives the instruction to move towards that aim by means of reasoned reflection on the particular objects and on the categories of nature and mind, the proper Yoga doctrine of Patañjali is engaged to reach this centre without such meditation, vehemently and at once.' ('Second Article'; trans. Herring 1995: 37).

27 'When using the term *penances* for those exercises we attribute to them a quality they do not involve and thus changes their meaning ('Second Article'; trans. Herring 1995: 59).

28 Hegel writes, 'Hence the Bhagavad-Gītā as such is to be understood as the passing on of this wisdom to the nation whereby what otherwise would stay unknown, and inaccessible to the people is being made generally known,– in an adequate way, that is to say in a poetic work. Both the national epics of India provide the Indians with what Homer's epics provided for the Greeks: the instruction about their religion, for there is no other source for these peoples. Religious cult in itself is not instructive. The Greek poets, too, who according to the famous passage of Herodot had presented to the Greeks their gods, could already rely on myths, traditions, cults, mysteries, etc.; but to the Indian poets the Vedas were a much more solid foundation' ('Second Article'; trans. Herring 1995: 102–3).

29 Other examples include 'old classical Upanishads' (Müller 1919: 94)'; 'old or classical Upanishads' (114); 'so-called classical Upanishads' (220); 'classical Upanishads' (236, 314, 373).

30 When discussing the *sūtras* as 'the first attempts at literary writing in India', he asserts that 'every classical scholar knows that there always is a long interval between an epigraphic and a literary employment of the alphabet' (Müller 1919: 218).

31 The late eighteenth and early nineteenth centuries also saw a relationship between classical religion and 'the classics' i.e. classical languages. For a discussion, see Smith (1982: 102–3) and Davis (2015: 89).

32 Garbe is, here, using 'pure' *Sāṃkhya* to refer to the standalone and systematized work *Sāṃkhyakārikā* and not the integrated discussions of Sāṃkhya in texts such as the *Gītā* or 'Śāntipārvan'.

33 The German neoclassical veneration of ancient texts began early. Opitz translated Seneca and Sophocles and in his *Buechlein von der Deutschen Poeterei* (1624) proclaimed the necessity of being versed in Latin and Greek books in order to learn the correct way of writing. Gottsched's *Versuch einer kritischen Dichtkunst vor die Deutschen* (1730) 'provides an ample and well-formulated introduction to all the more stereotyped facets of neo-classicism, from close attention to detail to the stoical practice of virtue, imagination being given a wide berth' (Secretan 1973: 71). Lessing's *Laokoon* (1766) compared painting and poetry and Winkleman's dictum was that ancient Greek art is 'Edle Einfalt und Stille Grösse' (noble simplicity and tranquil stateliness) – referring here to Winkleman's *Geschichte der Kunst des Altertums* (1764). Goethe's work developed in the direction of the neoclassical, e.g. *Iphigenie auf Tauris* (1779), and Hölderlin's *Hyperion* novel focused on ancient Greece (1797–9).

34 See Anquetil-Duperron's translation, discussed above.

35 Not only Jones but also the emerging Romantic movement was searching for more raw power to move on from 'polite neoclassicism' (Mulholland 2013: 23). As a consequence of increasing European overseas territorial expansion in the eighteenth century, there was a gradual cultural shift from classical to vernacular literacies – and overseas oral traditions were being used to invigorate a stagnating (self-cannibalizing) European poetry (Mulholland 2013: 157). Yet, despite Jones's favourable attitude to Hindu literary texts, the imperialist assessment of religion as 'primitive' is nonetheless reflected in his 'On the Primitive Religion of the Hindus', unfinished due to his death in 1794.

36 i.e. cessation, isolation, yoga of action, eightfold yoga, non-cognitive concentration, seedless concentration, equanimity, one-pointed mental focus, the concentration of the cloud of dharma.

37 For a discussion of the post-Enlightenment rationalist taxonomy of religions, see, for example, Smith (1982 and 2004). Within the nineteenth-century orientalist taxonomies of religion, it was Buddhism that was first promoted to the ranks of Christianity and Mohameddanism (as Islam was then called). However, Hinduism and its subclass yoga spent longer languishing in the category of 'primitive', 'natural' and 'non-rational religion'. Since Buddhism was viewed as a redeeming counterpart to the excesses of Hinduism, a separation was created between Buddhist rationalism

(which indicated Theravāda Buddhism and not Mahāyāna Buddhism, which included yogācāra) and Hinduism (with its yoga 'mysticism').

38 This long-standing characterization of Theravāda as 'earlier' and Mahāyāna as 'later' forms of Buddhism is no longer seen as accurate.

39 For the supplementary portion of the *Yogācārabhūmiśāstra* the situation is even more dire since some 90 per cent of the *Viniścayasaṃgrahaṇī* is only available in Tibetan and Chinese translations, 'Only a few sections or passages of this part of the YoBh are already available in critical editions and translations' (Delhey 2013: 532). Some improvement is imminent, however, in that further portions of the *Viniścayasaṃgrahaṇī* have been discovered in Lhasa (Delhey 2013: 510).

40 Scholars of Indian Brahmanical traditions tend to be trained in Sanskrit, Pāli, Prakrit and perhaps also Tibetan – but not necessarily Chinese.

41 The most recent attempt to give an overview of the corpus in terms of manuscripts, editions, translations and scholarship is by Delhey (2013).

42 The Chinese rendering is the *Yúqié shīdì lùn* (T1579), made by Xuanzang's 'translation bureau' in the seventh century CE, and the Tibetan edition exists in the *bstan 'gyur* and could hence be dated from the ninth century CE onwards (Delhey 2013: 507 fn 29 and fn 30).

43 Today, the Kashi Prasad Jayaswal Research Institute in Patna.

44 This is evident in Dasgupta's 1921 volume, in which his footnotes frequently point out that this can be understood in relation to Spinoza, William James, Christian saints, Plotinus, Schelling, etc.

45 In the preface to the revised edition of volume 2, which is dated to 1926, Radhakrishnan acknowledges that he has found the writings of Deussen and Keith helpful. We may therefore speculate that Radhakrishnan picks up on this term from Keith's 1925 publication (discussed below) – but until I see Radhakrishnan's 1923 manuscript, I cannot verify whether Radhakrishna's 1923 publication contains the prior usage of 'classical yoga'.

46 See, for example, Hopkins, who states, 'The second form of Yoga was simply *dama*, control of sense and thought, intense concentration of mental activity acquired by quietism. It is this which is common to the practice of Buddhism and Brahmanism alike' (Hopkins 1901: 336).

47 See Chapter 4 for more discussion on this point.

48 This description is discussed in various Upaniṣads and also in the *Bhagavad Gītā* and interpreted as a metaphor for the metaphysical principles of *prakṛti* and *puruṣa* in Sāṃkhya.

49 For example, Keith argues against Garbe's view that Plotinus derives his 'belief of the turning away of the mind from things of the sense and the achievement of a condition of union with the divine in ecstasy' from the parallel concept of *prātibha*, 'intuitive knowledge' of the Yogasūtra (3.33)' (Keith 1925).

50 *darśanam na samam tayoḥ* (*Mahābhārata* 12.300.8–9).
51 He also sums up the section as 'Discovery of the Origin of the Classical Yoga Doctrine of Transcendent God: Abandonment of the Upaniṣadic Identity of Jîva and Brahman' (Modi 1932: 81).
52 Müller makes some forward-thinking comments that are still, unfortunately, applicable today on how the study of philosophy in general should include Indian thinkers as part of the standard course of study.

Conclusion

1 Indology, the study of the historical civilizations of South Asia, is here styled with a small 'i' to denote that historically it had less to do with geographic 'India' than a colonialist outsider European attitude and ideology towards India. A parallel can be seen in choices to refer to orientalism as a cultural ideology rather than a geographical description of 'the Orient'. Indology is distinct as a humanities discipline, particularly in continental Europe, whereas in the UK, for instance, it has often been renamed as part of area studies, e.g. South Asian studies. See Chapter 5 for a discussion of the orientalist and colonial foundations of indology.
2 For a recent discussion of neoliberal yoga, see Jain (2020).
3 These include organizations with Indian figureheads and roots – such as Sivananda Yoga, The Yoga Life Institute, or Sadhguru's Isha Foundation: https://sivanandalondon.org/our-learning-centre/ (accessed 6 November 2020); https://www.yogalifeinstitute.com/books/0111181111a_hdr/ (accessed 12 May 2021); or https://isha.sadhguru.org/global/en/s?sq=classical&s=0&l=10&gs=0&gl=2&t=0 (accessed 6 November 2020). It also includes organizations led by Westerners who may identify as renouncers or *sannyasin*s – such as the Australian College of Classical Yoga which brands itself as 'Original, Classical, Authentic': https://classicalyoga.com.au/swami-shantananda/ (accessed 6 November 2020).
4 Often 'classical yoga' is used in a vague way as part of branding nous, e.g. an organization called 'Spirit of Yoga' in Spain offers a training programme titled 'Classical and Authentic Yoga Teacher Training' or a school in the UK is titled The Classical Yoga School: http://youareyoga.com/; http://www.cysyogateachertraining.com/ (accessed 6 November 2020). Another example in New York can be found here: http://www.brooklynyogaschool.com/classical-yoga (accessed 6 November 2020).
5 Although without a convincing explanation as to why, 'content of the intervention was based on Patanjal Yogadarshan. That is why the word classical has been used as Patanjal Yogadarshan is considered as the classical scripture on yoga' (Karmalkar and Vaidya 2017: 431). What is presented as 'classical yoga' is, however, a rather

free and anachronistic interpretation covering five practices: shavasana, meditative movements (like thoracic twisting), meditative asanas, pranayama and chanting of omkar (Karmalkar and Vaidya 2017: 431).

6 The authors state, 'If yoga is performed in a classical way, it touches all the aspects of human existence starting from physical to psychological to spiritual' (Karmalkar and Vaidya 2017: 431).

7 The type of nuanced problematization of historical definitions that is encouraged in humanities studies on yoga is not easily incorporated into biomedical research models.

8 To expand this point: 'The concept of Antiquity has been elaborated by European classicists to account for the singularity of the traditions coming down from Greece and Rome. While those societies certainly differed from other ancient cultures, just as they differed from earlier Archaic Greece and Rome, radical attempts were made to distinguish them from others not so much on the basis of the economy as of the political system and the ideology – for example, democracy and freedom found in Europe as distinct from tyranny and despotism supposedly prevalent in Asia' (Goody 2006: 289).

9 See, for instance, the long-standing revisionist history of David Frawley's 'Vedic Yoga' (https://www.vedanet.com/vedic-yoga-the-oldest-form-of-yoga/ (accessed 6 November 2020)) or the increased popularity of trends in Vedic chanting in yoga classes, e.g. http://sarahryanyoga.co.uk/vedic-chanting/.

10 The transliterated 'shastra yoga' without diacritics makes the same point.

11 We might here question whether Halbfass is also imposing classical criteria onto the Indian doxographical worldview.

12 It has been argued that the word *sutta* in the Buddhist *sutta* genre was derived from Vedic *sūkta* (hymn) and not *sūtra* (thread/aphorism), and so, like the *sūkta*s, the Buddhist *sutta* genre is characterized by extolment and hyperbole and not conciseness (e.g. Norman 2006: 135).

13 The term classist here refers to the inherent inequality of social class systems, and points to the intersection of such classism with the hegemony of classicism.

14 PYŚ 2.30–3; see also Maas's discussion of YS 3.51 in Maas (2014: 73).

15 One might consider whether there was a social class distinction between those who practised yoga and those who more singularly practised *tapas* (austerities).

16 Constructed by the Indian doxographers.

17 These are details in the 'Naiṣkramyabhūmi' section of the *Śrāvakabhūmi* discussed in Kragh (2013: 115–18).

Appendix 1

1 Other common titles for the *Bhāṣya* include the *Vyāsabhāṣya*, *Yogabhāṣya* and (its own self-given title) *Sāṃkhyapravacana-bhāṣya*.

2 Most scholars have regarded the *Bhāṣya* as separately authored from the *Yogasūtra* and have attributed its authorship to Vyāsa, dating the commentary to around the fifth to sixth century CE. In Larson's view, the *Bhāṣya* may have been composed by the Sāṃkhya author Vindhyavāsin and reflects polemical interaction with Buddhist thinkers (Larson 2012: 74). Whicher argues that the *Bhāṣya* was authored separately and later by Vyāsa, and postdates the *Sāṃkhyakārikā* (Whicher 2000:49). Gelblum and Pines speculate that the *Bhāṣya* that we have today may not be the original version (Gelblum and Pines 1989). This is suggested by discrepancies in two later renderings of the *Bhāṣya*. First, the *Bhāṣya* cited in Śaṅkara's *Vivaraṇa* commentary is not the same as that traditionally named as Vyāsa's. Second, al-Bīrūnī's (973–1050 CE) Arabic translation, the *Kitāb Pātañgal*, albeit an abridgement, seems to refer to a different commentary than the one we have. Angot states that Vyāsa's commentary replaced an earlier, ecumenical commentary and that Vyāsa's *Bhāṣya* is a response by Brahmins to attacks from Jains and Buddhists (Angot 2012). Angot further drives a wedge between the two texts by asserting that Patañjali's references in the first three *pāda*s of the *Yogasūtra* neglect the Vedas entirely and that Vyāsa's *Bhāṣya* draws on the *Purāṇas* (Angot 2012). Raveh writes of the 'gap' between Patañjali and Vyāsa, most notably in the *Bhāṣya*'s elision of explanations of some of the *siddhi-sūtra*s in the 'Vibhūti Pāda' (Raveh 2012: 12).

3 Several scholars have pointed out that Vyāsa is, most likely, not a proper name as it literally means 'compiler' or 'arranger' and is thus either a misattribution, misrendering or a corruption (Larson 2012: 74; Maas 2013). Burley adds that Vyāsa must be taken as a legendary figure, since it is also to him that the Vedas, *Mahābhārata*, *Purāṇas* and *Brahmasūtra* are also attributed (Burley 2007: 29).

4 We see this convention reflected in the other two main texts under consideration in this study. Together, the *Abhidharmakośakārikā* and the *Abhidharmakośakārikābhāṣya* are regarded as a unitary composition and referred to as the *Abhidharmakośabhāṣya*, authored by Vasubandhu. Similarly, the *Yogācārabhūmiśāstra* is presented as a unitary text comprised of core teachings called *bhūmis* (foundations) and accompanied by an auto-commentary of sorts (also called the supplementary section), the *Saṃgrahaṇī*.

5 The arguments as to whether or not the *Vivaraṇa* can be attributed to Śaṅkara and dated this early are controversial. For the claim that the *Vivaraṇa* was a *c.* eighth-century composition by Śaṅkara, see Leggett (1990) and Harimoto (1999). For the counterargument that the text is as late as the eleventh to fourteenth century, see Gelblum (1992), Rukmani (2001) and Larson and Bhattacharya (2008).

Appendix 2

1 Cited in Patton (2008: 49).
2 For a different account of *upacāra* in relation to Abhidhamma access concentration, see Gethin (2007: 333–5).
3 Covill refutes the argument that there is evidence of *alaṃkāra-śāstra* in the works of Aśvaghoṣa. She argues that theories of stylistic device did not exist in the early centuries of the Common Era (Covill 2009).
4 For overviews of general studies of metaphor in Buddhist scholarship, see Covill (2009: 25–30) and Tzohar (2018: 3–7). For an overview of studies of metaphor in Vedic and early Hindu studies, see Patton (2008: 49–51).

Bibliography

Primary

Abhayaśekharasūri, A. V. (ed.) (2009) *Yogaviṃśikā of Haribhadra with Commentary by Yaśovijaya in Hāribhadrayogabhāratī*, 3rd edn. Dholakā: Divyadarśana.

Āgāśe, K. (ed.) (1904) *Vācaspatimiśraviracitaṭīkāsaṃvalitavyāsabhāṣyasametāni Pātañjalayogasūtrāṇi, Tathā Bhojadevaviracitarājamārtaṇḍābhidhavṛttisametāni pātañjalayogasūtrāṇi. sūtrapāṭhasūtravarṇānukramasūcībhyāṃ ca Sanāthīkṛtāni.* Poona: Ānandāśrama.

Angot, M. (trans.) (2012) *Le yoga-sutra de Patanjali: Le Yoga-Bhasya de Vyasa avec des Extraits du Yoga-Varttika de Vijnana-Bhiksu.* Paris: Les Belles Lettres.

Āraṇya, H. (trans.) (1983) *Yoga Philosophy of Patanjali.* Translated by P. Mukherji. Albany: SUNY.

Asaṅga (1998) *Srāvakabhūmi: The First Chapter, Revised Sanskrit Text and Japanese Translation, ed. Śrāvakabhūmi Study Group (The Institute for Comprehensive Studies of Buddhism, Taisho University).* Tokyo: Institute for Comprehensive Studies of Buddhism, Taisho University (Taisho University Sogo Bukkyo Kenyujo, 4).

Asaṅga (2007) *Śrāvakabhūmi: The Second Chapter with Asamāhitā Bhūmiḥ, Śrutamayī Bhūmiḥ, Cintāmayī Bhūmiḥ, Revised Sanskrit Text and Japanese Translation, ed. Śrāvakabhūmi Study Group.* Tokyo: International Institute for Buddhist Studies (Taisho University Sogo Bukkyo Kenyujo, 18).

Ballantyne, J. R., and Sastri Deva, G. ([1852] 1971) *Yoga-sutra of Patanjali.* India: Indological Book House.

Bangali, B. (trans.) (1976) *Yogasutra of Patanjali with the Commentary of Vyasa.* Delhi: Motilal Banarsidass.

Belvalkar, S. (ed.) (1954) *The Sāntiparvan: In the Mahābhārata, for the First Time Critically Edited. Volumes 14–16.* Poona: Bhandakar Oriental Research Institute.

Bhattacharya, V. (1957) *The Yogācārabhūmi of Ācārya Asanga: The Sanskrit Text Compared with the Tibetan Version.* Calcutta: University of Calcutta.

Bolle, K. (ed.) (1979) *The Bhagavadgītā.* Berkeley: University of California Press.

Bryant, E. (trans.) (2009) *The Yoga Sutras of Patanjali.* New York: North Point Press.

Cleary, T. (trans.) (1995) *Buddhist Yoga.* Boston: Shambala.

Conze, E. (1954) *Buddhist Texts through the Ages.* Oxford: Bruno Cassirer.

Deleanu, F. (ed.) (2006) *The Chapter on the Mundane Path (Laukikamārga): A Trilingual Edition (Sanskrit, Tibetan, Chinese), Annotated Translation and Introductory Study* (2 vols). Tokyo: International Institute for Buddhist Studies.

Delhey, M. (ed.) (2009) *Samāhitā Bhūmiḥ: das Kapitel über die Meditative Versenkung im Grundteil der Yogācārabhūmi*. Vienna: Arbeitskreis für Tibetische und Buddhistische Studien, Universität Wien.

Edgerton, F. (trans.) (1965) *The Beginnings of Indian Philosophy: Selections from the Rig Veda, Atharva Veda, Upanisads, and Mahābhārata*. Cambridge, MA: Harvard University Press.

Engle, A. (trans.) (2016) *The Bodhisattva Path to Unsurpassed Enlightenment: A Complete Translation of the Bodhisattvabhūmi*. Translated by A. Engle. Boulder, CO: Snow Lion.

Fausbøll, V. (ed.) (2000) *The Jātaka: Together with Its Commentary Being Tales of the Anterior Births of Gotama Buddha. Volume 1*. Oxford: Pali Text Society.

Gaṅgānāṭha Jhā (trans.) (1984) *The Nyāya-Sūṭras of Gauṭama: With the Bhāṣya of Vāṭsyāyana and the Vārṭika of Uḍḍyoṭakara. Volume IV*. Delhi: Motilal Banarsidass.

Halbfass, W. (1988) *India and Europe: An Essay in Understanding*. New York: SUNY.

Hardy, E. (ed.) (1901) *Dhammapala's Paramattha-Dīpanī Part IV: Being the Commentary on the Vimana-Vatthu*. London: Pali Text Society.

Harimoto, K. (ed.) (2014) *God, Reason, and Yoga: A Critical Edition and Translation of the Commentary Ascribed to Śaṅkara on Pātañjalayogaśāstra*. Hamburg: University of Hamburg.

Hirakawa, A. (1963) *Index to the Abhidharmakośabhāṣya (P. Pradhan Edition). Volume 1*. Tokyo: Daizo Shuppan.

Horner, I. B. (trans.) (1963–4) *Milinda's Questions: Translated from the Pali*. Sacred Books of the Buddhists, volumes 22–3. London: Luzac.

Horner, I. B. (trans.) (1975) *Chronicle of Buddhas (Buddhavaṁsa) and Basket of Conduct (Cariyāpiṭaka)*. Sacred Books of the Buddhists, volume XXXI: The Minor Anthologies of the Pali Canon, Part III. London and Boston: Pli Text Society

Hume, R. (trans.) (1931) *The Thirteen Principal Upanisads*, 2nd rev. edn. Great Britain: Oxford University Press.

Jacobs, G. A. (1963) *A Concordance to the Principal Upnishads and Bhagvad Gītā* [*sic*]. Delhi: Motilal Banarsidass.

Jain, S. (trans.) (1992) *Reality: English Translation of Shri Pujyapada's Sarvarthasiddhi*. Madras: Jwalamalini Trust.

Jayawickrama, N. A. (ed.) (1974) *Buddhavaṃsa and Cariyāpiṭaka*. PTS Text Series, 166. London: Pali Text Society.

Joshi, S. D., and Roodbergen, J. A. F. (trans.) (2003) *The Aṣṭādhyāyī of Pāṇini: With Translation and Explanatory Notes*. Delhi: Sahitya Akademi.

Lamotte, E. (trans.) (1935) *Saṃdhinirmocana Sūtra: L'Explication des Mysteres*. Paris: Librairie d'Amérique et D'Orient.

Lamotte, E. (ed.) (1998) *Karmasiddhiprakaraṇa: The Treatise on Action by Vasubandhu*. Translated by Pruden, L. Berkeley, CA: Asian Humanities Press.

Leggett, T. (trans.) (1990) *The Complete Commentary by Sankara on the Yoga Sutras: A Full Translation of the Newly Discovered Text*. London: Kegan Paul International.

Lilley, M. (ed.) (1925–7) *The Apadāna of the Khuddaka Nikāya: Parts I and II*. Oxford: Pali Text Society.

Maas, P. (ed.) (2006) *Samādhipāda. Das erste Kapitel des Pātañjalayogaśāstra zum ersten Mal Kritisch Ediert*. Aachen: Studia Indologica Universitatis Halensis (GeisteskulturIndiens. Texte und Studien, 9).

Morris, R. (ed.) (1885) Aṅguttara-nikāya. *Volume 1*. London: Pali Text Society.

Mitra, R. (trans.) (1883) *The Yoga Aphorisms of Patanjali: With the Commentary of Bhoja Raja and an English Translation*. Calcutta: Royal Asiatic Society of Bengal.

Ñāṇamoli, B. (trans.) (2010) *The Path of Purification (Visuddhimagga) by Bhadantācariya Buddhaghosa*. Colombo: Buddhist Publication Society.

Olivelle, P. (trans.) (1998) *The Early Upaniṣads: Annotated Text and Translation*. New York: Oxford University Press.

Powers, J. (trans.) (1995) *Wisdom of Buddha. The Saṃdhinirmocana Sūtra*. Berkeley, CA: Dharma.

Pradhan, P. (ed.) (1975) *Abhidharmakośabhāṣyam of Vasubandhu*. Patna: K. P. Jayaswal Research Centre.

Pruden, L. (trans.) (1988–90) *Abhidharmakośabhāṣyam of Vasubandhu: Translated into French by Louis de La Vallée Poussin. English version by Leo M Pruden* (4 vols). Translated by L. Pruden. Berkeley, CA: Asian Humanities Press.

Radhakrishnan, S. (1929) *Indian Philosophy: Volumes 1 and 2*, rev. edn. London: George Allen & Unwin.

Rahder, J. (ed.) (1926) *Daśabhūmikasūtra*. Leuven: JB Istas.

Rahder, J. (ed.) (1928) *Glossary of the Sanskrit, Tibetan, Mongolian and Chinese Versions of the Daśabhūmika-Sūtra*. Paris: Librairie Orientaliste Paul Geuthner.

Rhys Davids, C. A. F. (ed.) (1975) *The Visuddhimagga of Buddhaghosa*. London: Pali Text Society.

Rhys Davids, T. W. (trans.) (2000) *Buddhist Birth Stories: The Oldest Collection of Folklore Extant*. London: Routledge.

Richard, T. (trans.) (1907) *Guide to Buddhahood: Being a Standard Manual of Chinese Buddhism*. Shanghai: Christian Literature Society.

Roebuck, V. (trans.) (2000) *The Upaniṣads*. London: Penguin Books.

Rukmani, T. S. (trans.) (1981–9) *Yogavārtikka of Vijñānabhikṣu: Text, with English Translation and Critical Notes along with the Text and English Translation of the Pātañjala Yogasūtra and Vyāsabhāṣya* (4 vols). New Delhi: Munshiram Manoharlal.

Rukmani, T. S. (trans.) (2001) *Yogasūtrabhāṣyavivaraṇa of Śaṅkara: Vivaraṇa Text with English Translation, and Critical Notes along with Text and English Translation of Patañjali's Yogasūtras and Vyāsabhāṣya. Volumes 1 and 2*. New Delhi: Munshiram Manoharlal.

Sastri, T. (ed.) (1984) *The Nyāyasutras with Vātsyāyaṇa's Bhāsya*. Delhi: Sri Satguru.

Sastri, R., and Krishnamurthi, S. R. (eds) (1952) *Pātañjalayogasūtrabhāṣya Vivaraṇaṃ of Śaṅkara-Bhagavat Pāda*. Madras: Government Oriental Manuscripts Library.

Savitarkā Savicārā Bhumistṛtīyā. Digital Sanskrit Buddhist Canon: http://www.dsbcproject.org/canon-text/book/341 (accessed 30 August 30 2018).

Senart, E. (ed.) (1882–97) *Le Mahāvastu: Text Sanscrit Publié pour la Première Fois et Accompagné d'Introductions et d'un Commentaire par E. Senart*. Paris: Imprimerie Nationale.

Shastri, S. D. (ed.) (1998) *Abhidharmakosa & Bhasya of Acarya Vasubandhu with Sphutartha Commentary of Acarya Yasomittra* (2 vols). Varanasi: Bauddha Bharati.

Shukla, K. (ed.) (1973) *Sravakabhumi of Acarya Asanga*. Patna: KP Jayaswal Research Institute.

Suzuki, D. T., and Idzumi, H. (eds) (1934) *The Gandavyuha Sutra*. Kyoto: Sanskrit Buddhist Texts.

Thakur, A. (ed.) (1997) *Gautamīya Nyāyadarśanam with Bhāṣya of Vātsyāyana and the Vārtika of Uddyotakara*. New Delhi: Indian Council of Philosophical Research.

Thera, N., and Bodhi, B. (eds) (1999) *Aṅguttara-nikāya. Numerical Discourses of the Buddha: An Anthology of Suttas from the Anguttara Nikāya*. Walnut Creek, CA: AltaMira Press.

Trenckner, V. (ed.) (1962) *The Milindapañho: Being Dialogues between King Milinda and the Buddhist Sage Nāgasena. The Pāli Text*. London: Luzac.

Trenckner, V., Anderson, D., and Smith, H. (1924–48) *A Critical Pāli Dictionary. Volume 1*. Copenhagen: Royal Danish Academy of Sciences and Letters.

Trenckner, V., Anderson, D., and Smith, H. (1960) *A Critical Pāli Dictionary. Volume 2*. Copenhagen: Royal Danish Academy of Sciences and Letters.

Vasu, S. R. (ed.; trans.) (1980) *The Ashṭāhdyāyī of Paṇini. Volumes 1 and 2*. Delhi: Motilal Banarsidass.

Walters, J. (trans.) (2017) *Legends of the Buddhist Saints*. Jonathan S Walters and Whitman College. Available at http://www.apadanatranslation.org.

Wayman, A. (ed.) (1960) *Analysis of the Śrāvakabhūmi Manuscript*. Berkeley: University of California Press.

Wogihara, U. (ed.) (1930–6) *Bodhisattvabhūmi: A Statement of Whole Course of the Bodhisattva (Being Fifteenth Section of Yogācārabhūmi)*. Tokyo: Taisho College.

Wogihara, U., and Tsuchida, C. (1934) *Saddharmapuṇḍarīka-sūtram*. Tokyo: Bibliotheca Buddhica.

Willis, J. D. (1979) *On Knowing Reality: The Tattvārtha Chapter of Asaṅga's Bodhisattvabhūmi*. New York: Columbia University Press.

Woods, J. (trans.) (1914) *The Yoga-System of Patañjali […] and the Comment Called Yoga-Bhāṣya Attributed to Veda-Vyāsa and the Explanation Called Tattva-Vaiśāradī of Vācaspati Miśra*. Cambridge, MA: Harvard Oriental Series.

Woodward, F. L. M. and Hare, E. M. (1973) *Pāli Tipiṭakaṁ Concordance. Volume II*. London: London and Boston.

Wynne, A. (trans.) (2009) *Mahābhārata Book Twelve. Peace: Volume Three, The Book of Liberation*. New York: New York University Press and the JJC Foundation (Clay Sanskrit Library).

Secondary

Adam, M. (2002) *Meditation and the Concept of Insight in Kamalaśīla's Bhāvanā-kramas*. McGill, unpublished PhD dissertation.

Adluri, S. (2017) 'Yoga in the Viṣṇu Purāṇa', *Journal of Indian Philosophy* 45: 381–402.

Akira, H. (1990) *A History of Indian Buddhism: From Śākyamuni to Early Mahāyāna*. Translated by Groner, P. Reprinted 1998. Buddhist Tradition Series. Delhi: Motilal Banarsidass.

Allchin, F. R. (1995) *The Archaeology of Early History Asia: The Emergence of Cities and States*. Cambridge: Cambridge University Press.

Allon, M. (1997) *Style and Function: A Study of the Dominant Stylistic Features of the Prose Portions of Pāli Canonical Sutta Texts and their Mnemonic Function*. Studio Philologica Buddhica: Monograph Series, XII. Tokyo: International Institute for Buddhist Studies.

Allott, N. (2010) *Key Terms in Pragmatics*. London: Continuum.

Alter, J. (2004) *Yoga in Modern India: The Body between Science and Philosophy*. Princeton, NJ: Princeton University Press.

Anacker, S. (1984) *Seven Works of Vasubandhu: The Buddhist Psychological Doctor*. Delhi: Motilal Banarsidass.

App, U. (2011) *The Birth of Orientalism*. Pennsylvania: University of Pennsylvania Press.

Aramaki, N. (2013) 'Two Notes on the Formation of the Yogācārabhūmi Text-Complex', in *The Foundation for Yoga Practitioners: The Buddhist Yogācārabhūmi Treatise and Its Adaptation in India, East Asia, and Tibet*. Harvard Oriental Series. Cambridge, MA: Harvard University Press.

Armpong-Nyarko, K., and De Datta, S. (1991) *A Handbook for Weed Control in Rice*. Manila: International Rice Research Institute.

Asad, T. (1993) *Genealogies of Religion: Discipline and Reasons of Power in Christianity and Islam*. Baltimore: John Hopkins University Press.

Bader, J. (1990) *Meditation in Śaṅkara's Vedānta*. New Delhi: Aditya.

Bailey, G., and Mabbett, I. (2003) *The Sociology of Early Buddhism*. Cambridge: Cambridge University Press.

Bakker, H. (1982) 'On the Origin of Sāṃkhya Psychology', *Wiener Zeitschrift für die Kunde Südasiens* 26: 117–48.

Balcerowicz, P. (2008) 'Some Remarks on the Opening Sections in Jaina Epistemological Treatises', in Slaje, W. (ed.), *Śāstrārambha: Inquiries into the Preamble in Sanskrit*. Göttingen: Deutsche Morgenländische Gesellschaft.

Baldick, C. (2001) *The Concise Oxford Dictionary of Literary Terms*. Oxford: Oxford University Press.

Barthélemy Saint-Hilaire, J. (1852) *Premier Mémoire sur le Sânkhya*. Paris: Insitut Nationale de France.

Basham, A. L. (1975) *A Cultural History of India*. Oxford: Clarendon Press.

Beardsley, M. (1958) *Aesthetics: Problems in the Philosophy of Criticism*. New York: Harcourt Brace.

Bedekar, V. M. (1960–1) 'The Dhyānayoga in the Mahābhārata (XII.188)', *Bharatiya Vidya (Munshi Indological Felicitation Volume)* 20–1: 115–25.

Bedekar, V. M. (1968) 'Yoga in the Mokṣadharmaparvan of the Mahābhārata', in Beiträge zur Geistesgeschichte Indiens: Festschrift für Erich Frauwallner, aus Anlass seines 70. Geburtstages, ed. G. Oberhammer (= Wiener Zeitschrift für die Kunde Sud- und Ostasiens und Archiv für Indische Philosophie 12–13: 43–53).

Bellwood, P. (2004) *First Farmers: The Origins of Agricultural Societies*. London: Blackwell.

Belvalkar, S. K., and Ranade, R. D. (1926) *A History of Indian Philosophy. Volume 2*. Poona: University of Bombay.

Bhushan, N. (2011) *Indian Philosophy in English from Renaissance to Independence*. Oxford: Oxford University Press.

Birch, J. (2011) 'The Meaning of *Haṭha* in Early Haṭhayoga', *Journal of the American Oriental Society* 131 (4): 527–54.

Birch, J. (2019a) 'The Amaraughaprabodha: New Evidence on the Manuscript Transmission of an Early Work on Haṭha- and Rājayoga', *Journal of Indian Philosophy* (47) 5: 947–77.

Birch, J., and Singleton, M. (2019b) 'The Yoga of the Haṭhābhyāsapaddhati: Haṭhayoga on the Cusp of Modernity', *Journal of Yoga Studies* (2) 1: 3–70.

Black, M. (1962) *Models and Metaphors: Studies in Language and Philosophy*. Ithaca, NY: Cornell University Press.

Böhtlingk, O., and Roth, R. (1865–8) *Sanskrit-Wörterbuch: Fünfter Theil*. St Petersburg: Buchdruckerei Der Kaiserlichen Akademie Der Wissenschaftern.

Boucher, D. (2008) *Bodhisattvas of the Forest and the Formation of the Mahayana: A Study and Translation of the Rāṣṭrapālaparipṛccha-sūtra*. Honolulu: University of Hawaii Press.

Brinton, L. (2003) 'Historical Discourse Analysis', in Schiffrin, D., Tannen, D., and Hamilton, H. (eds), *The Handbook of Discourse Analysis*. Malden, MA: Blackwell.

Brockington, J. (2003) 'Yoga in the Mahābhārata', in Carpenter, D., and Whicher, I. (eds), *Yoga, the Indian Tradition*, 13–24. London: RoutledgeCurzon.

Brockington, J. (2005) 'Epic Yoga', *Journal of Vaishnava Studies* 14 (1): 123–38.

Bronkhorst, J. (1981) 'Meaning Entries in Pāṇini's Dhātupāṭha*', *Journal of Indian Philosophy* 9: 335–57.

Bronkhorst, J. (1983) *The Two Traditions of Meditation in Ancient India*. Delhi: Motilal Banarsidass.

Bronkhorst, J. (1985) 'Patañjali and the Yoga Sūtras', *Studien zur Indologie und Iranistik* (10): 191–209.

Bronkhorst, J. (1993) *The Two Sources of Indian Asceticism*. Berne: Peter Lang.

Bronkhorst, J. (2006) 'Systematic Philosophy between the Empires', in Olivelle, P. (ed.), *Between the Empires: Society in India 300 BCE to 400 CE*. New York: Oxford University Press.

Bronkhorst, J. (2007) *Greater Magadha: Studies in the Culture of Early India*. Leiden: Brill.

Bronkhorst, J. (2012) *Absorption: Human Nature and Liberation*. Paris: UniversityMedia

Buescher, H. (2008) *The Inception of Yogācāra-Vijñānavāda*. Vienna: Verlag der Österreichischen Akademie der Wissenschaften.

Burley, M. (2007) *Classical Sāṃkhya and Yoga: An Indian Metaphysics of Experience*. London: Routledge.

Buswell, R. (1992) 'The Path to Perdition', in Buswell, R., and Gimello, R. (eds), *Paths to Liberation: The Mārga and Its Transformations in Buddhist Thought*. Honolulu: University of Hawaii Press (Studies in East Asian Buddhism, 7).

Buswell, R., and Gimello, R. (eds) (1992) *Paths to Liberation: The Mārga and Its Transformations in Buddhist Thought*. Honolulu: University of Hawaii Press.

Cantú, K. (2021) 'Sri Sabhapati Swami: The Forgotten Yogi of Western Esotericism', in Pokorny, L., and Winter, F. (eds), *The Occult Nineteenth Century: Roots, Development, and Impact on the Modern World*. London: Palgrave Macmillan.

Chan, Y. (2013) 'An English Translation of the *Dharmatrāta-Dhyāna-Sūtra* with Annotation and a Critical Introduction'. Doctoral dissertation, unpublished, University of Hong Kong.

Chakrabarti, D. K. (1995) *The Archaeology of Ancient Indian Cities*. Delhi: Oxford University Press.

Chakravarti, P. (1975) *Origin and Development of the Sāṃkhya System of Thought*. Delhi: Oriental Books Reprint Corporation.

Chapple, C. (2003) *Reconciling Yogas: Haribhadra's Collection of Views on Yoga with a New Translation of Haribhadra's Yogadrstisamuccaya*. New York: SUNY.

Clarke, J. J. (1997) *Oriental Enlightenment: The Encounter between Asian and Western Thought*. London: Routledge.

Colebrooke, T. H. (1858) *Essays on the Religion and Philosophy of the Hindus*. Leipzig: F. A Brockhaus; London: Williams & Norgate.

Colebrooke, T. H. (1873) *Miscellaneous Essays: A New Edition with Notes. Volume 1*. Ludgate Hill: Trübner.

Collins, S. (1982) *Selfless Persons: Imagery and Thought in Theravāda Buddhism*. Cambridge: Cambridge University Press.

Collins, S. (2010) *Nirvana: Concept, Imagery, Narrative*. Cambridge: Cambridge University Press.

Comeau, L. (2020) *Material Devotion in a South Indian Poetic World*. Bloomsbury Studies in Material Religion. London: Bloomsbury Academic.

Coomaraswamy, A. K (1909) 'Indian Nationality' in Bhushan 2011.
Conrad, S. (2016) *What Is Global History?* Princeton, NJ: Princeton University Press.
Conze, E. (1967) *Buddhist Thought in India: Three Phases of Buddhist Philosophy*. Ann Arbor: University of Michigan Press.
Cousins, L. (1992) 'Vitakka/Vitarka and Vicāra: Stages of Samādhi in Buddhism and Yoga', *Indo-Iranian Journal* 35: 137–57.
Cousins, L. (1996) 'The Origins of Insight Meditation' in Skorupski, T. (ed.), *The Buddhist Forum: Volume IV. Seminar Papers: 1994–1996*. London: School of Oriental and African Studies.
Covill, L. (2009) *A Metaphorical Study of Saundarananda*. Delhi: Motilal Banarsidass.
Cox, C. (1992) 'Attainment through Abandonment: The Sarvāstivādin Path of Removing Defilements', in Buswell, R., and Gimello, R. (eds), *Paths to Liberation: The Mārga and Its Transformations in Buddhist Thought*. Honolulu: University of Hawaii Press (Studies in East Asian Buddhism, 7).
Cox, C. (1995) *Disputed Dharmas: Early Buddhist Theories on Existence: An Annotated Translation of the Section on Factors Dissociated from Thought from Saṅghabhadra's Nyāyānusāra*. Studio Philologica Buddhica: Monograph Series, XI. Tokyo: International Institute for Buddhist Studies.
Crangle, E. F. (1994) *The Origin and Development of Early Indian Contemplative Practices*. Wiesbaden: Harrassowitz Verlag.
Darling, G. (1987) *An Evaluation of the Vedāntic Critique of Buddhism*. Delhi: Motilal Banarsidass.
Dasgupta, S. (1922) *A History of Indian Philosophy. Volume 1*. Delhi: Motilal Banarsidass.
Davids, T. W. R., and Stede, W. (1998) *The Pali Text Society's Pali-English Dictionary*. Oxford: Pali Text Society.
Davidson, R. (1985) 'Buddhist Systems of Transformation: Āśraya-Parivṛtti/Parāvṛtti among the Yogācāra'. Phd Dissertation. Berkeley: University of California Press.
Davidson, R. (2002) *Indian Esoteric Buddhism: A Social History of the Tantric Movement*. New York: Columbia University Press.
Davidson, R. (2010) 'The Place of Abhiṣeka Visualization in the Yogalehrbuch', in Franco, E., and Zin, M. (eds), *From Turfan to Ajanta: Festschrift for Dieter Schlingloff on the Occasion of his Eightieth Birthday*. Rupandehi, Nepal: Lumbini International Research Institute.
Davies, J. (1894) *Hindu Philosophy: The Sānkhya Kārikā of Iśwara Krishna*, 2nd edn. London: Kegan Paul, Trench, Trübner.
Davis, R. H. (2015) *The Bhagavad Gita: A Biography*. Princeton, NJ: Princeton University Press.
De Michelis, E. (2005) *A History of Modern Yoga: Patanjali and Western Esotericism*. London: Continuum.
Deignan, A. (2005) *Metaphor and Corpus Linguistics*. Amsterdam: John Benjamins (Converging Evidence in Language and Communication Research, 6).

Deleanu, F. (2012) 'Far from the Madding Strife for Hollow Pleasures: Meditation and Liberation in the Śrāvakabhūmi', *Journal of the International College for Postgraduate Buddhist Studies* 16: 1–38.

Deleanu, F., Hori, S., Maithrimurthi, M., and von Rospatt, A. (eds) (2016) *Lambert Schmithausen: Collected Papers. Volume 1 1963–1977*. Studio Philologica Buddhica: Monograph Series, XXXIVa. Tokyo: International Institute for Buddhist Studies.

Delhey, M. (2013) 'The Yogācārabhūmi Corpus: Sources, Editions, Translations, and Reference Works', in Kragh, U. T. (ed.), *The Foundation for Yoga Practitioners: The Buddhist Yoācārabhūmi Treatise and Its Adaptation in India, East India, and Tibet*. Cambridge, MA: Harvard University Press.

Demiéville, P. (1951) 'La Yogācārabhūmi de Saṅgharakṣa', *Bulletin du l'École Française d'Extrême-Orient* XLIV (2): 339–436.

Deussen, P. (1914) *Allgemeine Geschichte der Philosophie I, 3: Die Nachvedische Philosophie der Inder*. Leipzig: F.A. Brockhaus.

Dhammajoti, K. L. (2009) *Sarvāstivāda Abhidharma*. Hong Kong: University of Hong Kong.

Doniger O'Flaherty, W. (1983) 'Introduction', in Doniger O'Flaherty, W. (ed.), *Karma and Rebirth in Classical Indian Traditions*, ix–xxv. Delhi: Motilal Banarsidass.

Drewes, D. (2010) 'Early Indian Mahāyana Buddhism II: New Perspectives', *Religion Compass* 4 (2): 66–74.

Drewes, D. (2018) 'The Forest Hypothesis', in Harrison, P. (ed.), *Setting Out on the Great Way: Essays on Early Mahāyāna Buddhism*. Sheffield: Equinox.

Duerlinger, J. (2003) *Indian Buddhist Theories of Persons: Vasubandhu's 'Refutation of the Theory of a Self'*. London: RoutledgeCurzon.

Dundas, P. (1992) *The Jains*. London: Routledge.

Dundas, P. (2006) 'A Non-Imperial Religion? Jainism in Its "Dark Age"', in Olivelle, P. (ed.), *Between the Empires: Society in India 300 BCE to 400 CE*. Oxford: Oxford University Press.

Dutt, N. (1978) *Buddhist Sects in India*. Delhi: Motilal Banarsidass.

Eco, U. (1979) 'The Semantics of Metaphor' in *The Role of the Reader*. Bloomington: Indiana University Press.

Edgerton, F. (1953) *Buddhist Hybrid Sanskrit Grammar and Dictionary*. New Haven, CT: Yale University Press.

Egge, J. (2013) 'Theorizing Embodiment: Conceptual Metaphor Theory and the Comparative Study of Religion', in Pathak, S. (ed.), *Figuring Religions: Comparing Images, Ideas and Activities*. New York: SUNY.

Eliade, M. (1958) *Yoga: Immortality and Freedom*. New York: Bollingen Foundation.

Eltschinger, V. (2017) 'Why Did the Buddhists Adopt Sanskrit?', in *Open Linguistics* 3: 308–26.

Endo, K. (2000) 'Prasaṃkhyāna in the Yogabhāṣya', in Mayeda, S. (ed.), *Japanese Studies on South Asia*, 3. New Delhi: Manohar.

Esler, D. (2016) 'Traces of Abhidharma in the *bSam-gtan mig-sgron* (Tibet, Tenth Century)', in Dessein, B., and Teng, W. (eds), *Text, History, and Philosophy: Abhidharma across Buddhist Scholastic Traditions*. Leiden: Brill.

Fauconnier, G., and Turner, M. (2003) *The Way We Think: Conceptual Blending and the Mind's Hidden Complexities*. New York: Basic Books.

Fernandez, J. (1991) *Beyond Metaphor: The Theory of Tropes in Anthropology*. Stanford: Stanford University Press.

Feuerstein, G. (1979) *The Yoga-Sūtra of Patañjali: A New Translation and Commentary*. Kent: Dawson.

Fitzgerald, J. (2012) 'A Prescription for Yoga and Power in the Mahābhārata', in White, D. G. (ed.), *Yoga in Practice*, pp. 43–57. Princeton, NJ: Princeton University Press.

Flores, R. (2008) *Buddhist Scriptures as Literature: Sacred Rhetoric and the Uses of Theory*. Albany: SUNY.

Fludernik, M. (2011) *Beyond Cognitive Metaphor Theory: Perspectives on Literary Metaphor*. London: Routledge.

Fogelin, L. (2015) *An Archaeological History of Indian Buddhism*. Oxford: Oxford University Press.

Forsten, A. (2006) *Between Certainty and Finitude: A Study of Laṅkāvatārasūtra Chapter Two*. Brunswick: Transaction (Rutgers University).

Franco, E. (2017) 'Vasubandhu the Unified. Review Article of Jonathan C. Gold, Paving the Great Way. *Vasubandhu's Unifying Philosophy*', *Journal of Indian Philosophy* 45 (5).

Franco, E. (ed.) (2013) *Periodization and Historiography of Indian Philosophy*. Vienna: Publications of the De Nobili Research Library.

Frauwallner, E. (1951) *On the Date of the Buddhist Master of the Law*. Rome: Is.M.E.O.

Frauwallner, E. (1958) 'Die Erkenntnislehre des Klassischen Sāṃkhya-Systems', in *Wiener Zeitschrift für die Kunde Süd- und Ostasiens* 2: 84–139.

Frauwallner, E. (1971) 'Abhidharma-Studien III. Der Abhisamayavādaḥ', *Wiener Zeitschrift für die Kunde Südasiens* 15: 69–102.

Frauwallner, E. (1973) *History of Indian Philosophy*. Delhi: Motilal Banarsidass.

Frauwallner, E. (1995) *Studies in Abhidharma Literature and the Origins of the Buddhist Philosophical Systems*. Translated from the German by Sophie Franic Kidd. SUNY: New York.

Frazier, J. (2014) *Categorisation in Indian Philosophy*. Farnham, Surrey: Ashgate (Dialogues in South Asian Traditions).

Freschi, E., and Maas, P. (eds) (2017) *Adaptive Reuse: Aspects of Creativity in South Asian Cultural History*. Wiesbaden: Harrassowitz Verlag.

Gadamer, H. (2004) *Truth and Method*. New York: Continuum.

Ganeri, J. (2011) *The Lost Age of Reason: Philosophy in Early Modern India 1450–1700*. Oxford: Oxford University Press.

Garbe, R. (1897) *Sāṃkhya und Yoga*. Strassburg: KJ Trübner.

Garfield, J., and Westerhoff, J. (2015) *Madhyamaka and Yogācāra: Allies or Rivals?* Oxford: Oxford University Press.

Gelblum, T. (1992) 'Notes on an English Translation of the Yogasūtrabhāṣyavivaraṇa', *Bulletin of the School of African and Oriental Studies* 55 (1): 76–89.

Gelblum, T., and Pines, S. (1989) 'Al-Bīrūni's Arabic Version of Pātañjali's Yogasūtra: A Translation of the Second Chapter and a Comparison with Related Texts', *BSOAS* 2 (LII): 265–305.

Gethin, R. (1998) *The Foundations of Buddhism*. Oxford: Oxford University Press.

Gethin, R. (2007) *The Buddhist Path to Awakening*. Oxford: Oneworld.

Ghosh, A. (1973) *The City in Early Historical India*. Simla: Institute of Advanced Study.

Gibbs, R. (2017) *Metaphor Wars: Conceptual Metaphors in Human Life*. Cambridge: Cambridge University Press.

Gokhale, P. (2020) *The Yogasūtra of Patañjali: A New Introduction to the Buddhist Roots of the Yoga System*. Delhi: Routledge India.

Gold, J. C. (2015) *Paving the Great Way: Vasubandhu's Unifying Buddhist Philosophy*. New York: Columbia University Press.

Goldmann, L. (1980) *Essays on Method in the Sociology of Literature*. Translated by Boelhower, W. St Louis: Telos Press.

Gombrich, R. (1988) *Theravada Buddhism: A Social History from Ancient Benares to Modern Colombo*. London: Routledge.

Gombrich, R. (1996) *How Buddhism Began: The Conditioned Genesis of the Early Teachings*. London: Athlone.

Gonda, J. (1956–7) 'Professor Burrow and the Prehistory of Sanskrit', in *Lingua* 6: 287–300.

Gonda, J. (1965) *Change and Continuity in Indian Religion*. London: Mouton.

Goody, J. (2006) *The Theft of History*. New York: Cambridge University Press.

Griffiths, P. (1986) *On Being Mindless: Buddhist Meditation and the Mind-Body Problem*. La Salle, IL: Open Court.

Gupta, B., and Copeman, J. (2019) 'Awakening Hindu Nationalism through Yoga: Swami Ramdev and the Bharat Swabhiman Movement', *Contemporary South Asia* 27 (3): 313–29.

Habermann, I. (2011) 'Reaching beyond Silence: Metaphors of Ineffability in English Poetry – Donne, Wordsworth, Keats, Eliot', in Fludernik, M. (ed.), *Beyond Cognitive Metaphor Theory: Perspectives on Literary Metaphor*. London: Routledge.

Hacker, P. (1972) 'Notes on the Māṇḍūkopaniṣad and Śaṅkara's Āgamaśāstravivaraṇa', in Ensink, J., and Gaeffke, P. (eds), *India Maior: Congratulatory Volume Presented to J. Gonda*. Leiden: Brill.

Hakayama, N. (2013) 'Serving and Served Monks in the Yogācārabhūmi', in Kragh, U. T. (ed.), *The Foundation for Yoga Practitioners: The Buddhist Yogācārabhūmi Treatise and its Adaptation in India, East India, and Tibet*. Harvard Oriental Series. Cambridge, MA: Harvard University Press.

Halbfass, W. (1992) *On Being and What There Is: Classical Vaiśeṣika and the History of Indian Ontology*. New York: SUNY.

Hanson, E. F. (1998) 'Early Yogācāra and Its Relation to Nāgārjuna's Madhyamaka: Change and Continuity in the History of Mahāyāna Buddhism'. PhD dissertation, Harvard University.

Harimoto, K. (1999) 'A Critical Edition of the Pātañjalayogaśāstravivaraṇa, First Pāda, Samādhipāda with an Introduction'. PhD Thesis, University of Pennsylvania.

Harimoto, K. (2014) *God, Reason, and Yoga: A Critical Edition and Translation of the Commentary Ascribed to Śaṅkara on Pātañjalayogaśāstra*. Hamburg: University of Hamburg.

Hayes, G., and Timalsina, S. (2017) 'Introduction to "Cognitive Science and the Study of Yoga and Tantra"', in *Religions* 8: 1–11.

Harrison (2003) 'Mediums and Messages: Reflections on the Production of Mahāyāna Sūtras', *Eastern Buddhist* 35 (1–2): 115–51.

Hauer, J. W. (1958) *Der Yoga*. Stuttgart: W Kohlhammer Verlag.

Heesterman, J. C (1993) *The Broken World of Sacrifice: An Essay in Ancient Indian Ritual*. Chicago: University of Chicago Press.

Heiler, F. (1922) *Die Buddistische Versenkung: Eine Religionsgeschichtliche Versuchung*. Delhi: Gyan Books.

Herring, H. (ed.) (1995) *GWF Hegel: On the Episode of the Mahābhārata Known by the Name of the Bhagavad-Gitā by Wilhelm von Humboldt, Berlin 1826*. Translated by H. Herring. New Delhi: Indian Council of Philosophical Research.

Hiltebeitel, A. (2011) *Dharma: Its Early History in Law, Religion and Narrative*. Oxford: Oxford University Press.

Hirakawa, A. (1990) *A History of Indian Buddhism: From Śākyamuni to Early Mahāyāna*. Translated by P. Groner. Delhi: Motilal Banarsidass.

Hiriyanna, M. (1932) *Outlines of Indian Philosophy*. London: George Allen & Unwin.

Hilton, P. (2009) 'A Brief, Subjective History of Homology and Homotopy Theory in This Century', in Anderson, M., Katz, V., and Wilson, R. (eds), *Who Gave You the Epilson? and Other Tales of Mathematical History*. Spectrum: Mathematical Association of America.

Hopkins, E. W. (1901) 'Yoga-Technique in the Great Epic', *Journal of the American Oriental Society* 22.

Hwang, S. (2006) *Metaphor and Literalism in Buddhism: The Doctrinal History of Nirvana*. London: Routledge.

Irwin, W. (2004) 'Against Intertextuality', *Philosophy and Literature* (28): 227–42.

Jacobi, H. (1930) *Über Das Ursprüngliche Yoga System: Nachträge und Indices*. Hamburg: De Gruyter.

Jacobs, A., and Jucker, A. (1995) 'The Historical Perspective in Pragmatics', in *Historical Pragmatics: Pragmatic Developments in the History of English*. Amsterdam: John Benjamins.

Jacobsen, K. (2008) *Kapila, Founder of Sāṃkhya and Avatāra of Visṇụ: With a Translation of Kapilāsurisaṃvāda*. New Delhi: Munshiram Manoharlal.

Jain, A. (2020) 'Neoliberal Yoga', in Newcombe, S., and O'Brien-Kop, K. (eds), *The Routledge Handbook of Yoga and Meditation Studies*. London: Routledge.

Jaini, P. (1992) 'On the Ignorance of the Arhat', in Buswell, R., and Gimello, R. (eds), *Paths to Liberation: The Mārga and Its Transformations in Buddhist Thought*. Honolulu: University of Hawaii Press (Studies in East Asian Buddhism, 7).

Jakobsen, R. (1956) 'The Metaphoric and Metonymic Poles', in Jakobsen, R., and Halle, M. (eds), *Fundamentals of Language*. The Hague: Mouton.

Johl, S. (1980) *Irrigation and Agricultural Development*. Oxford: Pergamon Press.

Johnson, M. (2005) 'The Philosophical Significance of Image Schemas', in Hampe, B., and Grady, J. (eds), *From Perception to Meaning: Image Schemas in Cognitive Linguistics*. Berlin: Mouton de Gruyter.

Jones, W. (1799) *The Works of Sir William Jones in Six Volumes*. London: G G and J Robinson and R H Evans.

Jones, W. (1807) 'Extracts from the Vedas', in Shore, T., and Teignmouth, L. (eds), *Selected Works* XIII in *The Works of Sir William Jones, with The Life of the Author, by Lord Teignmouth* (13 vols). London: John Stockdale, John Walker.

Johnston, E. (1974) *Early Sāṃkhya: An Essay on Its Historical Development According to the Texts*. London: Royal Asiatic Society.

Johnson, K. A. (2011) '"Lisping Tongues" and "Sanscrit Songs": William Jones' Hymns to Hindu Deitie's', in *Translation and Literature* 20 (1): 48–60.

Jucker, A. (ed.) (1995) *Historical Pragmatics: Pragmatic Developments in the History of English*. Pragmatics & Beyond New Series. Amsterdam: John Benjamins.

Kaelber, W. (1989) *Tapta Mārga: Asceticism and Initiation in Vedic India*. Albany: SUNY.

Kamber, G., and Macksey, R. (1970) '"Negative Metaphor" and Proust's Rhetoric of Absence', *Comparative Literature* 85 (6): 858–83.

Karmalkar, S., and Vaidya, A. (2017) 'Effects of Classical Yoga Intervention on Resilience of Rural-to-Urban College Students', in *Indian Journal of Positive Psychology* 8 (3): 429–34.

Keith, A. B. (1918) *The Sāṁkhya System: A History of Samkhya Philosophy*. Calcutta: Association Press.

Keith, A. B. (1920) *A History of Sanskrit literature*. London: Oxford University Press.

Keith, A. B. (1925) *The Religion and Philosophy of the Veda and Upanishads. Volume 2*. Cambridge, MA: Harvard University Press.

Keith, A. B. (1932) 'Some Problems of Indian Philosophy', *Indian Historical Quarterly* 8 (3): 154–80

Kerr, J. (2020) 'Unsettling Gadamerian Hermeneutic Inquiry: Engaging the *Colonial Difference*', *Qualitative Inquiry* 26 (5): 544–50.

Khandalavala, K. (1991) *The Golden Age: Gupta Art: Empire, Province and Influence*. Bombay: MARG.

Killingley, D. (2017) 'The Upaniṣads and Yoga', in Cohen, S. (ed.), *The Upanishads: A Complete Guide*. London: Routledge.

King, R. (1999) *Orientalism and Religion: Postcolonial Theory, India and 'The Mystic East'*. New York: Routledge.

King, R. (2010) 'Colonialism, Hinduism and the Discourse of Religion', in Bloch, E., Keppens, M., and Hegde, R. (eds), *Rethinking Religion in India: The Colonial Construction of Hinduism*. London: Routledge.

King, R. (2011) 'Imagining Religions in India: Colonialism and the Mapping of South Asian History and Culture', in Dressler, M., and Mandair, A. (eds), *Secularism and Religion-Making*. Oxford: Oxford University Press.

Kiss, C. (2021) *Matsyendra's Compendium: Matsyendrasaṃhitā Volume I: A Critical Edition and Annotated Translation of Chapters 1–13 and 55* Collection Indologie, no. 146. Hatha Yoga Series, no. 1. Pondicherry: Institut Français d'Indologie/École française d'Extrême-Orient.

Klostermeier, K. (1986) 'Dharmamegha Samādhi: Comments on Yogasūtra IV, 29', *Philosophy East and West* 36 (3): 253–62.

Koelman, G. (1970) *Pātañjalayoga: From Related Ego to Absolute Self*. Poona: Papal Athenaeum.

Koeppen, C. F. (1859) *Die Religion des Buddha. Volume 2*. Berlin: Ferdinand Schneider.

Kövecses, Z. (2005) *Metaphor in Culture: Universality and Variation*. Oxford: Cambridge University Press.

Kövecses, Z. (2006) *Language, Mind, and Culture: A Practical Introduction*. London: Oxford University Press.

Kövecses, Z. (2010) *Metaphor: A Practical Introduction*. New York: Oxford University Press.

Kövecses, Z. (2015) *Where Metaphors Come From: Reconsidering Context in Metaphor*. Oxford: Oxford University Press.

Kövecses, Z. (2017) 'Conceptual Metaphor Theory', in Semino, E., and Demjén, Z. (eds), *The Routledge Handbook of Metaphor and Language*. London: Routledge.

Kragh, U. T. (2013a) *The Foundation for Yoga Practitioners: The Buddhist Yogācārabhūmi Treatise and Its Adaptation in India, East Asia, and Tibet*. Harvard Oriental Series. Cambridge, MA: Harvard University Press.

Kragh, U. T. (2013b) 'The Yogācārabhūmi and Its Adaptation', in *The Foundation for Yoga Practitioners: The Buddhist Yoācārabhūmi Treatise and Its Adaptation in India, East India, and Tibet*. Harvard Oriental Series. Cambridge, MA: Harvard University Press.

Kramer, J. (2012) 'Descriptions of "Feeling" (Vedanā), Ideation (Samjñā), and "the Unconditioned" (Asaṃskṛta) in Vasubandhu's Pañcaskandhaka and Sthiramati's Pañcaskandhakavibhāṣā', in Bareja-Starzynska, A., and Mejor, M. (eds), *Proceedings of the International Conference of Oriental Studies: Warsaw 2010*. Warsaw: Elipsa.

Krishan, Y. (1997) *The Doctrine of Karma: Its Origin and Development in Brāhmaṇical, Buddhist and Jaina Traditions*. Delhi: Motilal Banarsidass.

Kristeva, J. (1969) 'Le Mot, le Dialogue et le Roman', in Kristeva, J. (ed.), *Semiotiké: Recherches pour une Sémanalyse*. Paris: Edition du Seuil.

Kristeva, J. (1980) *Desire in Language: A Semiotic Approach to Literature and Art*. Oxford: Blackwell.

Kristeva, J. (1986) 'Word, Dialogue, Novel', in Moi, T. (ed.), *The Kristeva Reader*. Oxford: Blackwell.

Kritzer, R. (2005) *Vasubandhu and the Yogācārabhūmi: Yogācāra Elements in the Abhidharmakośabhāṣya*. Studio Philologica Buddhica: Monograph Series, 18. Tokyo: International Institute for Buddhist Studies.

Kumoi, S. (1997) 'The Concept of Yoga in the Nikāyas', in Kieffer-Pülz, P., and Hartmann, J. (eds), *Baudda Vidyāsudhākaraḥ: Studies in Honour of Heinz Bechert on the Occasion of his 65th Birthday*. Swisttal-Odendorf: Indica et Tibetica Verlag (Indica et Tibetica, 30).

Kunjunni Raja, K. (1977) *Indian Theories of Meaning*. Madras: Adyar Library and Research Centre.

Kunjunni Raja, K. (1990) 'Parisaṃkhyāna versus Prasaṃkhyāna in Śaṃkara's Philosophy', *Adyar Library Bulletin* 54: 191–6.

de La Vallée Poussin, L. (1936) 'Le Bouddhisme et le yoga de Patañjali', *Mélanges Chinois et Bouddhiques* 5: 232–42.

Lakoff, G., and Johnson, M. (1980) *Metaphors We Live By*. Chicago: University of Chicago Press.

Lakoff, G. (1987) *Women, Fire and Dangerous Things: What Categories Reveal About the Mind*. Chicago: University of Chicago Press.

Lakoff, G., and Turner, M. (1989) *More than Cool Reason: A Field Guide to Poetic Metaphor*. Chicago: University of Chicago Press.

Lakoff, G. (1991) 'Metaphor and War: The Metaphor System Used to Justify War in the Gulf', in *Peace Research* 23: 25–2.

Lamotte, E. (1974) 'Passions and Impregnations of the Passions in Buddhism', in Cousins, L., Kunst, A., and Norman, K. (eds), *Buddhist Studies in Honour of IB Horner*. Dordrecht: D Reidel.

Lamotte. E. (1988) *History of Indian Buddhism: From the Origins to the Śaka Era*. Translated by Webb-Boin, S. Louvain-La-Neuve: Institut Orientaliste.

Lang, K. (2003) *Four Illusions*. Oxford: Oxford University Press.

Larson, G. (1969) *Classical Sāṃkhya: An Interpretation of Its History and Meaning*. Delhi: Motilal Banarsidass.

Larson, G. (1989) 'An Old Problem Revisited, the Relation between Sāṃkhya, Yoga, and Buddhism', *Studien zur Indologie und Iranistik* 15: 129–46.

Larson, G. (2012) 'Patañjala Yoga in Practice', in White, D. G. (ed.), *Yoga in Practice*. Princeton, NJ: Princeton University Press.

Larson, G., and Bhattacharya, R. S. (eds) (1987) *Encyclopedia of Indian Philosophies, Volume IV. Sāṃkhya: A Dualist Tradition in Indian Philosophy*. Delhi: Motilal Banarsidass.

Larson, G., and Bhattacharya, R. S. (2008) *Encyclopedia of Indian Philosophies, Volume XII. Yoga: India's Philosophy of Meditation*. Delhi: Motilal Banarsidass.

Larson, G. (2018) *Classical Yoga Philosophy and the Legacy of Sāṃkhya with Sanskrit Text and English Translation of Pātañjala Yogasūtra-s, Vyāsa Bhāṣya and Tattvavaiśāradī of Vācaspatimiśra*. MLBD Classical Systems of Indian Philosophy. Delhi: Motilal Banarsidass.

Lindtner, C. (1995) 'Lokasaṃgraha, Buddhism and Buddhiyoga in the Gītā', in Narang, S. P. (ed.), *Modern Evaluation of the Mahābhārata: Prof. R. K. Sharma Felicitation Volume*. Delhi: Nag.

Lopez, D. (1992) 'Paths Terminable and Interminable', in Buswell, R., and Gimello, R. (eds), *Paths to Liberation: The Mārga and Its Transformations in Buddhist Thought*. Honolulu: University of Hawaii Press.

Lopez, D. (2001) *Buddhism: An Introduction and Guide*. London: Penguin.

Lotman, Y. (1976) *Analysis of the Poetic Text*. Ann Arbor: University of Michigan Press.

Lussier, M. (2006) *Romantic Dharma: The Emergence of Buddhism into Nineteenth-Century Europe*. New York: Palgrave.

Lusthaus, D. (2002) *Buddhist Phenomenology: A Philosophical Investigation of Yogācāra Buddhism and the Ch'eng Wei-shih lun*. London: RoutledgeCurzon.

Lusthaus, D. (2015) *What Is and Isn't Yogācāra*? Yogācāra Buddhism Research Association. Available at http://www.acmuller.net/yogacara/articles/intro.html (accessed 31 July 2018).

Maas, P. (2008a) 'Descent with Modification: The Opening of the Pātañjalayogaśāstra', in Slaje, W. (ed.), *Śāstrārambha. Inquiries into the Preamble in Sanskrit*. Wiesbaden: Harrassowitz.

Maas, P. (2008b) 'The Concepts of the Human Body and Disease in Classical Yoga and Āyurveda', *Wiener Zeitschrift für die Kunde Südasiens* 51: 123–62.

Maas, P. (2009) 'The So-Called Yoga of Suppression', in Franco, E. (ed.), *Yogic Perception, Meditation, and Altered States of Consciousness*. Vienna: Verlag der Österreichischen Akademie der Wissenschaften.

Maas, P. (2010a) 'On the Written Transmission of the Pātañjalayogaśāstra', in Bronkhorst, J., and Preisendanz, K. (eds), *From Vasubandhu to Caitanya: Studies in Indian Philosophy and Its Textual History*. Delhi: Papers of the 12th World Sanskrit Conference.

Maas, P. (2010b) 'Valid Knowledge and Belief in Classical Sāṃkhya-Yoga', in Balcerowitz, P. (ed.), *Logic and Belief in Indian Philosophy*. Warsaw: Warsaw Indological Studies (3).

Maas, P. (2013) 'A Concise Historiography of Classical Yoga', in Franco, E. (ed.), *Periodisation and Historiography of Indian Philosophy*. Vienna: University of Vienna.

Maas, P. (2014) 'Der Yogi und Sein Heilsweg im Yoga des Patañjali', in Steiner, K. (ed.), *Wege zum Heil(igen): Sakralität und Sakralisierung in Hinduistischen Traditionen?* Wiessbaden: Harrassowitz.

Maas, P. (2018) 'On the Relation of the *Pātañjalayogaśāstra* and the *Nyāyabhāṣya*'. Paper presented at the 17th World Sanskrit Conference on 10 July 2018. University of British Columbia, Vancouver, Canada.

Maas, P. (2020) 'Sarvāstivāda Buddhist Theories of Temporality and the Pātañjala Yoga Theory of Transformation (*pariṇāma*)', in *Journal of Indian Philosophy* 48 4.

Maithrimurthi, M. (1999) *Wohlwollen, Mitleid, Freude und Gleichmut: eine Ideengeschichtliche Untersuchung der vier apramāṇas in der Buddhistischen Ethik und Spiritualität von den Anfängen bis hin zum Frühen Yogācāra*. Stuttgart: Franz Steiner Verlag.

Malalasekera, G. P. (1938) *Dictionary of Pāli Proper Names. Volume 2*. London: John Murray.

Malinar, A. (2007) *The Bhagavadgītā: Doctrines and Contexts*. Cambridge: Cambridge University Press.

Malinar, A. (2012) 'Yoga and Yogin in the *Bhagavadgīta*', in Jezic, M., and Kokikallio, P. (eds), *Proceedings of the Fifth Dubrovnik Conference on the Sanskrit Epics and Purāṇas, August 2008*, Zagreb: Coration Academy of Science.

Mallinson, J. (2020a). 'Haṭhayoga's Early History: From Vajrayāna Sexual Restraint to Universal Somatic Soteriology' in Flood, G. (ed.), *The Oxford History of Hinduism: Hindu Practice*. Oxford: Oxford University Press.

Mallinson, J. (2020b) 'The Amṛtasiddhi: Haṭhayoga's Tantric Buddhist Source Text', in Goodall, D., Hatley, S., Isaacson, H., and Raman, S. (eds), *Śaivism and the Tantric Traditions: Essays in Honour of Alexis GJS Sanderson*. Gonda Indological Studies, volume 22. Leiden: Brill.

Mallinson, J., and Singleton, M. (2017) *Roots of Yoga: A Sourcebook from the Indian Traditions*. London: Penguin Classics.

Matilal, B. K. (1985) *Logic, Language and Reality: An Introduction to Indian Philosophical Studies*. Delhi: Motilal Banarsidass.

Matilal, B. K. (2001) 'Causality in the Nyāya-Vaiśeṣika School', in Perrett, R. (ed.), *Indian Philosophy: Metaphysics*. London: Garland.

Matsuda, K. (2013) 'Sanskrit Fragments of the Saṃdhinirmocanasūtra', in Kragh, U. T. (ed.), *The Foundation for Yoga Practitioners: The Buddhist Yogācārabhūmi Treatise and Its Adaptation in India, East India, and Tibet*. Harvard Oriental Series. Cambridge, MA: Harvard University Press.

Matsubayashi, M., Ryuji, I., and Toshio, N. (1968) *Theory and Practice of Growing Rice*. Tokyo: Fuji.

Mayrhofer, M. (1963) *Kurzgefaßtes Etymologisches Wörterbuch des Altindischen: A Concise Etymological Sanskrit Dictionary. Volume II*. Heidelberg: Carl Winter Universtitätsverlag.

McCartney, P. (2017) 'Politics beyond the Yoga Mat: Yoga Fundamentalism and the "Vedic Way of Life"', in *Global Ethnographic* 4: 1–18.

McGovern, W. M. (1977) *A Manual of Buddhist Philosophy. Volume 1: Cosmology*. San Francisco: Chinese Materials Centre.

McGraw, A. (2013) *Radical Traditions: Reimagining Culture in Balinese Contemporary Music*. Oxford: Oxford University Press.

McMahan, D. (2002) *Empty Vision: Metaphor and Visionary Imagery in Mahayāna Buddhism*. London: RoutledgeCurzon.

Meek, R. (2014) 'Intertextuality, Inner-Biblical Exegesis, and Inner-Biblical Allusion: The Ethics of a Methodology', *Biblica* 95(2): 280–91.

Mehta, J. L. (1985) *India and the West: The Problem of Understanding*. Chico: Scholars Press.

Mejor, M. (1999) 'There Is No Self (*Nātmāsti*): Some Observations from Vasubandhu's *Abhidharmakośa* and the *Yuktidīpikā*', in *Communication & Cognition* 32 (1/2): 97–126.

Mikogami, E. (1969) 'A Refutation of the Sāṃkhya Theory in the Yogācārabhūmi', *Philosophy East and West* 19 (4): 443.

Mirnig, N. 2019. 'Rudras on Earth on the Eve of the Tantric Age: The Śivadharmaśāstra on Creating Śaiva Lay and Initiatory Communities', in Nina, M., Rastelli, M. and Eltschinger, V. (eds), *Tantric Communities in Context*. Vienna: Austrian Academy of Sciences Press.

Modi, P. M. (1932) *Akṣara: A Forgotten Chapter in the History of Indian Philosophy*. Sri Satguru.

Mohanty, J. N. (2000) *Classical Indian Philosophy*. Lanham: Rowman and Littlefield.

Monier-Williams, M. (1899) *Sanskrit-English Dictionary: Etymologically and Philologically Arranged with Special Reference to Cognate Indo-European Languages*. Revised by Leumann, E., and Cappeller, C. Oxford: Clarendon Press.

Mukerji, A. C. (1938) 'Absolute Consciousness', in Bhushan 2011.

Mulholland, J. (2013) *Sounding Imperial. Poetic Voice and the Politics of Empire 1730–1820*. Baltimore: John Hopkins University Press.

Müller, M (1919) *Collected Works XIX: The Six Systems of Indian Philosophy*. London: Longmans, Green.

Muller, C. (2013) 'The Contribution of the Yogācārabhūmi to the System of the Two Hindrances', in Kragh, U. T. (ed.), *The Foundation for Yoga Practitioners: The Buddhist Yoācārabhūmi Treatise and its Adaptation in India, East India, and Tibet*. Cambridge, MA: Harvard University Press.

Nagao, G. (1991) 'Connotations of the Word Āśraya (Basis) in the Mahāyāna-Sūtrālaṃkara', in *Mādhyamika and Yogācāra: A Study of Mahāyāna Philosophies. Colelcted Paper of GM Nagao*. Delhi: Sri Satguru, Indian Books Centre (Bibliotheca Indo-Buddhica, 105).

Nicholson, A. (2010) *Unifying Hinduism: Philosophy and Identity in Indian Intellectual History*. New York: Columbia University Press.

Norman, K. R. (2006) *A Philological Approach to Buddhism*. Lancaster: PTS.

O'Brien-Kop, K. (2018) 'Classical Discourses of Liberation: Shared Botanical Metaphors in Sarvāstivāda Buddhism and the Yoga of Patañjali', *Religions of South Asia* 11 (2): 123–57.

O'Brien-Kop, K. (2020) 'Dharmamegha in Yoga and Yogācāra; The Revision of a Superlative Metaphor', *Journal of Indian Philosophy* 48 (4): 605–35.

Oberhammer, G. (1977) *Strukturen Yogischer Meditation*. Vienna: Verlag der Österrichischen Akademie der Wissenschaften.

Oberlies, T. (1998) *Die Religion des Ṛgveda. Erster Teil*. Vienna: Publications of the De Nobili Research Library.

Oguibenine, B. (1984) 'Sur le Term Yoga, le Verbe Yuj- et Quelques-uns de Leurs Dérivés dans les Hymnes Védiques', *Indo-Iranian Journal* 27: 85–101.

Oguibenine, B. (1998) *Essays on Vedic and Indo-European Culture*. New Delhi: Motilal Banarsidass.

Oldenberg, H. (1923) *Die Lehre der Upanishaden und die Anfänge des Buddhismus*. Göttingen: Vandenhoeck & Ruprecht.

Olivelle, P. (2004) *The Asrama System: The History and Hermeneutics of a Religious Institution*. Oxford: Oxford University Press.

Olivelle, P. (2005) *Language, Texts and Society: Explorations in Ancient Indian Culture and Religion*. Firenze, Italy: Firenze University Press.

Olivelle, P. (ed.) (2006) *Between the Empires: Society in India 300 BCE to 400 CE*. Oxford: Oxford University Press.

Ortner, S. (1973) 'On Key Symbols', *American Anthropologist* 75 (5): 1338–46.

Patton, L. (2008) '*Ṛṣis* Imagined across Difference: Some Possibilities for the Study of Conceptual Metaphor in Early India', *Journal of Hindu Studies* 1: 49–76.

Patton, L. (2013) 'Poetry, Ritual and Associational Thought in Early India and Elsewhere', in Patahak, S. (ed.), *Figuring Religions: Comparing Ideas, Images and Activities*. New York: SUNY.

Park, C. (2014) *Vasubandhu, Śrīlāta, and the Sautrāntika Theory of Seeds*. Vienna: University of Vienna.

Pejros, I., and Schnirelman, V. (1998) 'Rice in Southeast Asia: A Regional Interdisciplinary Approach', in Blench, R., and Spriggs, M. (eds), *Archaeology and Language: Archaeological Data and Linguistic Hypotheses*. Melbourne: University of Melbourne.

Pepper, S. (1942) *World Hypotheses*. Berkeley: University of California Press.

Petterson, B. (2011) 'Literary Criticism Writes Back to Metaphor Theory: Exploring the Relation between Extended Metaphor and Narrative in Literature' in Fludernik, M. (ed.), *Beyond Cognitive Metaphor Theory: Perspectives on Literary Metaphor*. London: Routledge.

Petrocchi, A. (2016) 'Early Jaina Cosmology, Soteriology, and Theory of Numbers in the *Aṇuoggadārāiṃ*: An Interpretation', *Journal of Indian Philosophy* 45: 235–55

Pollock, S. (2003) *Literary Cultures in History: Reconstructions from South Asia.* New Delhi: Oxford University Press.

Pollock, S. 2015. 'The Alternative Classicism of Classical India', Seminar 671 of India Seminar (July 2015), www.india-seminar.com. Available online at http://www.columbia.edu/cu/mesaas/faculty/directory/pollock_pub/The_alternative_classicism_of_classical%20India.pdf (accessed 31 July 2018).

Potter, K. (ed.) (1977) *The Encyclopedia of Indian Philosophies. Volume 2: Indian Metaphysics and Epistemology. The Tradition of Nyaya-Vaisesika up to Gangesa.* Princeton, NJ: Princeton University Press.

Potter, K. (1983) 'The Karma Theory and Its Interpretation in Some Indian Philosophical Systems', in Doniger O'Flaherty, W. (ed.), *Karma and Rebirth in Classical Indian Traditions.* Delhi: Motilal Banarsidass.

Potter, K., Buswell, R. E., Jaini, P. S., and Reat, N. R. (eds) (1996) *Encyclopedia of Indian Philosophies. Volume 7: Abhidharma Buddhism to 150 AD.* Delhi: Motilal Banarsidass.

Powers, J. (1993) *Hermeneutics and Tradition in the Saṃdhinirmocana Sūtra.* Leiden: Brill.

Proferes, T. (2007) *Vedic Ideals of Sovereignty and the Poetics of Power.* New Haven, CT: American Oriental Society.

Quijano, A. (2000) 'Coloniality of Power, Eurocentrism, and Latin America', in *Nepantla: Views from South* 1 (3): 533–80.

Radhakrishnan, S. (1923) *Indian Philosophy. Volume 1*, 2nd edn. New Delhi: Oxford University Press.

Radich, M. (2010) 'Embodiments of the Buddha in Sarvāstivāda Doctrine: With Special Reference to the **Mahāvibhāṣā*', in ARIRIAB XIII: 121–72.

Rahula, W. (1972) 'Vijñāptimātratā Philosophy in the Yogācāra System and Some Wrong Notions', *Middle Way: Journal of the Buddhist Society* 47 (3).

Ram-prasad, C. (2001) *Knowledge and Liberation in Classical Indian Thought.* Basingstoke: Palgrave Macmillan.

Rastelli, M. (2018) 'Yoga in the Daily Routine of the Pāñcarātrins', in Baier, K., Maas, P., and Preisendanz, K. (eds), *Yoga in Transformation: Historical and Contemporary Perspectives.* Vienna: Vienna University Press.

Raveh, D. (2012) *Exploring the Yogasūtra: Philosophy and Translation.* London: Continuum.

von Rau, W. (1957) *Staat und Gesellshaft im Alten Indien.* Wiesbaden: Otto Harrassowitz.

von Rospatt, A. (2013) 'Remarks on the Bhāvanāmayī Bhūmiḥ and Its Treatment of Practice' in Kragh, U. T. (ed.), *The Foundation for Yoga Practitioners: The Buddhist Yogācārabhūmi Treatise and Its Adaptation in India, East India, and Tibet.* Harvard Oriental Series. Cambridge, MA: Harvard University Press.

Richards, I. A. (1936) *The Philosophy of Rhetoric.* Oxford: Oxford University Press.

Roche, H., and Demetriou, K. (eds) (2017) *Brill's Companion to the Classics, Fascist Italy and Nazi Germany*. Leiden: Brill.

Rocher, R., and Rocher, L. (2012) *The Making of Western Indology: Henry Thomas Colebrook and the East India Company*. London: Routledge.

Ruegg, D. S. (1962) 'Notes on Vārṣagaṇya and the Yogācārabhūmi', *Indo-Iranian Journal* 6: 137–40.

Ruegg, D. S. (1967) 'On a Yoga Treatise in Sanskrit from Qïzïl', *Journal of the American Oriental Society* 87 (2): 157–65.

Rukmani, T. (2007) 'Dharmamegha-samādhi in the Yogasūtras of Patañjali: A Critique', *Philosophy East and West* 57 (2): 131–9.

Said, E. (1978) *Orientalism*. New York: Pantheon Books.

Salguero, C. P. (2014) *Translating Buddhist Medicine in Medieval China*. Philadelphia: University of Pennsylvania Press.

Salguero, C. P. (2017) *Buddhism and Medicine: An Anthology of Premodern Sources*. New York: Columbia University Press.

Samuel, G. (2008) *The Origins of Yoga and Tantra: Indic Religions to the Thirteenth Century*. Cambridge: Cambridge University Press.

Sanderson, A. (1994) 'The Sarvāstivāda and Its Critics: Anātmavāda and the Theory of Karma', in *Buddhism into the Year 2000: International Conference Proceedings*. Bangkok, LA: Dharmakāya Foundation.

Sanderson. A. (1995) 'Meaning in Tantric Ritual', in Blondeau, A. M., and Schipper, K. (eds), *Essais sur le Rituel III: Colloque du Centenaire de la Section des Sciences Religieuses de L'École Pratique des Hautes Études*. Bibliothèque de l'Ecole des Hautes Études, Sciences Religieuses, Volume CII. Louvain-Paris: Peeters.

Sanderson, A. (1999) (trans.) 'Yoga in Śaivism: The Yoga Section of the *Mṛgendratantra*: An Annotated Translation with the Commentary of Bhaṭṭa Nārāyaṇakaṇṭha' (unpublished draft) (available at academia.edu).

Sarbacker, S. R. (2005) *The Numinous and the Cessative in Indo-Tibetan Yoga*. Albany: SUNY.

Sattar, M., Sharma, S., and Pokharia, A. (2010) 'History of Rice in South Asia (Up to 1947)', in Sharma, S. (ed.), *Rice: Origin, Antiquity and History*. Enfield, NH: Science.

Sawyer, R. K. (2002) 'A Discourse on Discourse: An Archaeological History of an Intellectual Concept', *Cultural Studies* 16: 433–56.

Scharf, R. (1995) 'Buddhist Modernism and the Rhetoric of Meditative Experience', *Numen* 42 (3): 228–83.

Scharfe, H. (1999) 'The Doctrine of the Three Humors in Traditional Indian Medicine and the Alleged Antiquity of Tamil Siddha Medicine', *Journal of the American Oriental Society* 119: 609–29.

Schwab, R. (1984) *The Oriental Renaissance: Europe's Rediscovery of India and the East* 1680–1880. New York: Columbia University Press.

Schertzer, M. (1986) *The Elements of Grammar*. London: Collier Macmillan.

Schmithausen, L. (1967) 'Sautrāntika-Voraussetzungen im Viṃśatikā und Triṃśikā', *Zeitschrift für die Kunde Süd- und Ost-Asiens* 11: 109–36.

Schmithausen, L. (1973) 'Spiritual Practice and Philosophical Theory in Buddhism', in *German Scholars on India: Contributions to Indian Studies*. Varanasi: Chowkhamba Sanskrit Series Office.

Schmithausen, L. (1987) *Ālayavijñāna: On the Origin and Development of a Central Concept of Yogācāra Philosophy*. Studio Philologica Buddhica: Monograph Series, IVa and IVb. Tokyo: International Institute for Buddhist Studies.

Schmithausen, L. (2007) *Ālayavijñāna: On the Origin and the Early Development of a Central Concept of Yogācāra Philosophy, Reprint with Addenda and Corrigenda.* Tokyo: International College for Postgraduate Buddhist Studies.

Schmithausen, L. (2009) *Plants in Early Buddhism and the Far Eastern Idea of the Buddha-Nature of Grasses and Trees*. Lumbini: Lumbini International Research Institute.

Schmithausen, L. (2016) *Collected Papers. Volume 1: 1963–1977*, in Deleanu, F. (ed.). Tokyo: International Institute for Buddhist Studies.

Schlegel, F. (1849) *The Aesthetic and Miscellaneous Works of Friedrich von Schlegel.* Translated by E. J. Millington. London: Henry G Bohn.

Schlingloff, D. (ed. and trans.) (1964) *Ein Buddhistisches Yogalehrbuch*. Akademie Verlag (Sanskrittexte aus den Turfanfunde, 7).

Schopen, G. (2006) 'A Well-Sanitized Shroud: Asceticism and Institutional Values in the Middle Period of Buddhist Monasticism' in Olivelle, P. (ed.), *Between the Empires: Society in India 300 BCE to 400 CE*. Oxford: Oxford University Press.

Schreiner, P. (1999) 'What Comes First (in the Mahābhārata): Sāṃkhya or Yoga?' in *Asiatische Studien / Études Asiatiques* 53 (3): 755–77.

Searle, J. (1985) *Foundations of Illocutionary Logic*. Cambridge: Cambridge University Press.

Secretan, D. (1973) *Classicism*. London: Routledge.

Senart, E. (1900) 'Bouddhisme et Yoga', *Revue L'Histoire des Religions* 42: 345–64.

Serbaeva, O. (2020) 'Tantric Transformations of Yoga: Kuṇḍalinī in the 9th-10th Century', in Newcombe, S., and O'Brien-Kop, K. (eds.), *The Routledge Handbook of Yoga and Meditation Studies*. London: Routledge.

Seton, G. M. (2009) 'A Preliminary Study of The Meaning of "Yoga" in Sangharakṣa's Yogācārabhūmi and Its Context'. Unpublished MA Dissertation. University of California, Santa Barbara.

Shah, V. (2017) 'An Examination of Haribhadra's Aphoristic Text on Jain Yoga, the *Yogaviṁśikā* and Its Illumination in the Commentary of Yaśovijaya'. Unpublished MA Dissertation, University of Sydney.

Sharf, R. (1995) 'Buddhist Modernism and the Rhetoric of Meditative Experience', in *Numen* 42: 228–83.

Sharma, R. K. (1964) 'Elements of Poetry in the Mahābhārata', in *Classical Philology. Volume 20*. Berkeley: University of California Press.

Sharma, S. (2010) *Rice: Origin, Antiquity, and History*. New Hampshire: Science.

Shastri, S. D. (ed.) (1970) *Abhidharmakośa & Bhāṣya of Acharya Vasubandhu with Sphutārthā Commentary of Ācarya Yaśomitra Parts 1–4*. Varanasi: Bauddha Bharati.

Shaw, J. (2007) *Buddhist Landscapes in Central India: Sanchi Hill and Archaeologies of Religious and Social Change c. 3rd Century BC to 5th Century AD*. London: Routledge.

Silk, J. (1997) 'Further Remarks on the Yogācāra Bhikṣu', in Passadika, B., and Tampalawela Dhammaratana, B. (eds), *Dharmadūta: Melanges Offers au Venerable Thich Huyen-Vi a l'occasion de son Soixante-dixieme Anniversaire*. Paris: Editions You Feng.

Silk, J. (2000) 'The Yogācāra Bhikṣu', in *Wisdom, Compassion, and the Search for Understanding: The Buddhist Studies Legacy of Gadjin M. Nagao*. Honolulu: University of Hawaii Press.

Singleton, M. (2008) 'The Classical Reveries of Modern Yoga: Pataṇjali and Constructive Orientalism', in *Yoga in the Modern World: Contemporary Perspectives*. London: Routledge.

Singleton, M. (2010) *Yoga Body: The Origins of Modern Posture Practice*. New York: Oxford University Press.

Sinha, B. (1983) *Time and Temporality in Sāṃkhya-Yoga and Abhidharama Buddhism*. New Delhi: Munshiram Manoharlal.

Skilling, P. (2000) 'Vasubandhu and the Vyākhyāyukti Literature', *Journal of the International Association of Buddhist Studies* 23 (2): 297–350.

Skilling, P. (2013) 'Nets of Intertextuality: Embedded Scriptural Citations in the Yogācārabhūmi', in *The Foundation for Yoga Practitioners: The Buddhist Yoācārabhūmi Treatise and its Adaptation in India, East India, and Tibet*. Harvard Oriental Series. Cambridge, MA: London.

Skorupski T. (2009) 'Clouds, Their Emotions and Mysteries', in de Weck, Z. (ed.), *Cloud Choreography and Other Emergent Systems*. London: Parasol Unit/Koenig Books.

Smith, J. Z. (1982) *Imagining Religion: From Babylon to Jonestown*. Chicago: University of Chicago Press.

Smith, Jonathan Z. (1998) 'Religion, Religions, Religious', in M. Taylor (ed.), *Critical Terms for Religious Studies*. Chicago: University of Chicago Press.

Smith, J. Z. (2004) *Relating Religion: Essays in the Study of Religion*. Chicago: University of Chicago Press.

Sparham, G. (1993) *Ocean of Eloquence Tsong kha pa's Commentary on the Yogacara Doctrine of Mind*. New York: SUNY (Buddhist Studies).

Squarcini, F. (2016) *Patañjali Yogasūtra: A Cura di Federico Squarcini*. Torino: Giulio Einaudi.

Staiano-Daniels, L. (2011) 'Illuminated Darkness: Hegel's Brief and Unexpected Elevation of Indian Thought in On the Episode of the Mahābhārata known by the name Bhagavad-Gītā by Wilhelm von Humboldt', *The Owl of Minerva: Journal of the Hegel Society of America* 43(1–2): 75–99.

Stanford, W. (1936) *Greek Metaphor: Studies in Theory and Practice*. Oxford: Blackwell.

Stcherbatsky, T. (1991) *The Central Conception of Buddhism*. Delhi: Sri Satguru, Indian Books Centre.

Stein, B. (1998) *A History of India*. London: Blackwell.

Steiner, G. (1975) *After Babel*. Oxford: Oxford University Press.

Steinkellner, E. (1999) 'Die altesten Satze zur Theorie der Ehrnehmung in Indien: Eine Sammlung von Fragmenten des Klassischen Samkhya-systems', in Slunecker, T. (ed.), *Psychologie des Bewusstseins, Bewusstseins der Psychologie. Giseher Guttmann zur 65. Geburtstag*. Vienna: WUV.

Stevenson, A. (ed.) (2010) *Oxford Dictionary of English*. Oxford: Oxford University Press.

Stuart, D. (2013) *Thinking about Cessation: The Pṛṣṭhapālasūtra of the Dīrghāgama in Context*. University of Vienna: Arbeitskreis für Tibetische und Buddhistische Studien.

Stuart, D. (2015) *A Less Travelled Path: Saddharmasmṛtyupasthānasūtra Chapter 2: Critically Edited with a Study on Its Structure and Significance for the Development of Buddhist Meditation. Volumes 1 and 2*. Beijing: China Tibetology Publishing House and Austrian Academy of Sciences Press.

Strube, J. (2020) 'Yoga and Meditation in Modern Esoteric Traditions', in Newcombe, S., and O'Brien-Kop, K. (eds), *The Routledge Handbook of Yoga and Meditation Studies*. London: Routledge.

Sugawara, Y. (2013) 'The Bhāvanāmayī Bhūmiḥ: Contents and Formation', in Kragh, U. T. (ed.), *The Foundation for Yoga Practitioners: The Buddhist Yogācārabhūmi Treatise and its Adaptation in India, East India, and Tibet*. Harvard Oriental Series. Cambridge, MA: Harvard University Press.

Sundaresan, V. (1998) 'On Prasaṃkhyāna and Parisaṃkhyāna: Meditation in Advaita Vedānta, Yoga and Pre-Śaṃkaran Vedānta', *Adyar Library Bulletin* 62: 51–89.

Takeda, H., and Cox, C. (2010) 'Existence in the Three Time Periods: **Abhidharmamahāvibhāṣāśāstra*. (T.1545 pp 393a9–396b23), English Translation' in Nakasone, R. (ed.), *Memory and Imagination: Essays and Exploration in Buddhist Thought and Culture*. Kyoto: Nagata Bunshodo.

Tandon, S. N. (1995) *A Re-appraisal of Patanjali's Yoga-Sutras in the Light of the Buddha's Teaching*. Maharashtra: Vipassana Research Institute.

Teltscher, K. (1995) *India Inscribed: European and British Writing on India 1600–1800*. Oxford: Oxford University Press.

Thapar, R. (2003) *Early India: From the Origins to AD 1300*. London: Penguin.

Timalsina, S. (2016) 'A Cognitive Approach to Tantric Language', in *Religions* 7: 139–58.

Tripathi, G. C. (1997) 'Traces of Buddhist Thoughts in the Bhagavadgītā', *Annals of the Bhandarkar Oriental Research Institute* 78: 41–60.

Tubb, G., and Boose, E. (2007) *Scholastic Sanskrit: A Manual for Students*. New York: American Institute of Buddhist Studies, Columbia University.

Turner, R. L. (1966) *A Comparative Dictionary of the Indo-Aryan Languages*. London: Oxford University Press.

Turner, V. (1974) *Dramas, Fields and Metaphors: Symbolic Action in Human Society*. Ithaca, NY: Cornell University Press

Tzohar, R. (2018) *A Yogācāra Buddhist Theory of Metaphor*. Oxford: Oxford University Press.

Upadhyaya, K. (1971) *Early Buddhism and the Bhagavadgītā*. Delhi: Motilal Banarsidass.

Vajpeyi, A. (2017) 'Thinking and Counter-Thinking: On "Classical India"'. Guftugu. in. http://guftugu.in/2017/02/thinking-and-counter-thinking-on-classical-india/ (accessed 6 November 2020).

van der Veer, P. (2007) 'Global Breathing: Religious Utopias in India and China', *Anthropological Theory* 7 (3): 315–28.

Vasudeva, S. (2017) 'The Śaiva Yogas and Their Relation to Other Systems of Yoga', in *RINDAS Series of Working Papers: Traditional Indian Thoughts 26*.

Vega Moreno, R. E. (2007) *Creativity and Convention: The Pragmatics of Everyday Figurative Speech*. Amsterdam: John Benjamins.

Viefhues-Bailey, L. (2017) '"Religion" in Anglo-American (Analytical) Philosophy of Religion' in King, R. (ed.), *Religion, Theory, Critique: Classic and Contemporary Approaches and Methodologies*. New York: Columbia University Press.

Wagner, G. (2014) *Homology, Genes, and Evolutionary Innovation*. Princeton, NJ: Princeton University Press.

Waldron, W. (2003) *The Buddhist Unconsious: The Ālaya-vijñāna in the Context of Indian Buddhist thought*. London: RoutledgeCurzon.

Warder, A. K. (2000) *Indian Buddhism*, 3rd rev. edn. Delhi: Motilal Banarsidass.

Wayman, A. (1965) 'The Yogācāra Idealism', in *Philosophy East and West* 15 (1): 65–73.

Wezler, A. (1987) 'Zu der "Lehre von der 9 Ursachen" in Yogabhāṣya', in Falk, H. (ed.), *Hinduism und Buddhismus: Festschrift für Ulrich Schneider*. Freiburg: Heidwig Falk.

Whicher, I. (2000) *The Integrity of the Yoga Darśana: A Reconsideration of Classical Yoga*. Albany: SUNY.

White, D. G. (2009) *Sinister Yogis*. Chicago, IL: University of Chicago Press.

White, D. G. (2012) 'Introduction', in *Yoga in Practice*. Princeton, NJ: Princeton University Press.

White, D. G. (2014) *The Yoga Sutra of Patanjali: A Biography*. Princeton, NJ: Princeton University Press.

Whitney, W. D. (1881) 'On the So-Called Science of Religion', *Princeton Review* 57: 429–52.

Whitney, W. D. (1895) *The Roots, Verb-Forms and Primary Derivatives of the Sanskrit Language*. Reprinted 2008. New Delhi: DK Printworld.

Wiley, K. (2002) 'Extrasensory Perception and Knowledge in Jainism', in Balcerowicz, P. (ed.), *Essays in Jaina Philosophy and Religion*. Delhi: Motilal Banarsidass.

Wangchuk, D. (2007) *The Resolve to Become a Buddha: A Study of the Bodhicitta Concept in Indo-Tibetan Buddhism*. Studia Philologica Buddhica. Tokyo: International Institute for Buddhist Studies

Wilkins, C. (1785) *The Bhagavat-Geeta or Dialogues of Kreeshna and Arjoon in Eighteen Lectures with Notes*. London: C Nourse.

Willemen, C., Dessein, B., and Cox, C. (1997) *Sarvāstivāda Buddhist Scholasticism*. Leiden: Brill (Handbuch der Orientalistik).

Williams, P. (2001) *Mahāyāna Buddhism: The Doctrinal Foundations*. London: Routledge.

Wilson, H. W. (1837) *The Sankyakarika or Memorial Verses on the Sankhya by Thomas Colebrooke and the Bhashya or Commentary of Gaurapada*. Oxford: Oriental Translation Fund of Great Britain and Ireland.

Wiltshire, M. (1990) *Ascetic Figures before and in Early Buddhism: The Emergence of Gautama as the Buddha*. Berlin: Mouton de Gruyter.

Witzel, M. (2006) 'Brahmanical Reactions to Foreign Influences and to Social and Religious Change', in Olivelle, P. (ed.), *Between the Empires: Society in India 300 BCE to 400 CE*. Oxford: Oxford University Press.

Witzel, M. (2012) *The Origins of the World's Mythologies*. Oxford: Oxford University Press.

Woo, J. (2014) 'On the Yogic Path to Enlightenment in Later Yogācāra', in *Journal of Indian Philosophy* 41: 499–509.

Wujastyk, D. (2003) 'Introduction', in *The Roots of Ayurveda*. London: Penguin.

Wujastyk, D. (2012) 'The Path to Liberation through Yogic Mindfulness in Early Āyurveda', in *Yoga in Practice*. Princeton, NJ: Princeton University Press.

Wujastyk, D. (2018) 'Some Problematic Yoga Sutras and Their Buddhist Background', in Baier, K., Maas, P. and Presidendanz, K. (eds) *Yoga in Transformation: Historical and Contemporary Perspectives*. Vienna: Vienna University Press.

Yamabe, N. (1997) 'The Idea of Dhātu-vāda in Yogacara and Tathāgata-garbha Texts', in Hubbard, J., and Swanson, P. (eds), *Pruning the Bodhi Tree: The Storm over Critical Buddhism*. Honolulu: University of Hawaii Press.

Yamabe, N. (2003) 'On the School Affiliation of Aśvaghoṣa: "Sautrāntika" or "Yogācāra"?', *Journal of the International Association of Buddhist Studies* 26 (2): 225–54.

Yamabe, N. (2017a) 'Once Again on "Dhātu-vāda"', in *Critical Review for Buddhist Studies* 21: 9–43.

Yamabe, N. (2017b) 'On Bījāśraya: Successive Causality and Simultaneous Causality', in Kim, S., and Nagashima. J. (eds), *Śrāvakabhūmi and Buddhist Manuscripts*, 9–25. Tokyo: Nombre.

Yamabe, N. (2013) 'Parallel Passages between the Manobhūmi and the *Yogācārabhūmi of Saṃgharakṣa', in Kragh, U. T. (ed.), *The Foundation for Yoga Practitioners: The Buddhist Yogācārabhūmi Treatise and Its Adaptation in India, East Asia, and Tibet*, 596–737. Cambridge, MA: Department of South Asian Studies, Harvard University.

Yamabe, N. (2018) 'The *Tathatālambanapratyaya-bīja* Passage from the *Viniścayasaṃgrahaṇī* of the *Yogācārabhūmi*', seminar presented at SOAS University of London on 17 March 2018.

Yamashita, K. (1994) *Pātañjala Yoga Philosophy with Reference to Buddhism.* Calcutta: Firma KLM.

Yelle, R. (2013) *Semiotics of Religion: Signs of the Sacred in History.* London: Bloomsbury Academic.

Zyndenbos, R. (1983) *Mokṣa in Jainism According to Umāsvāti.* Wiesbaden: Franz Steiner Verlag.

Index

abandonment
  Buddhist-Hybrid 183 n.50
  nirvāṇa 45
  Nyāyasūtrabhāṣya 182 n.47
  Pātañjala 72, 107
  Sarvāstivāda 34, 184 n.56, 195 n.135
  Sautrāntika 72
  yoga 220 n.51
Abhidharma
  see Sarvāstivāda, Vaibhāṣika, Vasubandhu
Abhidharmakośabhāṣya 49–74
  see conceptual metaphor, *kleśa*, liberation, path, Sarvāstivāda, Sautrāntika, seed, Vaibhāṣika, Vasubandhu
affliction see *kleśa*
ākāra
  four *ākāras* (errors) in Buddhism 109–10, 207 n.15
ālayavijñāna 195 nn.134, 135, 198 n.8, 203 n.59
  metaphor 41, 192 n.114
  Saṃdhinirmocanasūtra 70, 92
  Sāṃkhya 16
  Sautrāntika 194 n.128
  Yogācārabhūmiśāstra 189 n.99, 191–2 nn.112, 115, 193 n.120
  Vasubandhu 194 n.127
  see also *āśrayaparāvṛtti* consciousness, seed, substratum
alchemy 172 n.35, 205 n.2
anātman 109, 213 n.60
aṅga
  ancillary or auxiliary 209 n.38
  limb 102, 139, 209 n.38
  see also *aṣṭāṅga yoga*
anger
  conceptual metaphor 24–5
  kleśa 40, 52, 56, 58, 84
  Jain 71
  Pātañjala 298 n.29
antarāya see obstacle
antidote *see* counterstate
anuśaya
  Abhidharmasāra 193 n.124
  etymologies 194 n.125
  kleśa 38, 181 n.39, 190 n.106, 194 n.131
  latent (dormant) 51, 62–9, 173 n.44, 190 n.107, 194 n.126
  Sautrāntika 190 n.105
Asaṅga see *Yogācārabhūmiśāstra*
āśraya see substratum
āśrayaparāvṛtti (transformation of the basis) 103, 193 n.121
āsrava (influx) 54, 57, 71, 180 n.33, 184 n.57, 193 n.125
aṣṭāṅga yoga 77, 100, 102, 130, 192 n.118, 206 nn.9–10
aśubha see contemplation
ātman (self) 33, 162 n.9, 186 n.77, 193 n.121
avidyā (nescience) 71, 109, 182 n.48, 187 n.80, 191 n.110, 192 n.113, 195 n.136, 209 n.33, 210 n.40, 213 n.57

Bhagavad Gītā 133, 216 nn.14, 20
  bhakti 30
  Hegel 217 nn.25, 28, 219 n.48
  kleśa 56, 182 n.46
  Sāṃkhya 8
  yoga 77, 114–15, 121–5, 138, 141, 146
bhāvanā see cultivation
bhūmi (foundation, stage)
  ground 58
  madhu-bhūmi 107
  Pātañjala yoga 107–8
  seven *bhūmis* 90
  ten stages (*daśabhūmi*) 35, 103–4, 199 n.20, 210 n.39
  see also Daśabhūmikasūtra; path; *Yogācārabhūmisūtra*
bīja see seed

blend
conceptual blend 54–6, 68, 170 n.17, 210 n.38
hyper-blend 54, 171 n.17
mega-blend, 171 n.17
bodhisattva 202 n.42, 203 nn.55, 59, 213 n.54
Maitreya 11
meditation 30, 65
path 81, 89–90, 210 n.41, 103, 108, 201 n.34
stage 138
yogācāra 80, 87
see also nirvāṇa, path (ten stages), *Yogācārabhūmiśāstra* (*Bodhisattvabhūmi*)
botanical imagery *see* seed
Brahmanism
classical yoga 138–40, 220 n.51
kleśa 53–4, 56, 62, 71, 194 n.130, 205 n.5
meditation 171 n.28
metaphor theory 157–8, 209 n.38
samādhi 3
Sāṃkhya 13
seed 186 n.77
smṛti 3
society 150–1
soteriology 27, 32–3, 56, 60, 102, 108, 168 n.66, 175 n.62, 176 n.79
sūtra 10, 129, 131, 149, 153
yoga 6–9, 19-22, 71, 77, 81, 102, 108, 121, 127–8, 133, 138, 219 n.46
yogācāra 133
Yogasūtra 116–17
brahmavihāras 98, 106, 212 n.48
Brahmins 3, 6, 11, 18, 20, 110, 164 n.26, 186 n.77, 202 n.44
classical 145
colonialism 121, 131
householder 55
yoga *see* Brahmanism
Yogasūtra 88, 100, 149–50, 152, 213 n.55, 222 n.2
Buddhabhadra 78
Buddhasena 78, 87, 201 nn.33, 44, 207 n.14, 209 n.32
buddhi 107
Buddhist yoga 2, 15, 19, 22, 93, 163 n.21, 168 n.71, 201 n.34
cessation (*nirodha*)
Buddhism 17, 184 nn.57–9, 189 n.98
cessative and numinous (Sarbacker) 5, 111, 176 n.81
cessative liberation 46, 57–9, 62–4, 72, 98, 103, 153, 176 n.80, 183 nn.51–2
concentration 14
etymologies 171 n.23
kleśa 57–9, 62–4, 72, 103
metaphor 25, 31, 44, 47–8
Yogasūtra 17, 97, 153, 175 n.69, 185 n.67, 189 n.97, 206 n.12, 211 nn.42–3
cittamātra (mind-only) 3, 12, 165 nn.36–40, 43
classical
aesthetics 128–31
classics 218 n.31
classism 149–50
colonialism 150, 153
comparison 122–8
fascism 145
Greek metaphor theory 22
Gupta *see* Gupta
Indian metaphor theory 22, 157–8
Indian philosophy 11
neoclassical 114–15, 128–9, 140–1, 144–5, 218 nn.33, 35
periodisation 117–20, 145, 147, 214 n.1, 215 n.9
soteriological metaphors 21
classical yoga 19–20, 82, 120–1, 123
Bhagavad Gītā 121-2, 124
category 113–17, 130–1, 135–6, 135–42, 143–9, 153
discourse 7, 62, 73, 114, 147
Hegel 124–5
orientalism 115
premises underpinning 116–17, 151–2
scholarship 2–7, 9
śāstra 75, 148–9, 152–3
cloud of dharma (*dharmamegha*) 28, 36, 47, 59, 70, 90, 103–4
cognitive linguistics 22, 169 n.5
cognitive metaphor 22, 25, 169 n.4, 170 n.11
Colebrooke, Thomas 114, 123–6, 134, 215 n.2, 216 n.21, 217 nn.23–4

Collins, Steven 34, 45, 171 n.24, 173 n.39, 176 n.71, 186 n.79, 190 n.103, 193 n.119
colonialism 116, 135, 146, 154, 161 n.3
concentration 8, 172 nn.32–5, 205 n.5
Buddhist 57, 137, 197 n.150, 223 n.2
cessative 14
cognitive 3, 30, 53, 59
diamond 35
metaphor 32, 172 n.35
non-cognitive 46, 63, 104
seed/seedless *see* seed
yogācāra 92, 104
Yogasūtra 104–6, 138, 153, 206 n.10, 207 n.13, 209 n.34
see also cessation, meditation, mind, *samādhi*
conceptual metaphor 6–7, 21–6, 28–35, 47, 73, 100-12, 151, 158
Abhidharmakośabhāṣya 49
āsravas 181 n.44
conventions 169 n.11, 177 n.2
kleśa 56, 61 *see also kleśa*
Lakoff and Johnson 169 n.5
neural theory 169 n.12
Pātañjala yoga 95
seed (*bīja*) 68 *see also* seed
see also counterstate
consciousness 176 n.79
Buddhism 187 n.80, 190 n.103, 191 n.111, 197 n.147
eight consciousnesses 12
kleśa 38
metaphor 187 n.79
puruṣa (Sāṃkhya) 33, 59, 121
storehouse (*ālayavijñāna*) 16, 41, 70, 92
Yogasūtra 59
yogācāra 87
see also *ālayavijñāna, cittamātra*
contemplation 60–1, 67, 83–4, 137, 185 n.65, 207 n.15
Abhidharmakośabhāṣya 57–8
aśubha (unattractive) 53, 83–4, 98–01, 109–10, 208 n.31, 213 n.58
Buddhist 209 n.33
Upaniṣads 29
yogācāra 89–91, 97–9, 107–9
Yogasūtra 58–60, 101, 105–7, 182 n.47, 206 n.10, 212 n.51, 213 n.55
see also *bhāvanā*, counterstate, path
counterstate (*pratipakṣa*) 91, 96–100, 205 nn.1, 4–5, 206 n.6, 207 n.23
antidote 53, 95–6, 99–101, 111, 205 nn.2–3, 5, 206 n.6, 207 nn.14, 18, 209 nn. 32–3, 210 n.40, 214 n.65
Bhāvanāmayī Bhūmiḥ 91–3, 204 n.67
ethical 100–1
Pātañjala yoga 95, 99–112, 206 nn.12–3, 208 n.29, 211 n.37, 212 n.51, 213 n.55
pratipakṣabhāvanā 91–112, 206 nn.11, 12, 207 n.16, 208 nn.25, 29
vipakṣa 92, 95–8, 207 n.21
yogācāra 103–5, 207 nn.14, 18, 208 n.24, 209 n.32, 212 n.49
see also path (sevenfold, ninefold)
cultivation (*bhāvanā*) 9, 174 n.41
botanical 22–3, 33–6, 44–5, 47, 172 n.35, 181 n.37
counterstate *see* counterstate
labour 42–5, 61
mental 34
meditative 22, 34
metaphor 33, 48, 55, 96
path of (*bhāvanāmārga*) 34–5, 62, 68, 184 n.64, 202 n.47, 210 n.39, 211 n.44
rice 36–42, 48, 72
soteriological 36
yoga 35
yogācāra 8, 84–8, 91–3, 97–9, 204 n.68
Yogasūtra 97, 100–3, 106–7, 206 n.12, 208 n.29

Damoduoluo chan jing see *Yogācārabhūmiśāstra*
darśana
darśanamārga see path
philosophy 116 n.1, 119, 123, 125, 131, 142, 148–9, 153
Dārṣṭāntika 52, 64, 86, 178 n.18, 179 nn.23, 25–6, 28, 187 n.79, 191 n.107
Daśabhūmikasūtra 12, 78, 90, 103, 165 n.42
ten stages *see* path
debate 7, 9–19, 27, 50, 52, 149, 164 nn.26, 29, 167 n.56, 179 n.30
decolonial 143, 150–4
defilement see *kleśa*

dharma
Buddhist 11, 50, 57, 92, 180 n.34, 195 n.134
cloud *see* cloud of dharma
impure 57, 184 n.57
Jain *dhyāna* 71
factor 13, 17, 50, 177 n.3, 183 n.53, 184 n.63, 191 n.112
seed 45
wheel 43, 92
yoga 11
dharmamegha see cloud of dharma
Dharmarakṣa 78
Dharmatrāta 5, 10, 78, 190 n.104, 199 nn.15, 17, 201 n.33
dhyāna 104, 137, 205 n.5
discriminating discernment (*vivekakhyāti*) 59–61, 103, 107, 162 n.7, 185 n.71, 188 n.87, 189 n.97, 211 n.42
disjunction (*viyoga*, *visaṃyoga*) 4, 57–64, 72, 184 nn.57–9, 185 n.64, 191 n.112
doṣa see fault

emptiness (*śūnyatā*) 84, 109–10, 138, 197 n.150, 200 n.32
epistemology 12, 16, 59, 109, 111, 120, 146, 154, 166 n.52
episteme 20, 73, 117, 150, 153, 166 n.53
Eurocentrism
classical 1, 143
episteme 150, 154
periodization 117–18, 147
philosophy 116 n.1, 119, 123, 125, 131, 142, 148–9, 153

fascism *see* classical
fault (*doṣa*) 53–4, 56, 71, 181 n.40, 205 n.5, 207 nn.15, 18
fire *see* seed (burnt)
foundation see *bhūmi*
four noble truths 17, 34, 57–8, 60, 89, 92, 107, 110, 184 n.58, 185 n.73, 204 n.69

Gadamer, Hans-Georg 150, 153–4
gradualism 35
Greek
aesthetics 128–9
comparison with 125, 216 n.15, 217 n.28
Indo-Greek debates 123–8
neoclassicism 129, 218 n.33
philosophy 115, 120–2, 140–1
Gupta
Chandragupta the Second 167 n.57
classical 119
'golden age' 114, 119–20
period 147–8
reign 21, 119–20, 150–1

Hegel, G. W. F. 124–5, 216 n.14, 217 nn.25–8
hermeneutics 113, 150–4
horse imagery 31, 80, 172 n.31

imperialism 120, 126, 141, 143, 146, 152, 218 n.35
neo-imperialism 152
Indocentrism 115, 117, 143
indology 118, 141, 143, 220 n.1
inference 36, 170 n.12, 189 n.93
insight (*prajñā*) 45–6, 57, 61, 138, 173 n.39, 183 n.51, n.53
samādhi 63
vipaśyana 35, 84, 164 n.32, 177 n.3, 213 n.60
intertextuality 6, 17–20, 49, 61, 73, 88, 147
Kristeva *see* Kristeva
isolation *see* kaivalya
īśvara
īśvarapraṇidhāna 105, 206 n.10, 211 nn.46–7
Pātañjala yoga 2, 5, 140, 196 n.136
Īśvarakṛṣṇa 14–16, 166 nn.50, 54

kaivalya (isolation) 64, 67, 72
chapter (*pāda*) 5
kleśa 61
Jain 171 n.21
ontology 33, 59, 186 n.75
Pātañjala yoga 130
karma 72
Bhagavad Gītā 182 n.46
cause 194 n.133
deposit 64, 70
fruition 168 n.69
imprint (impression) 63, 97 n.189, 195 n.135, 196 n.137
īśvara 195 n.136
Jain 71, 197 n.144
metaphors 42–3, 61–2, 68, 186 n.77, 190 n.111

Pātañjala yoga 36–7, 53, 69–70, 180 n.32, 185 n.67
'Śānti Parvan' 187 n.80
Sautrāntika 64, 67–8, 167 n.63, 191 n.112
theory 18, 37–40, 47–9, 52, 58–61, 154, 178 n.19, 190 n.101, 207 n.23
trace 70
yogācāra 80, 83, 91, 192 n.112, 196 n.142
see also substratum, *vāsanā*
kaṣāya see karma (Jain)
Kashmir 36–7, 50–1, 78, 82–3, 87
kleśa (affliction)
in *Abhidharmkośabhāṣya* 57–8, 61–3, 63–70, 72–3, 188 n.86, 189 n.98, 194 n.126, 195 n.135
bhūmi 103
Buddhist schemes 53–6, 177 n.6, 181 n.39, 184 n.56, 184 n.63, 190 n.107, 197 n.152, 209 n.34, 210 n.40
cessation 46, 183 n.52
elimination of 37, 96–100, 184 n.59, n.61, 191 n.110, 193 n.121, 197 n.151
ethics 180 n.33
growth patterns 47
kleśabīja see seed (of affliction)
metaphor 52–6
nescience 109, 192 n.113
in Pātañjala yoga 53, 58–61, 63–70, 72–3, 185 nn.67–8, 70, 189 n.97
poisons 53–5
primary *kleśa* 176 n.80, 181 n.37, 194 n.130, 197 n.152, 212 n.49
Sāṃkhya 56
soteriology 35, 198 n.153
translations of 52–3, 180 n.31
in *Yogācārabhūmiśāstra* 191 nn.109, 111, 207 nn.14, 18
see also anger; Brahmanism; conceptual metaphor; counterstate; fault; seed
Kristeva, Julia 163 n.13
kriyā yoga 59, 62, 73, 96–7, 103, 109, 206 n.10, 211 n.46

labour 42–8, 35–6, 176 n.79
Larson, Gerald 7, 12–15, 119, 161 n.5, 166–7 nn.52–6, 178 n.81, 222. n.2

liberation
Abhidharmakośabhāṣya 49–50, 52, 55, 184 n.64, 203 n.55
concepts 147, 171 n.22, 205 n.1
discourse 26, 58
existential 16
Jain 71–2, 197 nn.147–8
meditation 29
mental 90
metaphor 26, 28, 33, 36, 39, 42–8, 71–2, 197 n.150
Pātañjala yoga 59, 72–3
paths 18
renunciation 8
Saṃdhinirmocanasūtra 11
Sāṃkhya 111
Sautrāntika 62, 67, 70, 72–3
self 42
spiritual 9, 96
systems 18, 21, 99
Vedic 32
yoga 1, 5, 96
yogācāra 90, 92, 102, 195 n.135
see also cessative, counterstate, gradualism, *mokṣa*, nirvāṇa, path, subitism
limb see *aṅga*

Mahāyāna Buddhism *see* meditation, mind, *śāstra*, *Yogācārabhūmiśāstra*
manaskāra (mental orientation) 89–91, 107–8, 200 n.27, 203 n.57, 210 n.40
materiality 21–2
agriculture 36, 38
asceticism 46
bhāvanā 33–4, 48
bhūmi 34
colonialism 120
concentration 32
culture 150–1, 153, 169 n.2
definition 169 n.2
embodiment 149
evidence 149
food production 47
immateriality 28, 173 n.41
metaphor 29–31, 151
mills 44
mind 32, 63, 67
obstacle 99

pastoralism 31
rūpadhātu 183 n.52
yoga 149–50
see also labour, *prakṛti*
mārga see path
medicine
āyurveda 146, 215 n.3
medical discourse 53–4, 56, 205 n.5
metaphor 96, 101, 172 n.35, 180 n.35
yoga 205 n.2
see also fault (*doṣa*); counterstate (antidote)
meditation
Buddhist 2–3, 15, 65, 164 n.32, 169 n.73, 192 n.118, 201 n.35, 209 n.33, 213 n.56, 213 n.60
cessative 46–8, 183 n.52, 185 n.64
Jain 71–2, 197 n.147
Mahāyāna 8, 30, 89, 177 n.3
materiality 21
metaphor 23, 29–31, 38, 41
object 189 n.93
Pātañjala 15, 100, 148, 166 n.52, 185 n.70
practitioner 80–8, 150, 202 n.44
soteriology 8, 27–9
treatise, manual 77–9, 81, 84, 88, 113, 149
Upaniṣads 8
yoga 8, 21, 22, 46, 112, 116, 144, 205 n.5, 217 n.24
yogācāra 29–30, 77–90, 133, 208 nn.31–2
see also *aśubha*, Brahmanism, cessation, counterstate, cultivation (*bhāvanā*), contemplation, *dhyāna*, insight, *kaivalya*, liberation, *manaskāra*, mind, *samādhi*
metaphor *see* anger, blend, *bhūmi*, Brahmanism, cessation, classical, cloud of dharma, cognitive metaphor, concentration, conceptual metaphor, consciousness, cultivation, karma, *kleśa*, liberation, materiality, mill, mind, medicine, path, plant, roots, seed, weeds, wheel
metonymy 169 n.6
mill 43–4, 175 n.66
mind
citta 12, 57, 105, 106, 165 n.41, 180 n.34, 193 n.121
cognition 172
disjunction 72
Jain 197 n.144
kriyā yoga 62
metaphors 21, 29–31, 37–40, 46, 170 n.16, 175 n.69, 193 n.119, 195 n.135, 196 n.141
models 16, 121, 183 n.54, 189 n.97, 192 nn.112, 115
one-pointed 53, 85, 185 n.67
ontology 67–8, 70, 138
Pātañjala yoga 65, 70, 101, 106–7, 175 n.69
yogācāra 85, 87, 92, 101
see also *bhāvanā*, karma (imprints), *kleśa*, *cittamātra*, concentration, consciousness, *manaskāra*, materiality, meditation, *prakṛti*
Modern Indian Philosophy 135–41, 147
mokṣa (liberation) 21, 28, 158, 197 n.147
mokṣamārga 102–3, 211 nn.42–3
see also liberation, path

nirvāṇa 21
bodhisattva 213 n.54
metaphor 26, 29, 54–5, 171 n.24, 187 n.79
cessation 46, 57, 59
city of 45
Sautrāntika 64, 187 n.79
soteriology 61
two nirvāṇas 64
with remnant 64
without remnant 58, 64, 195 n.135
yogācāra 101
niyama 2, 100–1, 182 n.47

obstacles
five obstacles 204 n.62
meditation 91–3, 97–9, 205 n.4
metaphor 24, 95
nine obstacles 103–6
Pātañjala yoga 97, 103–6
removal 211 nn.44–7
yoga 99–100, 111, 149
yogācāra 204 n.73, 212 n.49–50

see also counterstate, *kleśa*
ontology see *kaivalya*, mind
orientalism 120, 128, 133, 135, 141, 218 n.37, 220 n.1
  classical yoga 114–15, 151–2
  indology 220
  neoclassical 128 *see also* classical (neoclassical)
  scholarship 128, 131, 135, 140

Patañjali
  authorship 215 n.9, 222 n.2, 155–6
  identity 6
  see also Vyāsa
Pātañjala yoga *see* abandonment, anger, *bhūmi*, conceptual metaphor, counterstate, *īśvara*, *kaivalya*, karma, *kleśa*, liberation, mind, obstacle, path, seed, *Pātañjalayogaśāstra*, *Yogasūtra*
Pātañjalayogaśāstra
  title and authorship 155–6
path (*mārga*) 77
  Abhidharmakośabhāṣya 38, 62–3, 68, 183 n.55, 184 n.58, 184 n.64, 209 n.37
  bodhisattva 89, 201 n.35, 210 n.41
  darśana and *bhāvanā* 34–5, 68, 173 n.44, 174 n.45, 180 n.34, 184 n.64, 185 n.73, 193 n.124, 195 n.135, 210 n.39, 213 n.56
  four noble truths 17
  eightfold path of Patañjali see *aṣṭāṅga yoga*
  gradualist 35, 174 n.47
  metaphors 21, 25, 29, 42, 95–108, 205 n.2
  mokṣamārga 102
  mundane (and supramundane) 38, 89, 91–2, 104, 107, 110, 202 n.47, 209 n.34, 212 n.54
  ninefold in Pātañjala yoga 105–6
  noble eightfold 109, 210 n.38
  Pātañjala yoga 53, 59, 73, 100, 103–8, 206 n.10
  Sarvāstivāda Abhidharma 50, 174 n.45, 184 n.64, 197 n.147, 198 n.153, 203 n.55, 210 n.39
  Sautrāntika 58
  sevenfold in Pātañjala yoga
  sevenfold in yogācāra 89–91, 93, 106–8
  sixfold in *Maitrī Upaniṣad* 77, 102, 139, 199 n.11
  tenfold path 93, 210 n.41
  threefold in Pātañjala yoga 96
  yoga 5, 95–108
  yogācāra 81, 87–93, 103, 164 n.30, 169 n.73, 193 n.121, 202 n.42
  see also *aṣṭāṅga yoga*, *bhūmi*, counterstate, cultivation, *kriyā yoga*, liberation, obstacles
periodization
  global history 117–20, 145, 215 n.8, 221 n.8
  see also classical, Eurocentrism, Gupta
plant 38, 40–2, 189 n.35
  attenuated
  cycle 23, 35, 49, 55, 61
  dharma 45
  metaphor 55, 61, 71, 181 n.44, 205 n.2
  propagation 58
  reproduction 174 n.58
  transplant 39–40
  see also cultivation, karma, labour, roots, seed (botanical; rice)
poison 53–5, 95, 99–100, 111, 180 n.35
  three 53–5, 181 n.40, 212 n.49
  see also *kleśa*
postcolonial 120, 141, 215 n.12
prajñā see insight
prakṛti (materiality)
  discernment 59, 109, 185 n.71
  isolation 33, 59
  mind 207 n.13
  unmanifest 17, 32, 167 n.60
  'Śānti Parvan' 186 n.77
  Sāṃkhya metaphysics 33, 196 n.139, 219 n.48
  yogācāra 196 n.143
  see also *kaivalya*
prasaṃkhyāna 56–69, 72, 182 n.47, 183 n.51, 185 nn.66, 69–72, 187 n.80, 189 n.97, 192 n.118
pratipakṣa see counterstate
pratisaṃkhyā 56–69, 72, 183 nn.51–3, 184 nn.56–8, 60–1
  pratisaṃkhyāna 57, 185 n.65
puruṣa see consciousness

Quijano, Anibal 154–4

Radhakrishnan, Sarvepalli 118, 137–42, 219 n.45
rice *see* seed
roots 38, 55
  cutting 47, 53, 176 n.80, 180 n.34, 197 n.151
  metaphor 53–4
  removing 61
  three 53
  unwholesome 53
  wholesome 180 n.34, 212 n.54, 213 n.56
  see also plant, poisons (three), weeds

ṣaḍaṅga yoga 77, 102, 139, 199 n.11
Saddharmasmṛtyupasthānasūtra 29, 78, 80, 83–6, 179 n.22, 200 n.28
Said, Edward 117, 128
samādhi
  afflictions 59
  cultivation 106
  defining 172 nn.32–3
  one-pointed 53
  metaphor 32
  Pātañjala yoga 185 nn.67–8, 70, 189 n.94, 206 nn.10, 13, 207 n.23
  path 35
  samādhipāda 105
  Saṃdhinirmocanasūtra 207 n.18
  seedless 63, 189 n.97, 192 n.118
  stages 3, 92, 104–5, 199 n.6
  synonyms 20
  translation 32
  yogācāra 207 n.23, 209 n.34
  see also cloud of dharma, concentration, insight, meditation, obstacles
Sāṃkhya
  Gauḍapāda 123
  Īśvarakṛṣṇa 14, 16, 166 nn.50, 54
  Kapila 122–3, 137, 166 n.51
  Sāṃkhyapravacanabhāṣya 14–5
  Sāṃkhyakārikā 8, 10, 13–16, 32, 56, 123, 137, 153, 164 n.29
  Śaṣṭitantra 10, 14, 16, 166 nn.49–50 and n.54, 176 n.81
  Śaṣṭitantravṛtti 166 n.54
  satkāryavāda 16–17, 167 n.60
  Vārṣagaṇya 4, 14–18, 166 n.49 and 54–5, 167 n.62–3
  Vindhyavāsin 14–15, 161 n.2, 164 n.29, 166 n.54, 167 nn.56, 58, 222 n.2
  Yuktidīpikā 166 nn.49, 55, 167 n.56
  see also *Yogasūtra*
saṃskāra see karma (imprint, impression)
Saṅgharakṣa 30, 35, 77–85, 112
'Śānti Parvan' 8, 56, 102, 140, 174 n.48, 186 n.77, 187 n.80
Sarvāstivāda
  temporality 5, 167 n.63
  yogācāra 15, 19, 79
  see also *Abihdarmakośabhāṣya*, path, Vaibhāṣika, Vasubandhu
śāstra
  doxography 11, 51, 75, 114, 116, 130–1, 135
  śāstra genre 113, 119, 148, 155, 214 n.1
  śāstra yoga 143, 148–53, 221 n.10
  sūtra genre 8, 10, 28, 50–1, 113, 129–31, 141, 149, 153, 221 n.12
  Yaska's *Nirukta* 148
  see also *Pātañjalayogaśāstra*, *Yogācārabhūmiśāstra*
Sautrāntika *see* abandonment, *anuśaya*, Dārṣṭāntika, karma, liberation, nirvāṇa, path, seed, substratum, Vaibhāṣika
seed (*bīja*)
  awake, awakened 65–6, 190 n.106
  bad 41, 55, 61
  botanical details 33, 49, 55, 186 n.76, 194 n.128
  burnt (scorched, parched) 37, 39, 41, 49, 62, 66–7, 95–6, 188 n.85, 189 n.97, 206 n.5, 211 n.42
  dormant *see* latent
  germination 41
  irrigation 36
  latent (dormant) 40, 64–6, 191 n.109
  metaphor 16, 30, 36, 42, 44–7, 55, 111, 186 n.77, 186 n.79, 187 n.80, 193 n.119
  nirbīja see seedless (below)
  ontology 16
  Pātañjala 65, 67–70, 72–3, 110, 189 n.93, 192 n.118, 206 nn.10, 13
  potential, potency 67, 191 n.112
  rice 36–41

Sautrānika theory of 62, 64, 66–7, 70–3, 180 n.34, 181 n.39, 186 n.78, 189 n.99, 190 n.105, 197 n.143
seedbed 38, 49, 69–70, 191 n.111, 196 n.137
seedless 46, 58, 63–4, 188 n.90, 189 n.94, 192 n.118, 206 nn.10, 13
seed of affliction (*kleśabīja*) 37–8, 49, 53, 55, 59, 61–6, 92, 190 nn.101, 103
sterilisation 37, 96
substratum 38, 47, 56
yogācāra 191 n.109, nn.111, 112, 194 n.127, 194 n.128, 196 n.142, 209 n.32
simile 29, 35, 52, 158, 169 n.3, 173 n.35, 179 n.25
six perfections 90, 103, 210 n.41
soteriology *see* Brahmanism, classical, cultivation, *kleśa*, meditation, liberation, *nirvāṇa*, metaphor, *mokṣa*, yogācāra
śramaṇa 37, 44–6, 151, 167 n.62
Śrāvakayāna Buddhism 5, 19, 50, 75, 80–2, 89–91, 200 nn.30–1, 201 nn.33, 35
stage see *bhūmi*
subitism 35
substratum 47–9, 56, 62, 68–72, 90
definitions 195 n.134
karma 192 n.113
kleśa 38
Sāmkhya 5, 16
Sautrāntika 193 n.121
yogācāra 195 n.135
śūnyatā see emptiness
synecdoche 29, 146

tapas 35, 62, 125, 188 nn.82–3, 197 n.147, 206 nn.5, n.10
trace see *vāsanā*
tridoṣa see fault

upāsana 29, 171 n.25

Vaibhāṣika 13, 82, 50–1, 177 n.6, 190 n.99, 203 n.55
Kashmir 82
kleśa 57, 60, 64, 181 n.39
root theory 180 n.34
and Sāṃkhya 13, 16–17
and Sautrāntika 16–17, 64, 67, 179 n.21
and yogācāras 82
Vajpeyi, Ananya 145, 149
vāsanā 70, 194 n.128, 196 n.137 *see also* karma (trace)
Vasubandhu 3–5, 9–15, 50–2, 67–8, 73–5, 103
vipakṣa see counterstate
vivekakhyāti see discriminating discernment, *prakṛti*
viṣa see poison
Vyāsa 6, 122, 155–6, 215 n.9, 222 nn.2–3
Vyāsabhāṣya 222 n.1

weeds 31, 38, 41, 176 n.80, 181 n.37
wheel 28, 42–4, 92, 175 n.63

Xiuxing dao di jing see *Yogācārabhūmiśāstra*

yama 2, 100–1, 182 n.47
yoga
canon 115–16, 135, 215 n.7
definition 7–9
Pāṇini's definition 8
Saṃdhinirmocanasūtra 11
verbal root √*yuj* 8
yogāntarāya see obstacles
yogamala 100
yogabhāvanā 89, 91–2, 97, 101, 111
see also abandonment, *Bhagavad Gītā*, Brahmanism, Brahmins, counterstate, dharma, liberation, materiality, medicine, meditation, obstacles, path, Sāṃkhya, *Yogasūtra*, *Pātañjalayogaśāstra*
yogācāra
distinction of yogācāra and Yogācāra 75, 79, 82, 198 n.1
masters 78, 80, 82–3, 85–8, 92, 104, 199 n.23
meaning 79–81
monk-yogin see *yogācāra bhikṣu*
practice 83–8
Sārvāstivāda 81–2
school of philosophy 5–6, 133, 137–8, 147, 163 n.21, 164 n.31, 178 n.16, 198 n.1
soteriology 88–93
yogācāra bhikṣu 84
yoggācariya 80, 200 n.26
yogasthāna (topic of yoga) 202 n.44

see also concentration, consciousness, contemplation, counterstate, cultivation, karma, *kleśa*, liberation, meditation, mind, nirvāṇa, obstacles, path, *prakṛti*, samādhi, Sautrāntika, seed, substratum, Vaibhāṣika, *Yogācārabhūmiśāstra*

Yogācārabhūmiśāstra
- Asaṅga 8, 12, 51, 75, 87, 93, 133–4, 143, 162 n.9, 178 n.14, 195 n.134, 202 n.52
- authorship 51, 198 n.6, 199 n.8
- *Bhāvanāmayī Bhūmiḥ* 85, 90–3, 97–8, 101, 104–5, 109, 112
- *bhūmi*s of 159
- *Bodhisattvabhūmi* 65, 77, 8–93, 97–8, 106–08, 132–4
- *Damoduoluo chan jing* 78, 199 nn.18, 20, 201 n.33
- proto-layers 77–9
- *Saṃdhinirmocanasūtra* 11–12, 70, 75–77, 81, 88, 92–3, 164 n.31, 191 n.112
- structure of 159–60
- *Śrāvakabhūmi* 52, 77–93, 97–112
- *Xiuxing dao di jing* 77–81
- **Yogācārabhūmi* 30, 35, 77–81, 112, 165 n.30, 199 nn.11–12, 16
- see also Saṅgharakṣa, *śāstra*, yogācāra

Yogasūtra 8, 14–15, 60, 113–4, 116–17, 120–30, 135–42, 151–3
- scholarship 2–7
- title 155–6
- translation 114
- *Yogasūtrabhāṣya* 14–15
- see also *bhūmi*, Brahmanism, Brahmins, cessation, classical yoga, cloud of dharma, concentration, consciousness, contemplation, counterstate, cultivation, *īśvara*, *kaivalya*, *kleśa*, meditation, mind, path, Patañjali, *Pātañjalayogaśāstra*, yoga (canon)